TECHNOLOGY FOR ADAPTIVE AGING

Steering Committee for the Workshop on
Technology for Adaptive Aging

Richard W. Pew and Susan B. Van Hemel, Editors

Board on Behavioral, Cognitive, and Sensory Sciences
Division of Behavioral and Social Sciences and Education

NATIONAL RESEARCH COUNCIL
OF THE NATIONAL ACADEMIES

D1737952

THE NATIONAL ACADEMIES PRESS
Washington, D.C.
www.nap.edu

THE NATIONAL ACADEMIES PRESS   500 Fifth Street, N.W.   Washington, D.C. 20001

NOTICE: The project that is the subject of this report was approved by the Governing Board of the National Research Council, whose members are drawn from the councils of the National Academy of Sciences, the National Academy of Engineering, and the Institute of Medicine. The members of the committee responsible for the report were chosen for their special competences and with regard for appropriate balance.

The study was supported by Contract No. N01-0D-4-02139, T.O. 94 between the National Academy of Sciences and the National Institutes of Health. The views, opinions and/or findings contained in this report and papers are those of the author(s) and should not be construed as an official NIH position, policy or decision unless so designated by other official documentation.

Library of Congress Cataloging-in-Publication Data

Workshop on Technology for Adaptive Aging (2003 : Washington, D.C.)
  Technology for adaptive aging / Steering Committee for the Workshop on Technology for Adaptive Aging ; Richard W. Pew and Susan B. Van Hemel, editors ; Board on Behavioral, Cognitive, and Sensory Sciences, Division of Behavioral and Social Sciences and Education.
     p. cm.
  "The project that is the subject of this report was approved by the Governing Board of the National Research Council, whose members are drawn from the councils of the National Academy of Sciences, the National Academy of Engineering, and the Institute of Medicine. The members of the committee responsible for the report were chosen for their special competences and with regard for appropriate balance."
     ISBN 0-309-09116-0 (pbk.) — ISBN 0-309-52923-9 (PDF)
     1. Aged—United States—Congresses. 2. Aged—Health and hygiene—United States—Congresses. I. Pew, Richard W. II. Van Hemel, Susan B. III. National Research Council (U.S.). Steering Committee for the Workshop on Technology for Adaptive Aging. IV. National Research Council (U.S.). Board on Behavioral, Cognitive, and Sensory Sciences. V. Title.
     HQ1064.U5W654 2003
     305.26'0973—dc22
                          2004001868

Additional copies of this report are available from National Academies Press, 500 Fifth Street, N.W., Lockbox 285, Washington, DC 20055; (800) 624-6242 or (202) 334-3313 (in the Washington metropolitan area); Internet, http://www.nap.edu.

Suggested citation: National Research Council. (2004). *Technology for Adaptive Aging.* Steering Committee for the Workshop on Technology for Adaptive Aging. Richard W. Pew and Susan B. Van Hemel, editors. Board on Behavioral, Cognitive, and Sensory Sciences, Division of Behavioral and Social Sciences and Education. Washington, DC: The National Academies Press.

THE NATIONAL ACADEMIES
Advisers to the Nation on Science, Engineering, and Medicine

The **National Academy of Sciences** is a private, nonprofit, self-perpetuating society of distinguished scholars engaged in scientific and engineering research, dedicated to the furtherance of science and technology and to their use for the general welfare. Upon the authority of the charter granted to it by the Congress in 1863, the Academy has a mandate that requires it to advise the federal government on scientific and technical matters. Dr. Bruce M. Alberts is president of the National Academy of Sciences.

The **National Academy of Engineering** was established in 1964, under the charter of the National Academy of Sciences, as a parallel organization of outstanding engineers. It is autonomous in its administration and in the selection of its members, sharing with the National Academy of Sciences the responsibility for advising the federal government. The National Academy of Engineering also sponsors engineering programs aimed at meeting national needs, encourages education and research, and recognizes the superior achievements of engineers. Dr. Wm. A. Wulf is president of the National Academy of Engineering.

The **Institute of Medicine** was established in 1970 by the National Academy of Sciences to secure the services of eminent members of appropriate professions in the examination of policy matters pertaining to the health of the public. The Institute acts under the responsibility given to the National Academy of Sciences by its congressional charter to be an adviser to the federal government and, upon its own initiative, to identify issues of medical care, research, and education. Dr. Harvey V. Fineberg is president of the Institute of Medicine.

The **National Research Council** was organized by the National Academy of Sciences in 1916 to associate the broad community of science and technology with the Academy's purposes of furthering knowledge and advising the federal government. Functioning in accordance with general policies determined by the Academy, the Council has become the principal operating agency of both the National Academy of Sciences and the National Academy of Engineering in providing services to the government, the public, and the scientific and engineering communities. The Council is administered jointly by both Academies and the Institute of Medicine. Dr. Bruce M. Alberts and Dr. Wm. A. Wulf are chair and vice chair, respectively, of the National Research Council.

www.national-academies.org

STEERING COMMITTEE FOR THE WORKSHOP ON ADAPTIVE AGING: FROM TECHNOLOGY TO GERONTOLOGY

RICHARD W. PEW (*Chair*), BBN Technologies, Cambridge, MA
SCOTT A. BASS, Dean of the Graduate School and Department of Sociology and Public Policy, University of Maryland, Baltimore County
JOSEPH F. COUGHLIN, AgeLab, Massachusetts Institute of Technology
MELISSA A. HARDY, Gerontology Center and Department of Human Development & Family Studies and Sociology, The Pennsylvania State University
ARTHUR F. KRAMER, Department of Psychology, University of Illinois, Urbana-Champaign
MARTHA E. POLLACK, Department of Electrical Engineering and Computer Science, University of Michigan
WENDY A. ROGERS, School of Psychology, Georgia Institute of Technology
RICHARD SCHULZ, University Center for Social and Urban Research and Department of Psychiatry, University of Pittsburgh
CHARLES T. SCIALFA, Department of Psychology, University of Calgary, Alberta
THOMAS B. SHERIDAN, emeritus, Departments of Engineering and Applied Psychology, Massachusetts Institute of Technology

SUSAN B. VAN HEMEL, *Study Director*
JESSICA G. MARTINEZ, *Senior Project Assistant*

Contents

Preface

This volume is the product of work by a steering committee appointed by the National Research Council (NRC) and of 16 workshop paper authors in response to tasking from the sponsor, the National Institute on Aging (NIA) office of Behavioral and Social Research (BSR).

In September 2001, the NRC entered into a contract with the NIA BSR to conduct workshops on applications of technology to the needs of an aging population. The initial plan envisioned two workshops that would bring together experts, first in behavioral sciences and later in technology, to discuss the needs of older Americans today and in the next few decades and to look at current and emerging technologies to see how they might fill some of these needs. The task also included identifying and discussing those factors in society and the economy that might act as facilitators or barriers to the development, marketing, or use of technological solutions.

BSR saw the workshops as one means of addressing some concerns about federal programs intended to foster the transfer of technology from the laboratory to the marketplace. They were especially interested in the Small Business Innovation Research (SBIR) program, which provides grants and contracts to small businesses for product and services research and development with the goal of having the private sector complete the development process and bring the products or services to market. For several years the NIA, like other federal agencies with significant extramural research programs, has been required to set aside a percentage of research funding for SBIR and related programs, but the programs at NIA have been less successful than desired in meeting their goals, judging by available outcome measures. The workshop project was intended to help NIA obtain a better return on their SBIR investments by identifying promising areas of technology that could be developed for application to the needs of the older population.

The NRC assembled a steering committee of 10 experts in various subject areas related to the science of aging and the potential applications of technology to the problems and needs of older Americans. The steering committee then selected the experts to participate in the workshop and write the papers presented in this volume. (Biographical sketches of the steering committee members are included in Appendix B.)

WORKSHOP PLANNING

At its first meeting in May 2002, the steering committee decided to combine the originally proposed two 1-day workshops into a single 2-day event. The steering committee selected two overview topics and six major "life domains" to be addressed. The overview topics were changes with aging, and methodology and measurement issues, designed to avoid the need for specific topic authors to address these generic areas. The life domains selected for the workshop were communication, employment, health, learning, living environments, and transportation.

For each topic, the steering committee decided to select a team of two authors. For changes with aging, one author was to deal with cognitive, sensory, and attentional changes and the other with perceptual-motor and related changes. In the end these two topics were addressed in separate papers. The authors for methodology and measurement issues were to be experts in the research issues of measurement, techniques of data collection, research design, and data analysis, with particular emphasis on research with older adults and studies of change. (Biographical sketches of the workshop authors are included in Appendix B.)

For each of the six life domains, one author would have special expertise in the behavioral and social characteristics of the older population in that domain, and the other would have more knowledge of technology as applied to that domain. A steering committee member was assigned responsibility for each topic to serve as liaison with the steering committee, to foster cooperation between authors, and to provide critical feedback as the work progressed.

The steering committee was responsible for the selection of authors and for the topic statements that provided the charge to each pair of authors. By the fall of 2002 authors were under contract and developing outlines for all of the papers. The steering committee reviewed all outlines received and provided feedback to the authors through their liaisons. First drafts of many papers and presentations were received in time to provide feedback before the workshop.

Two primary authors (George Stelmach and Jacqueline Dunbar-Jacob) chose to add additional co-authors. Four of the original authors were unable to complete their assignments, but we would like to acknowledge their contributions to the workshop. The late Patricia Waller had agreed to be an author of the transportation paper but was forced to withdraw because of her final illness. We greatly regret her loss, both for this project and for the transportation research community. Joachim Meyer kindly agreed to replace Dr. Waller as author. Brian Repa delivered the presentation on transportation at the workshop and contributed ideas to the paper, but is not an author of the final paper. In the case of the learning paper, both Sherry Willis and James Sullivan presented at the workshop, with input from Gerhard Fischer, but Drs. Sullivan and Fischer were unable to participate in the completion and revisions of the paper.

THE WORKSHOP

The workshop was held on January 23 and 24, 2003, at the National Academy of Sciences in Washington, DC. Steering committee liaisons served as discussants for the papers, along with two outside discussants invited to address economic factors related to the health and employment topics. In addition to the presenters and the steering committee, there were approximately 40-50 attendees over the course of the two days. (The guests who registered and attended are listed in Appendix A.) These included government personnel, researchers, business people, members of the caregiving professions, representatives of advocacy and service organizations, and others. Interesting issues were raised in discussion sessions, and many attendees praised the workshop for bringing together people from disciplines and interest groups that seldom communicate with each other, thereby raising awareness of the opportunities for cooperation.

Part I of this volume is the report of the steering committee, based on the workshop papers and discussion and on its own deliberations. Parts II and III present revised and edited versions of the papers presented at the workshop.

The committee would like to acknowledge the contributions of a number of people who helped us to complete the work reported here. In addition to the steering committee members who served as discussants at the workshop, Jonathan Skinner and Joseph Quinn served as invited discussants for the Health and Employment papers, respectively. We are grateful for their participation and for the insights they contributed. We wish to thank Richard Suzman, our sponsor, and his staff at the NIA BSR program office for their guidance and assistance, especially in the planning of the workshop. At the NRC, Susan B. Van Hemel was the study director for this project. Special thanks are due to Christine Hartel, director of the

Board on Behavioral, Cognitive, and Sensory Sciences, for her guidance and support, to Elaine McGarraugh and Christine McShane for editing the manuscript, and to Jessica Gonzalez Martinez, our dedicated project assistant. Wendy Keenan and Deborah Johnson also provided invaluable help with the January 2003 workshop.

Part I, the steering committee's report of the workshop, has been reviewed in draft form by individuals chosen for their diverse perspectives and technical expertise, in accordance with procedures approved by the Report Review Committee of the NRC. The purpose of this independent review is to provide candid and critical comments that will assist the institution in making the published report as sound as possible and to ensure that the report meets institutional standards for objectivity, evidence, and responsiveness to the study charge. The review comments and draft manuscript remain confidential to protect the integrity of the deliberative process. Parts II and III, the workshop papers, were reviewed by the steering committee. Their authors are responsible for their content.

We thank the following individuals for their participation in the review of Part I of this report: Laura L. Carstensen, Department of Psychology, Stanford University, Lona H. Choi, Spry Foundation, Washington, DC, James L. Fozard, Florida Gerontological Research and Training Services, Palm Harbor, FL, Daryle Gardner-Bonneau, Bonneau and Associates, Portage, MI, Denise G. Park, Department of Psychology, University of Illinois at Urbana-Champaign.

Although the reviewers listed above have provided many constructive comments and suggestions, they were not asked to endorse the content of the document, nor did they see the final draft of the report before its release. The review of this report was overseen by William Howell of Arizona State University. Appointed by the NRC, he was responsible for making sure that an independent examination of this report was carried out in accordance with institutional procedures and that all reviewers' comments were considered carefully. Responsibility for the final content of this report, however, rests entirely with the authors and the institution.

Richard W. Pew, *Chair*
Steering Committee for the Workshop on
Technology for Adaptive Aging

TECHNOLOGY FOR ADAPTIVE AGING

Executive Summary

The Workshop on Technology for Adaptive Aging was designed to identify high-payoff areas in the development of technological devices that assist people who are aging normally, as well as those with disabilities and impairments. From the many candidate domains identified as important in the daily life of older adults, the steering committee focused on six: communication, employment, health, learning, living environments, and transportation. This volume consists of commentary by the steering committee on the workshop topics together with the complete set of papers presented.

CHANGES WITH AGING

The life-span effects of aging include changes in sensory, perceptual, and motor performance and in cognitive functioning and the ability to operate in the world. While much is known about changes that can be measured in tightly controlled laboratory tasks and environments, less is known about the implications of these changes for everyday tasks and activities under natural conditions. The steering committee recommends National Institute on Aging support of research designed to develop such knowledge, to support design of technologies that will be useful and usable for older adults.

There is a need to develop research designs and measurement and analysis techniques to enable more naturalistic studies of proposed and emerging technologies for older adults. In particular, longitudinal studies

1

are needed to learn about how use and acceptance of technologies evolves over time. The steering committee recommends support of such methodological work by the National Institute on Aging.

TECHNOLOGY IN DAILY LIFE

Many factors could potentially affect the acceptance and success of any new technology for older adults. The steering committee developed a list of such factors for consideration when applicable in each of the selected domains: access, cohorts, culture and language, customization, expectations, legal constraints, stereotyping, privacy, safety, training, trust, usability, and control, autonomy, and dignity.

Communication Exciting possibilities exist for new technologies to support older adults and their caretakers and to enable the maintenance of social contacts for those whose mobility is reduced. Technology developers must understand the special communication needs and the cognitive, affective, and sensory characteristics of older people and take these into account in developing technology for this population. Three major barriers impede communication with and for older adults: overaccommodation to aging, word retrieval, and multitasking; each has implications for the design of communication technology for older adults. Specific technologies of interest include "mobile communication and computing devices" or MCCDs, which can combine features currently available in mobile telephones, personal digital assistants, and more. The challenges involved in designing MCCDs to be acceptable to and usable by aging users include usability, the need for adaptive interfaces, and privacy concerns. Development of successful technology solutions will require cooperative work by technologists and behavioral and social scientists.

Employment Recent and predicted future changes in career and retirement patterns in American society and in the age-related demographics of the U.S. population have implications for the development of technological innovations. The size of the older population will increase rapidly as the baby boomers age, with a concomitant reduction in the proportion of younger adults. The research literature documents age-related changes in abilities and work performance, as well as in occupational trends. Technology has specific effects on work and especially on older workers, with significant differences in cohort responses to new technology. Technology can help older workers remain employed and maintain or upgrade their skills, as well as support the transition to retirement, through adaptive interfaces and other means of supporting computer input and output, software to provide planning and cueing assistance, and health monitoring devices. Research is needed on behavioral, social, and technological issues relating to older workers, particularly given the many influences that are converging to require society to develop new responses to the employment and retirement issues of these workers.

Health Systems have been developed for monitoring the health of older adults in their homes and for enabling independent living for as long as possible. Changing views of healthcare see it less as a way to respond to disease than as an attitude of "How can we help you live your life well?" A transition in healthcare delivery systems is taking place, from today's clinic-centered model to a community-centered model, with the maintenance of good health as a primary goal. There is a large literature on aging and health that describes the changes in health status that commonly accompany aging. One important development is that of "tele-health" systems, which can be embedded in a person's living environment. Useful technologies include wireless broadband, microelectronic mechanical systems, lab-on-a-chip devices, and activity sensors. It is essential to develop the software needed to transform the huge amounts of data generated by these systems into information useful to healthcare workers, caregivers, and clients. New technology must be developed in ways that avoid information overload, provide useful outputs, and respond to ethical, acceptability, and liability concerns, especially those related to privacy.

Learning occurs in different learning settings, and there is a large literature on the learning characteristics of older adults, particularly in the context of on-line learning and information retrieval situations. How developers present on-line instruction has implications for older learners, and how older adults currently use technology has implications for their technology-related learning needs. Developers need to ensure that learning technologies for older adults take account of the learners' changing abilities and preferences, as well as of individual differences that increase with age.

Living Environments Functional changes in their abilities often motivate older people to choose environments in which more assistance is available. As in the health domain, in-home monitoring and assistive technologies to support independent living are of great interest. Specific technologies include cognitive orthotics, such as various types of reminder systems, to support the independence of those with memory impairment or other cognitive deficits, and systems to monitor biological and other activity, which raise both privacy and data reduction issues. Social communication aids include regularly updated profiles of the older adult's status on various monitored variables, which are represented visually in the caregiver's environment. The challenges to developing successful technology in this area include cost, ease of use, reliability, and privacy.

Transportation The automobile is not the only transportation mode available to older adults, but because it is so important to most people in America, the steering committee concentrated on issues involving personal automobiles, older drivers, and their driving safety. The special characteristics and needs of older drivers include behavioral, cognitive, and sensory changes that can affect their behavior and their ability to use technology effectively. Adaptive technologies include vehicle control devices, like adaptive cruise control, rear-view cameras, and backup proximity warnings; driving assistance devices, such as navigation and traffic information systems; and "infotainment" and comfort devices, including entertainment, Internet access, and communications systems. Technology developed for use in the automobile should be designed to be appropriate to the needs of older drivers. The issues include physical, visual, auditory, and cognitive design, as well as design of the driving environment; examples abound of unintended bad outcomes of well-intentioned but poorly designed and tested technology. Driver training could be required to ensure that new technologies are used properly and return the intended benefits. The steering committee emphasizes the call for user-centered design.

LESSONS FROM THE WORKSHOP

Although a goal of the workshop was to list technologies that are ready for transition to commercialization, what actually transpired was the identification of opportunities and the need for further focused multidisciplinary collaboration among three groups: (1) specialists in the disciplines related to aging, (2) specialists in user-centered design, and (3) technologists who wish to foster product development for the market provided by the growing population of older adults.

Rather than letting the initiative of individual investigators define the research agenda and market forces alone drive the development of product requirements, research and development should be driven by in-depth analysis and understanding of the needs, capacities, and limitations of the aging population across all six domains. In the field of human factors engineering or user-centered design, there are well-developed methodologies that support consideration of the user throughout the product development process. When applied to the development of technological support for older adults, these methods include systematic observation of older adults' behavior in their working, living, and recreational environments to establish their requirements and the constraints on potential products. The methods include the interactive development and quantitative evaluation of prototype products and services during the formative stages of development. They include systems analysis studies of the larger context in which products will be introduced to look for cost-effective gains and unintended consequences.

The National Institute on Aging is well positioned to support studies that bring about this multidisciplinary focus and that apply the kinds of methodologies that will ensure development of technologies truly useful to the aging population. Projects could be specifically targeted for collaboration between major U.S. corporations interested in tapping into the market created by the aging population and specialists interested in developmental aspects of aging.

This multidisciplinary focus should also be brought to the education and training world. University faculty and graduate students from laboratories for aging could be supported for sabbaticals, summer positions, and internships in industrial settings. Reciprocally, specialists from industry could be sponsored for leaves to interact in university laboratories.

Finally, there is an urgent need to hasten the development of infrastructure to support the kinds of technology of interest to the older population. This is especially true for communications technology. Many of the developments for support of the elderly at home require high-bandwidth communication access and wireless networking in the home. While these developments are widely forecast, they will be slower to be achieved, especially at a cost that the older adults can afford.

It was clear throughout the workshop that technological opportunities abound and that it is the responsibility of the kinds of specialists who attended to ensure that the most valuable, accessible, cost-effective, and user-centered alternatives are developed. The welfare and happiness of future cohorts of the population depend on it.

Part I

Steering Committee Report

1

Introduction and Overview

PROJECT BACKGROUND

It is becoming well known, as we will document later, that the proportion of the population older than age 65 in the United States is increasing at a rapid rate, that increased life expectancy means that a larger segment of this population is over age 85, and that the great majority of older adults choose to continue to live at home rather than be in assisted living facilities or in nursing homes. In American culture, it is both socially valuable and cost-effective to support the independence of this aging population in as many of the aspects of their lives as possible, whether by supporting their continued employment, independent living and healthcare arrangements, access to transportation, or educational enrichment. Many experts predict that technology can and will play an important role in supporting the independence of older adults, but to date there has been only modest evidence that this potential is being realized. The Workshop on Technology for Adaptive Aging was held to further understand the reasons why more progress has not been made and to stimulate further advances.

The Need

Each year the Administration on Aging of the U.S. Department of Health and Human Services publishes a report entitled *A Profile of Older Americans*. The facts in Box 1-1 are taken from the 2002 edition of that report.

BOX 1-1
Some Demographic Facts About Older Americans

A. Population

- The older population (65+) numbered 35.0 million in 2000 (the most recent year for which data are available), an increase of 3.7 million or 12.0 percent since 1990.
- About one in every eight, or 12.4 percent, of the population is an older American.
- The number of Americans aged 45-64—who will reach 65 over the next two decades—increased by 34 percent during the 1990-2000 decade.
- Persons reaching age 65 have an average life expectancy of an additional 17.9 years (19.2 years for females and 16.3 years for males).
- Older women outnumber older men at 20.6 million older women to 14.4 million older men.
- By the year 2030, the older population will more than double to about 70 million.
- The 85+ population is projected to increase from 4.2 million in 2000 to 8.9 million in 2030. Members of minority groups are projected to represent 25 percent of the older population in 2030, up from 16 percent in 2000.

B. Living Arrangements

- About 30 percent (9.7 million) of noninstitutionalized older persons live alone (7.4 million women, 2.4 million men).
- Almost 400,000 grandparents aged 65 or older had the primary responsibility for their grandchildren who lived with them.

C. Income

- The median income of older persons in 2001 was $19,688 for males and $11,313 for females. Real median income (after adjusting for inflation) fell by 2.6 percent for older people since 2000.

It is clear that the population of aging (age 65 and older) adults in the United States is entering a period of rapid growth, as baby boomers age and life expectancy increases. The large growth expected in the "oldest old" will pose special challenges.

Given the importance and high costs of healthcare for older adults, applications of technology that could improve health maintenance and healthcare, or reduce the associated costs, would be especially valuable.

Many needs of older adults would seem to be amenable to technological solutions. What has been lacking to date is a coherent effort simultaneously to understand these needs and bring together that understanding with the expertise both to design solutions and to successfully bring them to market. The workshop was an effort to begin to do just that.

- The Social Security Administration reported that the major sources of income for older people were
  -Social Security (reported by 90 percent of older persons),
  -income from assets (reported by 59 percent),
  -public and private pensions (reported by 41 percent), and
  -earnings (reported by 22 percent).
- About 3.4 million older persons lived below the poverty level in 2001. The poverty rate for persons 65+ continued at a historically low rate of 10.1 percent. Another 2.2 million older adults were classified as "near poor" (income between the poverty level and 125 percent of this level).

D. Health, Healthcare, and Disability

- In 2000, among those 65-74 years old, 26.1 percent reported a limitation caused by a chronic condition. Almost half (45.1 percent) of those 75 years and over reported they were limited by chronic conditions.
- The percentages with disabilities increase sharply with age. Almost three-fourths (73.6 percent) of those aged 80+ report at least one disability.
- Older people had about four times the number of days of hospitalization (1.8 days) as the under-65 population (0.4 days) in 2000, and their average length of stay was greater as well. Older persons averaged more contacts with doctors in 2000 than did persons of all ages (7.0 contacts versus 3.7 contacts).
- In 2000, older consumers averaged $3,493 in out-of-pocket healthcare expenses, whereas the total population averaged $2,182 in out-of-pocket costs. Older Americans spent 12.6 percent of their total expenditures on health, more than twice the proportion spent by all consumers (5.5 percent).

NOTE: Principal sources of data for the *Profile of Older Americans* are the U.S. Bureau of the Census, the National Center on Health Statistics, and the Bureau of Labor Statistics. The profile incorporates the latest data available but not all items are updated on an annual basis.
SOURCE: Administration on Aging, Profile of Older Americans (2002).

Selection of Topics

At our first meeting, the steering committee discussed several ways of organizing the workshop content and agreed to assign papers based on domains, or areas of function and activity, that we identified as important in the daily life of older adults. Many candidate domains were proposed, and we eventually selected six: communication, employment, health, learning, living environments, and transportation.

The changes people undergo as they age, specifically cognitive and sensory changes and changes in motor performance, were seen as applicable to all of the domains, so we decided to assign these as "overview" papers, eliminating the need for each domain-specific paper to address them. In addition, we decided to assign a paper on methodological issues in research on aging and technology, another topic applicable to all specific research areas.

There is a great deal of excellent research on technology applications for older adults being performed in Europe, Asia, and elsewhere. However, the limited resources for the workshop led the steering committee to select mostly American researchers as authors, and thus the work of researchers in the United States is emphasized in this report. Research conducted in other countries is frequently cited in the workshop papers, and some authors have worked with foreign scientists, both here and abroad.

KEY ISSUES FOR THE ACCEPTANCE OF TECHNOLOGIES

As the steering committee continued to explore the topics and issues to be addressed in a workshop, we identified a series of issues that, if not addressed effectively, might pose barriers to the acceptance and therefore the success of a technology in the marketplace. First we considered a series of potential barriers to acceptance of the technology from the perspective of the aging population themselves. These are issues that could affect potential users' motivation or willingness to try or use a technology, their ability to use it effectively and be satisfied with the results, or other aspects of their interaction with technologies. All workshop authors were asked to address these issues in their papers to the extent that they were relevant. This discussion of potential barriers is not intended to discourage investments in technology, but rather to highlight for innovators not familiar with the literature on the aging population the interesting challenges that are there to be conquered.

Control, Autonomy, Agency, Dignity

One of this country's founding principles is the primacy of individual liberty, the inalienable right of the individual to be free to choose. Embedded in this notion is the belief that individuals can, in fact, make independent choices, that we know our own minds, and that we can initiate effective action to bring about a desired outcome without directly harming others. In the arena of aging, these issues are complicated by the onset of certain diseases, such as dementias, and by the life-and-death context in which certain types of decisions are made. Technology will not be used or accepted if it does not respect these individual rights and allow a person to age with dignity.

Customization

Universal design, that is, the design of products and environments to be usable by all people to the greatest extent possible without the need for adaptation or specialized design, is now a national goal. Universal design incorporates the concept of customization in the sense that it specifies design requirements that allow adjustment of information presentation and response modes to accommodate those with differing abilities and preferences. However, there are also individual differences among the aging population that transcend universal design criteria. In the field of aging especially, universal design, while important, is not sufficient because there are many special requirements. Large print does not help the individual with impaired cognitive function who has difficulty remembering the first part of a sentence coherently with the concluding part. Aids for this limitation would be disruptive for more cognitively normal individuals. We need to understand how to take account of the range of abilities, needs, and desires of older users to ensure that the technology can adapt to their individual differences.

Culture and Language

Applications of new technologies are designed to appeal to potential users. They will not be accepted if they confuse or alienate individuals on the basis of their cultural or language norms. Designs, descriptions, written instructions, and advertisements, for example, present the technology in a particular way. Depending on the cultural diversity of the potential user group, an approach that may appeal to one subgroup may discourage or turn off another. Thus it may be imperative to consider different designs and approaches for different cultural contexts.

Expectations and Stereotyping

As people age, their expectations of themselves and others may change. These expectations can present major barriers to the acceptance of new technologies. Recent literature has suggested that older adults both stereotype themselves and are stereotyped by others (e.g., with respect to speed of movement, memory, sensory function) and that this stereotyping can often be detrimental to their motivation or performance. There are great individual differences in how people adjust their expectations and in the affect associated with these changes. Also, each individual brings to a technology unique expectations for its performance based on knowledge, beliefs, and experience with that and similar technologies. Expectations need to inform the design and application of technological solutions and the way in which they are marketed and introduced to potential users.

Privacy

Privacy issues have been a focus of growing concern as new information technologies gain more widespread use. Whenever use of a technology involves communicating information of a personal nature, it directly affects the acceptance of a technology. Apprehension that private information (e.g., health, financial, or personal data) may be captured by persons or organizations for uses other than those intended by the user, without the user's knowledge or consent, is one of the unintended consequences of improving the flow of information necessary for sound decisions. For example, a technological application, such as a medical monitoring system, may require that users provide information they regard as sensitive and would rather not share. Systems need to be developed, applied, and marketed with the assurance that an appropriate level (and perception) of privacy will be maintained. The factors that influence individual privacy concerns also need to be better understood.

Safety

It seems obvious that no technology should be made available to seniors if it presents an unreasonable risk of danger or harm to its user, whether in normal operation or as a result of the failure or malfunction of a technology in use. From the perspective of the user, even the perception of risk presents a barrier to acceptance. Nevertheless, some technologies that are now being made available to consumers could pose safety problems, especially for older users. One example is the attention distraction implicit in the proliferation of information displays (navigation aids, restaurant listings, Internet access) now being introduced in automobiles. Issues of safety in design must be addressed as well as methods of conveying hazards to older users through instruction and warning systems.

Training

How much training is required to make use of a technology? If it is excessive, the technology may be improperly used or not used at all. Thoughtful design of training is especially important for older adults. Good training motivates and empowers people to use technology; poor training may discourage them. Training must be appropriate to its audience's knowledge, skills, and abilities, as well as to what the audience wants and needs to learn. With a DVD player a failure to do this may be only an annoyance, but with a glucose monitoring system it can have life-threatening consequences.

There are special considerations in designing appropriate instructional materials and programs for this audience that go beyond universal design to take account of perceptual and cognitive aging. It is particularly important to minimize the need for dividing attention across instructional materials, make appropriate use of memory aids so that working memory is not overburdened, and provide fundamental knowledge that older users may lack.

Trust

The degree of trust the older person places in another person, a device, a service, a procedure, or a system may be measured by expressed or observed satisfaction, acceptance, or willingness to use. Typically, trust increases as individuals accumulate exposure, familiarity, and a history of successful use of a technology. However, trust can be weakened or destroyed by unreliability, unpredictability, or excessive complexity. Distrust may lead to lack of acceptance or reliance on the technology. There is also the potential for "over-trust," or an inappropriate dependence on technology, which could have serious consequences if the technology fails.

Usability

There are countless examples in which a lack of product usability has led to a failure of a product in the marketplace. The barriers to successful usability among older adults are even higher than for the general population. Many factors (e.g., preference, ease and speed of learning, success probability when experienced) are important in determining the ease with which users can learn and use a product. Training, usability, and customization are mutually interactive. Improved usability results in reduced need for training, while additional customization may make effective usability more challenging and require more extensive training. Keeping technological supports simple and easy to use should be integral to meeting the needs of the aging population.

ISSUES FOR THE SUCCESSFUL INTRODUCTION OF NEW TECHNOLOGIES

In addition to potential barriers from the user's perspective, many other considerations can limit the likelihood that new technologies will successfully make the transition from research into marketable products. Here we consider the practical and economic issues that are potential barriers to the introduction of new technology in this domain.

Technology Transfer from Research to Manufacturing

Researchers who have ideas for useful products for older adults and who develop a product through the prototype stage may underestimate the time and cost to bring a new idea to market. Having a good idea that "works" at the laboratory prototype stage is only the very beginning of a progression of efforts necessary to get a product into the hands of a user at an affordable price. These costs include the need to engineer for reliability and safety as well as for manufacturability. If one starts with a laboratory prototype, the development path will be somewhat different depending on the extent to which novel hardware is involved.

Consider first a product that is primarily software. After user testing and refinement of the prototype, there will be a point at which the decision to actually produce a product will be made. This will be based on input and analysis from the marketing and sales organizations, from the development team who must estimate the development cost and schedule, and from a variety of other sources. Factors to be considered are reliability, safety, production cost, potential for market penetration, and so on. The outcome of this stage is not only the go-no-go decision, but also definitions of the target market, a concept of operation, a financial pro forma (estimating the magnitude of the return on investment as a function of time), hardware and operating systems to be supported, production software language, target performance specifications, and initial requirements documents that specify what features will and will not be included.

The next stage is detailed design of the software during which the detailed requirements are fleshed out, an architecture defined, and software specifications written. When this stage is complete, the actual coding can begin and, ideally in parallel with software development, technical documentation should be developed. However, the process is far from complete when the coding is done.

A lengthy process of testing ensues, including repeatedly exploring each aspect of the functionality to ensure that it is operating as intended and then testing the product and the documentation to ensure that they meet usability, performance, and safety goals. Usability testing is especially important when the market is the aging population. Product testing concludes with a phase of "beta testing," in which the product is released selectively to potential market segments for prerelease evaluation. Meanwhile, marketing and sales are operating in parallel with the developers to formulate the distribution, marketing, and advertising plans.

When the product involves significant manufactured hardware, many of the same steps are accomplished, but there are added decisions about produceability and ease of manufacturing as well as the specification and design of the entire manufacturing process, including the design and construction of production and assembly lines. There is an entire design and development process associated with manufacture that is accomplished in concert with the actual product development process.

Reflection on this complex of processes reveals just what a significant decision it is to begin product development, because it sets in motion a very large commitment to follow through to successful deployment. It illustrates why there have to be large segments of the aging population for whom the product is attractive before a new product decision is undertaken. At the same time, we should not lose sight of the fact that future generations will be much more computer savvy than today's older adults, and they may present a considerably larger and more stable market for technological support as they reach senior status.

Legal Constraints

If there are liability issues associated with the use of a given technology, they will have serious consequences for the willingness of manufacturers to offer the technology, as well as for user acceptance. These issues may affect the manner in which a technological solution should be designed, used, marketed, and supported. For example, what are the implications of an "easy-to-use" glucose monitor that is used improperly and gives erroneous readings, leading to adverse health effects?

The Market Is a Moving Target

Gerontologists use the term *cohort* to refer to a birth cohort, those people born at approximately the same historical time. Older people in a particular cohort may have a different reaction to technological innovation because they have had different opportunities to learn about and use various technologies. For example, those currently over age 70 may have completed their working years without ever having learned to use computers or a cellular phone. Those now about to retire have had very different experiences, and one can expect that future cohorts will have still different experiences and perspectives to consider. A product developer needs to take account of the fact that the target audience is not static, but changing as new cohorts move into senior status.

Defining Products That Can Be Customized

In addition to changes with cohort, as noted above customization may be needed to overcome barriers to individual differences in the acceptance of technology. This need for customization may become a barrier to the development and marketing of products for an older market, because highly adaptable products may be more expensive to design and manufacture than one-size-fits-all products. Some products and systems are likely to require skilled personnel to install or prepare them for use by the individual consumer and to periodically readjust them to the customer's changing needs.

Economics of the Marketplace

Manufacturers are loath to begin development of a new product unless there is a clear and sufficiently large market because development costs must be underwritten by and amortized over projected sales. All the planning and other costs of the marketing itself, including advertising, packaging, instructional literature, distribution, warranties, and product liability, must be recovered. There is a role for the government in supporting some of these development costs in the interest of seeing desirable products reach the marketplace.

Sources of Funding

The discussion of funding at the workshop focused mainly on sources of funding associated with medical and health-related technologies. Many products will find a ready market among seniors. However, there are also technology products that meet unique needs, but for which the relatively small market either will not justify the required commercial investment or will result in unrealistic cost to the consumer. There are basically four alternative ways to underwrite these investment costs: (1) The government may directly contribute to the development costs through grants or contracts. (2) The government may subsidize the cost to the consumer through programs such as Medicare and Medicaid. (3) Private health insurance companies may justify reimbursing the cost by demonstrating reduced costs for hospitalization or reduced requirements for medication. (4) In a limited number of cases, the individual consumers may be able to afford the technology.

This issue was discussed at the workshop by Jonathan Skinner of Dartmouth College. If the government reimbursed for such devices, there would be great industry interest. The government can use the argument that, even if a product or service is not profitable, it should be supported because it saves lives. However, government reimbursement for medical and assistive devices is very limited, and many of the innovations being discussed for future development will cost much more than those available today. If use of new devices in home healthcare reduced the incidence or cost of hospital visits, both the government and private health insurance providers could justify covering the cost, but, according to Skinner, so far there has been no study completed that indicates that home healthcare actually does reduce hospital visits. In summary, there is a need to evaluate technology in comprehensive studies that examine the dollar costs, the impact on other types of healthcare costs, and the value to patients.

STEERING COMMITTEE COMMENTARY ON THE WORKSHOP

The body of the workshop proceedings consists of nine papers that address the role of technology in supporting individuals as they adapt to the changing needs and abilities associated with aging and in ameliorating the barriers to acceptance of the technology from as broad a perspective as possible. The steering committee's commentary on each paper reflects the discussion at the workshop. For references supporting this material, the reader is referred to the papers themselves. First we consider the three invited papers that provide a background for the discussion of the role of technology.

Overview Papers

Changes with Aging

The authors of the first two papers provide a summary of what is known about the life-span effects of aging on sensory, perceptual, and motor performance and on cognitive functioning and the ability to operate in a world involving social interaction, in which individual intentions, the demands of multiple external tasks, and feedback come together to produce behavior.

The paper on "Cognitive Aging" by K. Warner Schaie and the paper on "Movement Control in the Older Adult" by Caroline J. Ketcham and George E. Stelmach provide the theoretical and empirical context for the current knowledge and future projections that appear in the other papers. As in any research arena, there are gaps in the knowledge base concerning changes across the adult life span in perception, cognition, and motor control. Several of these "knowledge gaps" merit brief comment.

First, although knowledge of age-related changes in circumscribed cognitive processes (e.g., attention, working memory, perceptual speed) is sufficient, in many cases, for application to the design and evaluation of technology aids, there is a need for research that examines the manner in which different processes interact across the adult life span (e.g., the manner in which attention influences memory and vice versa). Clearly, additional research is required to explore potential changes in these important interactions and the manner in which they impact the design of technologies and technology aids for older adults.

Second, the great majority of current knowledge about cognitive aging has been obtained in well-controlled but relatively impoverished laboratory tasks and environments. However, technological solutions to age-related changes in cognition will be realized in complex environments, making it necessary to determine whether the laboratory-based research findings "scale-up" to the kinds of environments in which people live their lives. This scaling-up process is clearly beginning to occur to a limited extent in the human factors community and must increase in the near future.

Third, as is evident from the Schaie and the Ketcham and Stelmach papers, researchers already know a great deal about cognitive and motor changes across the life span. This information has, in turn, been used to design a number of different interventions that have shown promising improvements in a variety of perceptual, cognitive, and motor processes of older adults. Interventions have, thus far, included intellectual training, physical fitness training, and nutritional interventions. Clearly this theoretically based trend in interventions needs to continue and expand with the use of new technologies that enable the measurement of behavior and inferences about cognition in complex tasks and environments. Research is also needed on the mechanisms that underlie the beneficial effects of such interventions, the impact of multiple coordinated interventions on the cognitive vitality of older adults, and the ways in which technology can support the beneficial effects of these interventions.

Fourth, in recent years the study of changes in human brain physiology and structure has blossomed with the development of new neuroimaging technologies, such as positron emission tomography, functional magnetic resonance imaging, and near-infrared optical imaging. These technological developments have enabled scientists to understand, in a way not previously possible, the changes in brain function and structure that underlie changes in cognition across the adult life span. We believe that the information garnered from the application of this technology in theoretically driven studies is crucial to the development and extension of the understanding of the impact of current and future technologies on the cognitive vitality of older adults.

Methodological and Measurement Considerations

A number of questions that focus on ways to develop scientific evidence to support the efficacy of new technologies are addressed in the methodology paper by Christopher Hertzog and Leah Light. People today expect technology to compensate for their frailties and offer them improvement in their circumstances or, at the very least, a slowing in the rate of decline. But which of these outcomes is the most appropriate, and how is that choice determined? It is not difficult to think of ways in which improvement should be self-evident. People can do things they could not do before. They can do things better, more quickly, more easily, with less pain. They can do them by themselves. But to determine whether the rate of functional decline is slowing requires choosing a point of comparison other than one's own prior behavior or experience. The question "How would I be doing if I did not have the use of this technology?" is answerable through a controlled comparison to someone else with like limitations but without the technology. Comparable to clinical trials for new medical treatments, a technological placebo is required.

But have scientists developed and tested the necessary measures not only to assess the impact of a specific technology, but also to compare across technologies? One of the measures most often used to assess technologies is speed—can the person do things faster than before? Whereas speed has been emphasized as an outcome in evaluating technologies relevant to the workplace, it is less clear how speed should be weighed as one outcome among many. For example, if use of a technology does not increase the speed of production but does reduce the wear and tear on workers, produce less stress, or reduce certain types of injuries, how do researchers assess the overall impact of its use? If they rely on a cost-benefit analysis, how do they assess all costs and benefits within a single metric, especially when either the costs or the benefits may occur over a protracted time frame?

To the extent that measures of accuracy are used, researchers too often rely on the summary measure—was the response correct or incorrect?—rather than analyzing the process that led to the outcome and determining where in that process the sequence of events may have departed from what it should have been. When looking at measures of overall satisfaction or quality of life, researchers often rely on measures that are likely to be confounded with more generally attributable sources of contentment or discontent, or on measures that are relatively crude, making it difficult to determine whether any meaningful change did, in fact, occur. Finally, when evaluating technology relative to the goal of enhanced autonomy, are researchers also assessing how the replacement of human contact by technological capability may impact other areas of a person's life?

Clearly, adaptive technologies—those that accommodate a variety of user characteristics and often compensate for users' disabilities—offer some advantages. By extending the range of human performance, they allow older adults to reintegrate into their daily regimens routine tasks that have become too difficult for them. But the promise of independence involves a caution, because dependence is not being eliminated but rather redistributed among people and technology. Users may still need to depend on the reliability of the technology and on the people who service, repair, and update that technology. As this kind of technology is introduced, it is important to avoid severing the personal relationships that are important to the older population.

In the attempt to assess the impact of technology on people's lives, scientists must move beyond an individualistic research design that looks at the ramifications of technology use in isolation. They must be sensitive to the contextual factors of both environment and personal history. Whereas experimental studies allow the most leverage in assessing causal relationships, the limitations placed on generalization beyond the experimental design are troubling. People will be relying on these technologies in circumstances subject to far less control than a laboratory, and although it is possible to gain important insight from randomized experimental designs, experimental frameworks do not adequately substitute for more naturalistic assessments that allow the variability in environmental conditions and the influence of other persons to be considered. Furthermore, researchers must be sure that they are defining the unit of analysis appropriately. Are they assessing the impact on the individual? On the individual and the spouse? On the individual and the caregiver? People live in a complex social and environmental milieu. Therefore, part of the assessment should involve the impact of technology on these relationships and the possibility that technology can reshape and restructure these relationships in both positive and negative ways.

Researchers should also build dynamic assessment into their framework, allowing them to study the *process* of adaptation to a new technology. The impact of the technology is likely to develop with time, and these developmental processes may proceed at different rates and in many different ways, depending on the purpose of the technology, the individual using it, and the social and environmental context into which it has been placed. Dynamic analyses are more demanding in terms of measurement, data collection, and the skill level of the analyst; they can be more intrusive for the user; and they introduce additional complications into the sifting of information into categories of "error" and "real change."

Some adaptive technologies may allow the incorporation of monitoring capability directly into the device itself. Combining technological tools and measurement technology in the same device can produce a wealth of timed data that will track all sorts of indicators in real time. This wealth of information, however, requires analytic tools that are not currently well developed in the sciences. Other sciences are developing new analytic methods to work with new kinds of information, and behavioral scientists may benefit from advances made in these apparently unrelated fields.

The information flow in research on aging and technology is information about users as they live their lives. Quantum particles and genetic materials have no claim to privacy; people do. American society has greatly expanded its observations of individuals in public places in the interest of security. Will researchers also monitor people's activities in their own homes or in care facilities? How do researchers minimize the risks that can result from the failure of the technology without unacceptable intrusion into people's privacy? How do they understand and measure the construct of privacy itself?

Finally, the development of technology through private-sector research and design operations is inevitably linked to market dynamics. The size of the potential market and whether the device is affordable within that market are key issues that must be addressed in an encouraging way. The potential for technology to provide significant benefits to those with access to it raises ethical questions regarding the role of government in both the development and the distribution of these technologies. Should research into particular adaptive technologies be discouraged because those who need the innovation are a relatively small group, or because a larger group who could benefit from the advance cannot afford to purchase it? To what extent should market dynamics be allowed to shape development and access? Clearly, devices aimed at lucrative markets will be developed in any case. But the funding of research into technologies with potential applications to disadvantaged individuals also increases the upward cost pressure on government programs to make these technologies available on the basis of need. What is society willing to pay to provide wider access to these technologies? These are all questions that need to be discussed as scientists move forward with projects designed to build the knowledge base required to make these advancements a reality.

Domain-Specific Papers

We now discuss the papers that address the potential opportunities and impacts of a wide range of technologies on a spectrum of practical domains that the steering committee deemed important to the aging population. The topics are discussed in the order they appear in this volume.

Communication

Susan Kemper and Jose Lacal address the communication needs of older adults and emerging technical solutions for those needs. Communication may be between people, from a person to a system, or from a system to a person. Person-to-person communication is one of the most common methods of transmitting information, whether by face-to-face conversation, by a telephone or other telecommunication method; through writing on paper, electronic mail, or text messaging; or through symbolic means with icons, symbols, or pictograms.

Communication is also a key component of technology use—the user has to tell a system what to do (e.g., make the house warmer) or the system has to tell the user something (e.g., blood glucose level is in the normal range). Person-system communication may consist of spoken messages, button presses, or text entry, and the system may communicate back by spoken, text, or symbolic messages.

In addition to basic activities of daily living (e.g., bathing and toileting), successful independent living requires the capability to carry out instrumental activities of daily living such as managing a medication regimen, maintaining the household, and preparing adequately nutritious meals. Such instrumental activities of daily living are dependent on successful communication between people and/or systems. In addition, many older adults engage in what have been referred to as enhanced activities of daily living, involving the ability and willingness to adapt to changing environments, to accept new challenges, and to engage in lifelong learning. These enhanced activities of daily living may be viewed more as luxuries than necessities, but they may be key to staying fully functional and maintaining a high quality of life. Such activities also involve communication at various levels.

Older adults may have communication difficulties because of agerelated changes in perceptual, cognitive, and motor function: Text is too small. Illumination is insufficient. Hearing loss limits speech understanding. Cognitive deficits, combined with degradation in perceptual-motor skill, limit access to people and events both in the immediate environment and in the wider world. At the same, time new technology, such as miniaturized and inexpensive sensors, computers, and high-bandwidth technology, has great potential to enhance the communication of older adults. This can take the form of two-way video and audio communication with loved ones or transportation providers; on-line shopping, education, or entertainment through the Internet; or automatic monitoring of location by security agencies and of health parameters by hospitals or physicians. In this paper the authors discuss the most critical problems in communication for older adults and the technologies currently available or on the horizon, both specific products and infrastructure, that show the most promise to cope with these problems. The authors consider the actions required to allow older adults to access, understand, accept, and trust these remedies so as to improve their quality of life.

For communication technologies to truly be successful in meeting the needs of older adults they must be developed with consideration for the cultural norms of the potential user group and an understanding of the fundamental age-related barriers to communication. For example, speech comprehension may be improved somewhat by making the message louder and slower. However, as the authors of the communication paper argue, such changes will be insufficient to ensure the success of communication technologies. Researchers on cognitive aging have shown that there are other important variables that are relevant to the design of speech communication systems, such as prosody, working memory, and the pros and cons of "elderspeak." The practical relevance of these findings must be conveyed to technology designers.

This domain exemplifies the importance of translational research—designers have to know what the researchers on cognitive aging know, and the researchers should know more about the trends in technology design and be able to provide guidance about capabilities and limitations of older adults. Prototype technologies must be tested with the target user population, who may be suffering from hearing deficits, working memory declines, attention deficits, and arthritis. In addition, the specific communication needs of older adults can serve as the impetus for development, provided that designers are informed of these needs.

Employment

The two papers on learning and employment, out of necessity, examine a younger elder population in their 50s, 60s, and 70s. In particular, Sara Czaja and Phyllis Moen, in their paper on employment, examine the "younger old," a vast majority of whom are fully able to carry out the responsibilities associated with an active lifestyle, but who traditionally have exited from the work force. Retirement in America, although no longer mandatory, begins at an age as early as the late 50s, is prevalent at age 62, and is the norm by age 65. In this paper the authors focus on this younger old group.

Many of the other papers in this volume examine the realities of aging today based on research involving persons born in the 1910s, 1920s, and, to a lesser extent, the 1930s. As researchers look at the issues associated with work and the influence of technology on people's working lives, they will be looking at very different populations, those born in the 1940s and 1950s, with different life experiences and expectations than those born in the earlier part of the twentieth century. America's baby boom generation—those born between 1946 and 1964—are today's older workers approaching the traditional retirement age.

Many scholars and journalists have pointed out that the events and circumstances surrounding the establishment of retirement as an institution have changed or are about to change—its timing, its finality, and its all-or-none nature. Sociologist Matilda White Riley noted that often there is a structural lag that occurs between society's institutions and its evolving culture, forcing the institutions to play catch-up to the social behaviors. Retirement—formalized in the late nineteenth century and institutionalized with the passage of the Social Security Act in 1935—may be one of those institutions lagging behind social behavior. The paper on employment and technology acknowledges this impending change.

One of the many factors in the mix of influences on tomorrow's older working and retirement population is the pervasiveness of technology. Technology has already altered the use of time at work and the nature of labor; it has influenced the ability to respond to both acute and chronic diseases and has promoted lifestyle adjustments to accommodate changing bodies. And it will continue to do so. For the baby boom population weaned on technology, the capacity to ride the crest of change seems particularly evident. Although aspects of this change that is swiftly approaching have been discussed here and elsewhere, the combined effect of multiple factors is significant and has been referred to collectively by steering committee member Scott Bass as the "perfect storm." Like the perfect storm in nature, the entrance of the baby boom generation into later adulthood presents a confluence of independent variables playing off one another in perfect but dramatic harmony. This fact is highlighted early in the volume to point out that both aging and developments in technology are moving targets whose developments are rapidly evolving and changing. Figure 1-1 identifies 12 factors contributing to the upcoming dramatic change, and discussed below:

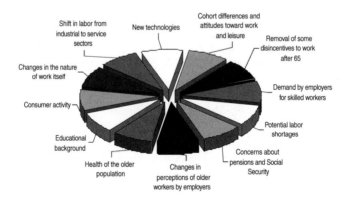

1-1

FIGURE 1-1 The perfect storm: factors converging to force changes in employment and retirement policy.

Cohort differences and attitudes toward work and leisure: In national surveys, baby boomers have indicated that they want to work after traditional retirement ages. About half have indicated that they need to work for the income and the other half indicated they wanted to work for the social contact and stimulation. Most said they are interested in part-time or seasonal work.

Removal of some of the disincentives to work after age 65: Historically, public policy encouraged those age 65 and older not to work, thereby making room for younger workers. Pensions and Social Security benefits were weighted to provide incentives for early retirement. For the most part, these incentives have been removed to make selection of the age of retirement neutral. In addition, Social Security earnings penalties for older workers have been reduced or eliminated.

Demand by employers for skilled workers: As productivity has become associated with working smarter, more efficiently, and drawing on new technologies, experienced and skilled workers are in demand. In selected industries, there are shortages of highly skilled workers. A scarcity of well-educated, skilled workers of any age sought by employers who are losing them to retirement would be unfortunate.

Potential labor shortages: Labor shortages are cyclical and are influenced by the overall economy. In times of economic expansion, even nontraditional labor markets are recruited, including retired workers. However, even in projections of most growth in the gross domestic product (around 3 percent per year), the demographics, which include smaller cohorts of skilled younger workers, point to selective labor shortages. Even in times of recession, there are sectors with labor shortages, such as nursing and teaching.

Concerns about pensions and Social Security: With the increase in longevity, older people will need resources to support themselves. Many are concerned that Social Security will be too little and too precarious to support their needs. In addition, pensions, particularly those invested in stocks, are subject to the ups and downs of the larger economy, possibly forcing older workers to consider working longer and later in life.

Changes in perceptions of older workers by employers: At one time, human resource managers voiced negative stereotypes of older workers. Recent surveys have shown that many of those negative images have faded and are being replaced by positive images of reliable and conscientious employees.

Health of the older population: Successive cohorts of older populations are healthier and less impaired than previous cohorts. Most older individuals of around age 65 are active and capable of full-time work.

Educational background: Younger cohorts of aging adults in the United States reflect higher educational attainment. Lifelong learning, once an unrealized concept, has become the expectation in the changing work-place. Strong basic skills are needed as a foundation for learning; new and novel skills are a consequence of new technologies and changing work patterns. Today's older workers are better prepared for lifelong learning and on-the-job retraining.

Consumer activity: The baby boomers have been robust consumers, setting trends and developing habits driven by consumption of quality goods and services. To support this habit as they age, baby boomers will need sufficient income to support the lifestyle to which they have become accustomed. This factor alone is a salient one in considering the need for income maximization among aging boomers.

Changes in the nature of work itself: Historically, labor relied on manual effort, was standardized, routine, and hierarchical, involved sequential decision making, necessitated high volume, and relied on basic skills. The nature of work itself has changed. The economy of the twenty-first century is much more dependent on services. With customization and atten-tion to detail that characterize transactions, collaborative planning and teamwork are needed, quality and high productivity are rewarded, and the workplace draws on higher order skills, such as problem solving, planning, innovation, and process efficiencies. It is these skills of the mod-ern economy in which experience and maturity are assets.

Shift in labor from industrial to service sectors: America was an indus-trial giant in the first half of the twentieth century. Associated with indus-trial might were environmental hazards, occupational risks, and costs of unionized labor. Today, industrial production has migrated to nations with lower labor costs and the capacity to make goods cheaply and effi-ciently. American strength now lies in the service sector, providing for the management of goods and services to customers. In labor involving brawn, older workers were disadvantaged; in labor involving services, older workers are competitive with younger counterparts.

New technologies: New technologies have changed the way informa-tion is organized, cataloged, and disseminated. They have influenced the way organizations do business and the way workers interact. Large num-bers of baby boomers are computer literate and are adaptable to ubiqui-tous computing environments. In addition, new technologies have provided greater access to mainstream occupations for people with dis-abilities and have given those with debilitating diseases or infirmities that might once have triggered a premature retirement decision the ability to continue or return to work.

Czaja and Moen's chapter examines the dynamic and changing envi-ronment surrounding work, technology, and cultural expectations. Their recommendations point out that much of the literature about aging and human performance has focused on cohorts who were born in the 1920s and 1930s and whose performance has been measured in laboratory studies at the upper boundaries of retirement age. The experiences of and attitudes toward work and retirement for those growing up in the Great Depression or during World War II are quite different from those of the emerging Vietnam-immersed baby boom cohort. Studies examining human performance in a laboratory setting of those in their 70s and 80s may be different from observing people in their 50s and 60s in their natural work setting, in which they have made adjustments to their work and the workplace has made adjustments for them. As a result, Czaja and Moen argue that there is "limited empirical data on the practical implications of aging for work activities." It is to this end that they make a recommendation for a research program to better understand the performance of current cohorts of older workers in actual working environments, rather than performance on laboratory-based tests.

A second area of research that Czaja and Moen call to our attention is a more detailed understanding of gradual age-related change in abilities associated with aging and the specific skill requirements of jobs in different sectors. Longitudinal research in this area would provide detailed insight into the concomitant effects of health, ability (at different ages), work force expectations and actual performance, influences of technology, uses of technology, changes in the workplace and jobs, and a variety of different employment sectors and their effects on different age, ethnicity, and gender subgroups over time.

Health

The paper by Eric Dishman, Judith Matthews, and Jacqueline Dunbar-Jacob discusses research in applications of technology, especially information technology, to health and healthcare. Older adults represent the largest consumers of healthcare resources in the United States. They are also the largest users of assistive devices, with more than half of all community-residing individuals age 85 and over using one or more devices. Inasmuch as health and functioning are key components of quality of life, technologies that address these concerns have the potential of significantly improving the quality of life of older individuals. The authors discuss current and emergent technologies designed to maintain and enhance the health of older adults. Examples of health-related technologies include monitoring devices, decision support systems, emergency response systems, sources of health-related information for consumers, as well as technologies designed to enhance patient and institutional compliance with treatment and lifestyle regimens. Several challenges face those who are developing new technological solutions for health and wellness.

Information overload. One of the hallmarks of current and emerging technology is its ability to provide vast amounts of information. For example, sensors and monitoring devices can inform caregivers or others about a person's location, what he or she is doing, and even their biological and physical functioning. Such information can be very useful in helping older patients evaluate their own status or in providing a relative or healthcare professional with assurances that all is well. However, information also has the potential for creating anxiety, distress, guilt, or, alternatively, a false sense of security. There may be too much information for an individual to process, leading to anxiety and distress. The information may be ambiguous or inconsistent, making it difficult to interpret, and it may even be unreliable. From a social perspective, the mere availability of monitoring technology may put pressure on older persons to be monitored when they wish not to be, and it can put pressure on family members to monitor their relatives in ways they may not wish to be monitored.

Need for data reduction and integration. The technical capacity now exists to generate vast amounts of data about older persons and their environment, but having data is not the same as having useful information. Success in developing hardware to generate data is not matched by a corresponding ability to convert data to useful information. In other words, the capacity of current hardware far exceeds the capacity of the available software. Thus, much more effort is needed in developing the means to reduce and integrate data to make it useful in decision making. Moreover, the data reduction and integration will vary for different users. An older person with some functional impairment is likely to need more data reduction and decision support than a family member or a healthcare professional.

Ethical, liability, and acceptability issues. For technology to be useful, it should facilitate decision making and ultimately impact behavior. This raises questions about who is responsible for wrong decisions or actions, particularly if they are the result of a technological failure.

The ubiquitous presence of sensing and monitoring devices has the potential of undermining privacy. Individuals may be monitored without their consent or awareness. Although this already happens in public spaces, what are the implications of being monitored in private spaces such as someone's home or office? A challenge is to develop technologies that also provide feedback to the person about what is being monitored and when.

New technology is often expensive. There are already large socioeconomic disparities in the health and well-being of older persons. Will the availability of useful but costly technology further widen the gap between people who do and do not have access to this resource?

Technology has the potential of undermining functioning in older persons. Most older individuals are very resilient and are able to develop compensatory adaptive strategies for dealing with life challenges. Technology that provides too much support has the potential of eroding these adaptive capacities. Successful technological supports will maximize people's independent functioning and perhaps sense and adapt to changes over time in their needs and abilities.

Learning

Learning will continue to play a vital role in the lives of tomorrow's elders. As described in the paper by Sherry Willis, there are three general arenas in which this learning will be carried out. First, having considerable leisure time as well as a desire for knowledge and information, older adults will be learning informally about matters, such as health and travel, that are important to their everyday lives. Second, older learners are expected to need training and retraining that will enhance their employability and work efficiency. Finally, and overlapping both of these domains, along with the rest of the population, older adults will be learning to use technologies to support a variety of activities, including learning about other matters.

The diverse learning needs of older adults make it likely that the nature of learning itself will be quite variable. Traditional, highly structured learning is exemplified by the numerous formal courses and training programs available on the World Wide Web. A very different model is the spontaneously organized, nonhierarchical community of learners, who meet virtually or in person to pursue a common interest or problem, often without a designated teacher. This latter approach to learning is often more motivating and effective. However, a suggestion that traditional learning environments should be eliminated ignores relations between task demands, learner characteristics, and the learning environment. That is, a student-centered approach to learning may be ideal for highly motivated and cognitively robust individuals who have general learning goals that emphasize problem solving over the performance of specific and concrete tasks. This same approach may not work at all for teaching entry-level computer skills to those with cognitive deficits and no background knowledge. The match among task demands, environmental affordances, and individual abilities is especially important when discussion centers on technology and the older learner.

There have been some remarkable recent efforts to clearly delineate the physical, perceptual, and cognitive requirements of technology-mediated tasks, such as banking and blood glucose monitoring. Similar research needs to be carried out on the use of the Internet, synchronous and asynchronous learning applications (e.g., NetMeeting, Vclass, and CentraOne), and immersive environments such as driving simulators. Some of the learning tasks enabled through these technologies are highly structured and linear, whereas others are ill defined. Only by clearly understanding the demands of these tasks can technologies be efficiently built to enable them for users of all ages.

Task demands can rarely be separated completely from the environments in which they are carried out, and this is certainly true in the area of technology for learning among older adults. Many of the technologies discussed in the paper by Willis have substantial divided attention, working memory, and task-switching requirements that can be reduced through intelligent design. Acknowledging the need for matching technology to the older learner, there have been several sets of guidelines for web-site development, in-vehicle telematics systems, and automated phone response systems. This research needs to be continued so that the older person is not left muddling through a learning tool that is filled with bells and whistles or heavy with content but cannot be used.

Learning environments can be optimized to task demands only when the understanding of user abilities is sufficient. Although there have been some attempts to find the predictors of individual differences in searching web sites and databases, these are small in number and do not extend to more complex learning tasks and applications. Researchers do not know if age-related changes in speed of processing, verbal and visual spatial memory, attention, and executive control account for individual differences in the performance of these tasks. Developing that knowledge base will help both designers and users.

There are two particularly interesting ways in which research could focus on individual differences that affect the older learner. The first concerns preferences for structure in learning. It may be that many older adults prefer highly structured tasks and environments, so that learner-centered and loosely organized materials are less effective. The second research area deals with mental models of technological entities. Engineers and software designers, as well as people who have grown up with technology, have highly detailed representations of such constructs as links and cookies, file management, logical structures, and so on. It is possible that imparting these models to older users will confuse them early in learning, but it may in the long run give them a better understanding of the technology that is being used to support their learning. If this makes learning less frustrating and more enjoyable, then everyone will benefit.

There is the persistent issue of cohort-based delay in exposure and access to technology. Certainly tomorrow's elders will comfortably and frequently use today's technologies, such as the web, automatic teller machines, and personal data assistants. They may not face the same barriers to access and use that challenge many older people today, although they will still be susceptible to age-related changes in movement control, perception, and cognition that impact interactions with technology. Moreover, technology will continue to develop, elders will continue to move out of educational and work settings, and thus future generations of older learners will still have to cope with technology lag. How learning experts and technology developers can reduce the effects of this lag is a central challenge, the solution to which will benefit not only older adults, but poor, disabled, and geographically isolated people.

Living Environments

In this paper, Ann Horgas and Gregory Abowd describe technology for use in an older adult's living environment. It includes a discussion of technology for such settings as assisted living and nursing homes, but, consistent with the fact that the vast majority of older adults live in their own homes, the focus is on technology for use in the home. A major goal of such technology is extending the period during which people can age in place, that is, remain safely in their homes. Toward this end, the technology helps compensate not only for motor and sensory deficits but also, importantly, for cognitive decline: there is a growing body of research that aims to develop cognitive aids to help ensure that older adults perform necessary routine daily activities. An additional key goal of the technology is to support the caregivers of older adults. In many cases, caregiving is provided by an aging spouse, while in many others, it is provided by adult children who do not reside with their parents. Cognitive aids can support this latter group by providing them with frequent, detailed information about their parents' activities and status. This in turn supports aging in place, because adult children are more satisfied with such living arrangements when they can monitor their parents' well-being.

The maturity of the technology described varies, from devices and systems that are nearly ready to be marketed to concepts and prototypes that are still in the design and development stages in the laboratory. Before becoming widely used, however, all the technology discussed must overcome four key challenges:

1. Cost. In most cases, the major expenses of the technologies described are not hardware-related, and when they are, these costs can be mitigated by economies of scale. Potentially more intractable expenses arise from the need to customize the technologies to individual users, a requirement that is closely related to the second challenge. Universal design principles do not apply in a straightforward manner to cognitive aids, since by definition these systems must represent the details of their users' daily activities.

2. Ease of use. It is essential that the technologies be made completely transparent to use, and, if the user is to install them, they need to be

transparent to install as well. One way to facilitate this is by customizing a system to a user's particular situation, but customization can be expensive. Advanced machine-learning techniques may help mitigate this problem by automating the customization process.

3. Reliability. Reliability is essential for technologies that are put into the home, where technical support staff are not immediately available. Although we are all familiar with the frustrating experience of dealing with unreliable software systems, we also deal daily with many instances of highly reliable technology. Cable television is one example. In addition, the design of "self-healing systems" is a very active current area of research, and there is similarly a large body of knowledge on the design of fault-tolerant systems. These and related engineering techniques will play a large role in the development of future technologies for the living environment.

4. Privacy. Many of the technologies described in this paper involve extensive monitoring of the routine daily activities of an older adult. Clearly, such monitoring raises important privacy concerns that will need to be addressed by technology designers to ensure that the rights and dignity of the users of the technology are respected.

Although these challenges are significant, it should not be forgotten that the technology that gives rise to them is being created to handle equally significant challenges that result from the dramatic demographic shifts currently under way. As the proportion of older adults skyrockets, there will not be enough younger adults to serve as full-time caregivers in the home, and technology will have to take up some of the slack. The technology discussed in this paper—if it is able to meet the four classes of challenges mentioned above—offers the hope of a better and safer quality of day-to-day life, in the home, for many older adults.

Transportation

The paper by Joachim Meyer starts from the assumption that transportation is more than getting from point A to point B. Mobility is an integral part of everyday independent living. In the United States, transportation is defined as "automobility," wherein more than 92 percent of the public choose the car as their primary mode of transport. The next wave of retirees, the baby boomers, have been defined by the automobile since their youth, and today as adults most live in the suburbs or rural areas where alternatives to the car are few or nonexistent. However, the natural aging process and age-related conditions may affect the capacity of older drivers to operate a vehicle safely and comfortably. Meyer discusses both the promise and the challenges associated with the introduction of new in-vehicle technologies to assist the older driver. Although the major focus is on the automobile because of its importance in American life, other modes of transport are also important to many seniors, and some discussion is presented concerning public transportation.

WHAT CAN BE LEARNED FROM THE WORKSHOP

The vision for the workshop was the identification of a list of exciting new technologies to support the aging population that could be recommended for immediate transition to application in the range of settings studied by the workshop participants. No such list was forthcoming from the invited papers or the workshop discussion. On one hand, we heard about the promising new directions in miniaturization, electronic connectivity, and software sophistication that would enable all kinds of communications aids and sensory instrumentation to enhance social support from relatives and peers, monitoring and control of health care and medication administration in the homes where seniors prefer to live independently, and potentially to enhance their instrumental activities of daily living and quality of life. On the other hand, in each domain we heard about the serious challenges that the development of truly useful technological support would encounter, from trust, privacy, and safety to acculturation, autonomy, and dignity. At this stage in the field, there is simply not enough mutual understanding between specialists in aging research and technology developers to enable sensible, prioritized development of such a list. Instead, in the paragraphs that follow we suggest the kinds of further developments that are required and some of the means to accomplish those developments that the steering committee considers to have the greatest potential to bring about the most useful and usable technological support of the aging population.

Multidisciplinary Focus

Although we of course already knew this at some level, the workshop strongly reinforced the fact that producing technology that is genuinely supportive of the aging population is a many-faceted problem that requires multidisciplinary effort across the developmental spectrum, from basic research to evaluation of operating products in use in the field. The nation's current approach, as it is with many problems, is to "let a thousand flowers bloom." However, in this domain, such an approach has the effect of letting available technology seek its own market, and as discussed above, there are too many reasons, involving both user acceptance and economic reality, why such an approach will facilitate only the most widely applicable technological supports.

There are many ways government agencies can play a role in promoting this kind of multidisciplinary collaboration. First, they could foster mutual education among industrial technologists and specialists in aging research in government and university laboratories. University faculty could be supported to spend summers or sabbatical leaves on site in industrial settings where potentially relevant technology is being developed. Graduate student training grants could be focused specifically on multidisciplinary training in laboratories conducting aging research, together with internships in industrial and field settings where potential technology interventions are being developed and evaluated. Specific work groups, workshops such as this one, and conferences could be sponsored to promote education across disciplines among established experts.

Second, government agencies could sponsor unconventional types of translational research and development that explicitly call for collaboration between technologists with ideas for product innovations and experienced specialists in research on aging. There is great interest among some of the major U.S. corporations in tapping into the growing market created by the aging population, but they lack the expertise needed to develop products that are truly responsive to the needs of the aging population. Program projects are an existing funding mechanism that is suitable for this purpose, but they would require that sufficient resources be committed to support both halves of the venture, the corporate developers and the specialists in gerontology. Thoughtful negotiation of the allocation of intellectual property rights is another prerequisite. Without this kind of support, it is unlikely that these sorts of collaborations will happen serendipitously.

Collaborative Ethnographic Studies

There is a need for research studies employing sophisticated, structured observation, taking the user's perspective in settings in which the aging population is found, in order to understand the real needs, the impact of the physical and social environment, and the range of individual differences that must be accommodated. Recently a new breed of ethnographers has become involved in collecting this kind of information for the design of computer-supported applications across a wide variety of settings. But without an understanding of the potential of technology, such studies will lack a focus. What is needed is collaborative research in realistic settings with observation and input from technologists who can educate the observers and the users about potential technical innovation and at the same time learn what the needs are and begin to shape the available technology to be responsive. It is difficult for users to articulate what will be useful to them without some examples of what is practical and feasible. With multiple prototypes to examine, they can interpolate and extrapolate from examples to recommend valuable innovations. Furthermore, this kind of human factors approach to a "requirements analysis" from the perspective of older users should become an integral part of the technology development process.

Formative Premarket Evaluation Studies

Another kind of study need spans the range from research to prototype application. Once a product idea has reached the prototype stage, there is a need for the equivalent of what in the software industry is called beta testing—that is, testing by the intended user population in real-life situations. This beta testing needs to be carried out by an interdisciplinary team that works in the aging user's environment, and it needs to include specialists who understand the aging population and specialists in the conduct of formative evaluation. Such evaluation is not directed at assessment of the final outcome but rather attempts to discover the modifications to the technology that will enhance its effectiveness. Such studies will also reveal potential behavioral changes required of the users themselves to make the technology successful. Speakers at the workshop identified the need for more advanced evaluative methodologies to support such studies. It was mentioned repeatedly that the goal is a change on some outcome that is important to the life of an individual—in the activities of daily living or their overall "quality of life"—but clear definitions or evaluative criteria are not available to assess these features. The problem is complicated further by the fact that the introduction of technology will represent a change agent that will cause the aging population to adapt and change. The measurement regimens needed to take account of these potential dynamics have yet to be developed, and should be a priority for the National Institute on Aging.

Systems Implementation Studies

There is a third kind of study that is needed to support technology transition into widespread use. It is the study of actual "pilot" systems implementation in the broader setting with the opportunity to observe the impacts across the organizations and agencies that will be impacted. It was suggested that technology might be a primary means for integrating healthcare delivery in hospitals and clinics with primary healthcare in the home, or eventually for permitting significantly more care to be provided in the home and less in traditional healthcare environments. It has even been suggested that a change is needed in the overall healthcare delivery model to make affordable healthcare available to older adults. If system changes such as these are to be effected—and there are opportunities to do so across the domains in which the aging population potentially will meet new technologies—there is a need for collaborative multidisciplinary "model implementation" studies among the organizations and agencies that will be impacted.

Technology transition can have impacts where they are least suspected. In a hospital in which computer-supported drug ordering was to be introduced, an interdisciplinary study was undertaken while the technology was being introduced to understand the broad potential positive and negative impacts of its introduction. The evaluation extended not only to the pharmacy and the doctors who would be using the system, but also to potential impacts throughout the hospital. Transitioning technology to the systems affecting the aging population will require the same kind of care in evaluation to ensure that the positive impacts outweigh the negative ones.

Improvements in Infrastructure

There is a need for substantial improvements in physical and electronic infrastructure before much of the potential of technological contributions can be achieved. The Americans with Disabilities Act and related legislation are making giant strides in improving physical accessibility in public spaces, but few new homes are being built with wheelchair access in mind and few existing private homes can accommodate even the most fundamental physical access needs without serious renovation.

Advanced communications technology was frequently mentioned in the workshop, not just by the speakers on that topic but also in the discussions of living environments, healthcare, and transportation. However, the application of communications technology presumes the availability of the infrastructure to support it. It was argued that broadband access can be assumed to be available in the home in the next few years, but at what cost, with what user interfaces, and with what technical support to the population that may already be having difficulty with the activities of everyday living?

It would also be useful to investigate ways to site or design environments suitable for older persons that encourage them to stay engaged in educational activities, stimulating leisure pursuits, or fitness activities. Some housing has been strategically placed near colleges or universities, where access to educational or intellectually challenging resources is easily available, but other approaches could also be considered.

Need for Training and Instruction

Although a goal of design may be to develop products that do not require training, this is probably an inappropriate goal. The best-designed product, especially if it is complex, is going to require some training. A better goal is to ensure that the documentation and instructional support that is provided with the product itself is well designed. Older adults are generally more willing to use technologies if training is provided, but we need to better understand their specific training needs—how, when, and if training for older adults should differ from training for younger or middle-aged adults.

A recurrent theme of the workshop reflected the importance of providing training and instruction for the use of technology by older adults. Manuals and on-line help systems are notoriously ineffective and difficult to use—this aspect of technology development often receives short shrift in the design process. Moreover, system error messages are often vague or confusing and sometimes misleading.

Users must be taught how to interact with the technology and to understand sufficiently well how the system works to be able to tell when it is not working properly. Training and instruction must be developed following instructional design principles, and such education must be tailored to usage patterns; that is, if a system is used infrequently, the instructions must be easily accessible and interpretable. If the consequences of misuse are extremely critical, users must be trained to the level of perfect performance. Issues of retention over time and the potential need for refresher training must also be addressed.

Future developments in this area should also focus on the potential for the technology itself to provide user training, sometimes referred to as "embedded training." The device could serve as a "coach" for the user by providing specific feedback and guidance when errors are made or introducing new features of the system only after the user becomes proficient with the basics.

Human Factors Tools and Techniques

The discipline of human factors is a multidisciplinary approach to design that puts the user at the center of the design process with the goal of developing safe, effective, and efficient user-system interactions. Within this discipline are tools and techniques that can be used to increase the likelihood that technologies will be designed to meet the needs of the users and that users will be able to safely and effectively use the technologies because they are designed well and accompanied by help systems, manuals, and instructions that are efficacious. Such tools and techniques include needs analysis to fully understand what the system should do and how it should do it; person analysis to recognize the capabilities and limitations of the target user population; task analysis to detail the components of tasks and ensure that the system functionality is appropriate, the expectations of the user are considered, and that error messages are clear at each point in the process; and instructional analysis to determine the form, content, and medium that will provide effective instructions for initial learning, retention over time, troubleshooting, and system maintenance.

The techniques of iterative, user-centered design and user testing provide methods of ensuring that systems will be usable. There are documented components to usability that provide guidance for design: learnability, efficiency, memorability, error avoidance, and satisfaction. Techniques such as rapid prototyping to develop mock representations of a product can be used to identify critical flaws early in the design process. Similarly, "wizard-of-oz" methods may be used to mimic what the system will do to measure user behaviors and expectation, prior to the expense of building the final product. Practitioners with these skills should be involved throughout the technology development process, whether it is the development of a single web site or the development of the smart home of the future.

SUMMARY

These are exciting times for researchers and practitioners who are interested in making a difference in the lives of aging citizens. As this workshop has attested, technological opportunities abound, and it is likely that, whether the multidisciplinary communities that have a stake in making them successful participate or not, many of these technologies will reach the marketplace and some of them will be imposed on the older population in the interests of efficiency and cost-effectiveness. It is up to the readers of this workshop report to make sure that these technologies are developed in ways that will ensure their success and to ensure that future cohorts of the population age with greater dignity, feelings of self-worth, accomplishment, and happiness.

Part II

Overview Papers

2

Cognitive Aging

K. Warner Schaie

DEFINITION OF COGNITIVE AGING

Research on cognitive aging is concerned with the basic processes of learning and memory as well as with the complex higher-order processes of language and intellectual competence or executive functioning. Much of the literature in this field has been concerned with explaining the mechanism of cognitive decline with advancing age. However, there has also been pervasive interest in issues such as compensation and the role of external support including external aids as well as collaborative problem solving. The study of cognitive aging has followed two rather distinct traditions. The first grew out of experimental child psychology, whereas the second derived from psychometric roots that included the assessment of intellectual competence and development in normal and abnormal populations.

Experimental Study of Memory Functions and Language

The literature on memory functions and language has been concerned with the identification of potentially causal variables that might be responsible for the memory loss and decline observed in many older adults in complex manipulation of language variables such as text processing. Conventional approaches in this literature involve the design of experiments that test for the effects of single variables in carefully controlled laboratory settings and that require only a limited number of subjects. Because there is often little interest in individual differences or population parameters, study participants are typically drawn from convenience samples (McKay and Abrams, 1996). In addition, this literature includes primarily age-comparative studies (see below for the implicit methodological problems inherent in such studies). Hence, little is known from this literature regarding the extent of individual differences or major types of differential patterns of cognitive aging, nor is it clear how findings generalize to broader or specialized populations.

The literature described above may suggest many hypotheses that would be useful for designing technical aids that could compensate in general for age-related changes. However, the literature is as yet too limited to be helpful in determining typologies of age changes that may be needed for customization of devices for optimal individual use.

Descriptive Study of Adult Intellectual Development

Many studies of adult intellectual development originated from the longitudinal follow-up of samples that were first assessed in childhood or adolescence. Other studies, however, represent carefully stratified samples from defined populations, first assessed at a particular life stage, whether in early adulthood or in early old age. Descriptive studies often began as cross-sectional inquiries that were expanded into long-term longitudinal studies. Longitudinal data were required because the interest here is typically in the study of individual differences in intraindividual change, or in the identification of typologies of individuals who follow different growth trajectories. Such studies frequently involve large samples, and they typically employ correlational or quasi-experimental approaches (Baltes and Mayer, 1999; Schaie, 1996b). This literature will be particularly helpful in predicting characteristics of future older adults as well as to provide an understanding of different patterns of age changes.

METHODOLOGICAL ISSUES

Two major methodological issues in cognitive aging research are whether one should employ age-comparative (between participants) or age-change (within participants) designs and how investigators should address the role of response speed.

Age-Comparative Versus Age-Change Designs

The bulk of reported findings from the experimental cognitive aging literature is based on age-comparative studies that usually contrast a group of young adults (typically college students) with convenience samples of community-dwelling older adults in their 60s and 70s. However, it is often unreasonable to assume that the two age groups can be adequately matched for other status variables that might provide rival explanations for any observed age difference on the dependent variable of interest. This internal validity threat (cf. Campbell and Stanley, 1966) creates particular problems for identifying the mechanisms that may be implicated in age-related decline from young adulthood into old age. Age-comparative designs are also inadequate in explaining individual differences in intraindividual age changes. The latter can be investigated only by means of longitudinal paradigms (Schaie, 1965, 1996a). The internal validity of longitudinal studies, moreover, can also be impaired by failure to attend to issues such as participant attrition, impact of history, and reactivity (practice) effects.

Data from cross-sectional and longitudinal studies have rather different implications for guiding the design of compensatory devices or interventions. Figure 2-1 provides an illustration of this for the case of age differences and age changes from 25 to 81 years for a measure of verbal meaning

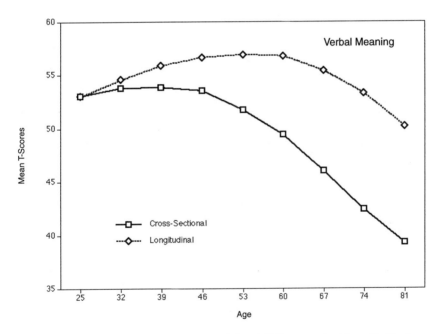

FIGURE 2-1 Comparison of cross-sectional age differences and longitudinal age changes on the Verbal Meaning Test. T-scores are standardized scores with a mean of 50 and a standard deviation of 10.
SOURCE: Adapted from Schaie (in press).

(vocabulary comprehension) from the Seattle Longitudinal Study (Schaie, in press; also see Schaie, 1996b). This figure shows steady negative cross-sectional differences from young adulthood to old age. However, the longitudinal (within-persons) data suggest that verbal meaning increases until late middle age and shows only modest decline thereafter. These findings can be interpreted to suggest that there is little age-related decline in verbal comprehension; but they also suggest that older persons may benefit from simplified (less esoteric) language in instruction manuals. Current older adults may be impacted by technological obsolescence that may not similarly impact future cohorts of older adults. In other words, cross-sectional data can be used to determine current differences in performance level for different age groups, but longitudinal data are required to predict within-individual changes with age.

The Role of Response Speed

Several theorists have suggested that general changes in the central nervous system are the primary common cause for the observed age-related declines in cognitive performance. An unbiased marker of such change might be the commonly observed increase in simple reaction time. Many published analyses show a substantial reduction in age differences, if some measure or measures of reaction time or perceptual speed is partialled out of the relation between measures of a cognitive process and chronological age (Madden, 2001; Salthouse, 1999). The average increase in many measures of reaction time is a factor of approximately 1.6 from the early 20s to the late 60s (Cerella, 1990). However, it is not clear whether the observed average increase in reaction time, although reliably demonstrable in the laboratory, is of significance in many or most tasks of daily living. Nevertheless, it is critical therefore in cognitive aging studies to disaggregate changes in speed of response from changes in accuracy of performance (cf. Willis, 1996; Willis and Schaie, 1986).

The literature also has many findings of a trade-off between accuracy and speed (cf. Ketcham and Stelmach, this volume; Salthouse, 1999). Given the need for accuracy in programming compensatory devices, it might therefore be desirable to increase response windows to facilitate better performance by individuals whose speed of reaction time has declined.

The Role of Individual Differences

Although empirical findings on age differences or age changes suggest virtually linear declines for many cognitive functions, it is difficult to reproduce linear decline patterns at the individual level. Indeed, it appears that there are many different aging patterns of which linear decline may be only a sparsely represented phenomenon. More common are stairstep patterns that reflect decline occurring in response to an unfavorable event (perhaps severe physiological insult or the loss of a spouse) followed by a period of stability at a lower level, with further decline upon the occurrence of other unfavorable events (cf. Schaie, 1989).

It has been shown that a significant percentage of individuals will remain stable over a 7-year period even at advanced ages and that a small percentage of individuals will even show a significant increase in performance levels. Figure 2-2 shows the percentage of community-dwelling individuals declining, remaining stable, or showing an increase in performances from ages 60 to 67, 67 to 74, 74 to 81, and 81 to 88 on the Verbal Meaning Test. Although there is a modest increase in the percentage declining over each older 7-year span, the largest proportion remains stable even into an advanced age (Schaie, in press; also see Schaie, 1989).

Recent advances in multilevel analyses and growth curve modeling provide new and exciting tools for the identification and analyses of typologies of cognitive aging patterns (cf. Rudinger and Rietz, 2001).

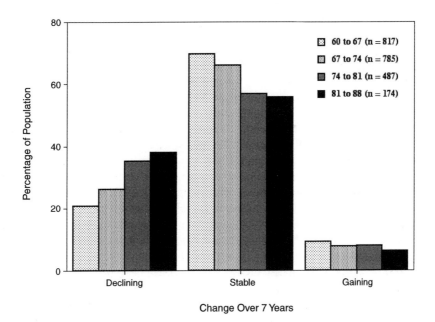

FIGURE 2-2 Percentage of individuals who decline, remain stable, or gain significantly on the Verbal Meaning Test (criterion for significant decline or gain is ±1 standard error of measurement).
SOURCE: Adapted from Schaie (in press).

Sensory-Perceptual Limitations in Older Adults

An important meta-issue in the study of aging and cognition addresses the extent to which the decline in cognitive processes in older adults can be attributed to changes in peripheral sensory functions. I briefly review here some of the major age-related declines in sensory-perceptual processes that aging researchers need to consider. For more extensive reviews, the reader is referred to Fozard and Gordon-Salant (2001) or Schieber (2003).

Vision

Anatomical changes. The size of the pupil declines with advancing adult age (*senile miosis*), and the lens becomes more opaque. This loss of transparency is particularly pronounced at short wavelengths (e.g., for blue light). Lenticular opacity and reduced pupil size result in less retinal illumination. Almost half of those over 65 years of age have sufficiently reduced lenticular transparency to be diagnosed as having cataracts. There is also some evidence of age-related photoreceptor and ganglion cell loss. Macular degeneration and glaucoma also impair vision in significant numbers of older persons.

Visual acuity. This is the indicator of how well fine spatial detail can be recognized. A distinction is made between near and far acuity. By age 40, difficulty is experienced focusing on printed text that is closer than about a foot, and by age 60 it becomes difficult for most people to focus on objects located within 3 feet. Decreases in both near and far acuity until around age 70 are usually due to refractive errors that can be corrected with eyeglasses or contact lenses. However, visual difficulties that remain after wearing eyeglasses increase sharply in the late 70s and 80s. Impaired visual acuity among those in the oldest groups is attributable to greater prevalence of diseases of the retina. Age-related deficits in visual acuity become more severe when there is low luminance or low-contrast stimuli. Figure 2-3 shows the age-related increase in the percentage of people requiring correction for visual defects and the percentage of those who suffer from cataracts, glaucoma, or other visual impairments (National Center for Health Statistics, 1994).

Dark adaptation and glare. Changing the level of illumination results in a significant reduction in visual sensitivity. There is some age-related slowing in the rate of dark adaptation, and older adults have more difficulty throughout the dark adaptation cycle. The rate of loss is greater for short-wavelength light (i.e., blue, green) due to the age-related yellowing of the lens.

Age-related decrements in visual function are also observed when glare is present. The aging lens scatters light across the retina decreasing the contrast of the retinal image. Visual difficulties due to glare increase

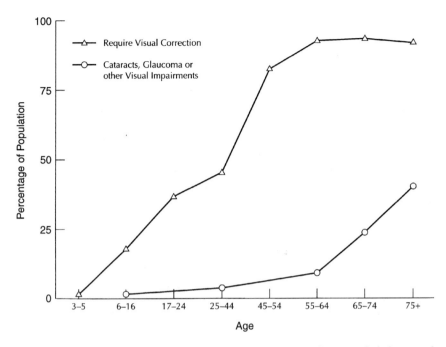

FIGURE 2-3 Percentage of people requiring corrections for visual defects and percentage of those who suffer from cataracts, glaucoma, and other visual impairments.
SOURCE: Schaie and Willis (2002); adapted from National Center for Health Statistics (1994).

markedly for low-contrast stimuli, and recovery time for lost visual sensitivity in response to glare also increases.

Color vision. Small age-related declines have been found in the ability to distinguish between similar hues past age 70. This phenomenon has been attributed to a differential loss of sensitivity in short-wavelength photoreceptors. Difficulties in color vision are greater under low light conditions, and age differences in blue-green color discrimination can be reduced at high levels of illumination. Color constancy mechanisms remain relatively intact in older adults, possibly minimizing performance decrements on real-world tasks.

Motion perception. Age-related decrements have been found in motion sensitivity and accuracy of speed perception although the nature and magnitude of these effects vary across different investigations. It has been suggested that these age-related losses may be mediated by neural rather than optical mechanisms. There are also age differences in thresholds for the detection of motion, as well as age differences in the ability to judge the apparent speed of automobiles (Fozard, 2000; Schieber, 2003).

Hearing

Anatomical changes. Changes in the outer ear include accumulations of earwax that block the auditory canal and a narrowing of the auditory canal. The joints connecting the bones of the middle ear often become less elastic with advancing age. In the inner ear there is age-related loss in the number of hair cells. This loss occurs principally among hair cells transmitting high frequencies. There is also an age-related reduction in the number of neurons in the auditory nerve and the auditory cortex.

Auditory sensitivity and discrimination. Age-related loss of sensitivity (presbycusis) particularly affects high-frequency sounds, requiring greater stimulus intensity for detection of a sound. Age-related hearing loss is more prevalent in males than in females in the current older population. This phenomenon has often been attributed to gender differences in workplace noise exposure. Loss of sensitivity proceeds at a pace of about 1 dB per year after age 60 and at 1.5 dB per year after age 80 in both genders.

Age-related decrements have also been found in the ability to discriminate small changes in the frequency or intensity of sounds during speech recognition and sound localization. Older adults are less able to discriminate between similar sounds that differ slightly in intensity or frequency. Age-related difficulties in frequency discrimination are greater with very brief tones, i.e., older persons in conversations have greater difficulty processing phonemes than syllables. There is also increasing difficulty in discriminating the arrival of sounds, especially for low-frequency sounds.

Speech recognition. Speech recognition for monosyllabic words at normal conversational levels has been found to decrease from almost 100 percent correct at age 30 to less than 60 percent correct for those 80-89 years of age. Particularly severe age-related decrements in speech intelligibility occur when there is background noise, echo, and time compression. Figure 2-4 shows the percentage decrement in speech intelligibility under various conditions from the 20s to the 80s (Bergman et al., 1976).

There is a question as to the relative contribution of peripheral versus central mechanisms in these decrements. Remediation of decrements in speech perception due to sensory factors would require interventions in signal processing, whereas decrements due to cognitive deficits would need to be addressed by comprehensive training approaches (see below). Decrements in understanding speech are lessened when stimulus intensity levels are increased and when speech stimuli are presented within "sentence" or "paragraph" contexts.

Advances in hearing-aid technology provide many ways of compensating for a variety of the hearing problems described above. However, the increasing miniaturization of these devices poses additional problems for

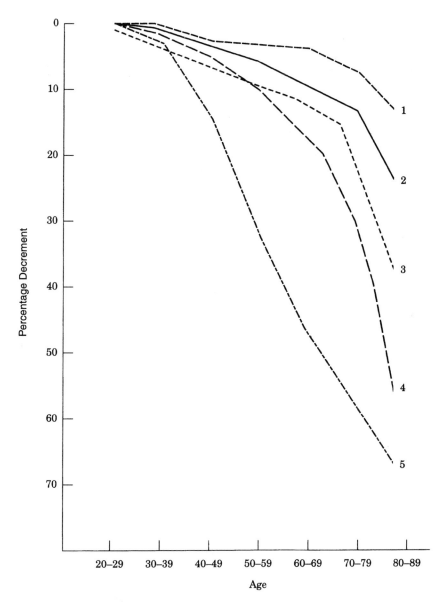

FIGURE 2-4 Percentage decline in speech intelligibility for various ages and listening conditions. Conditions are (1) normal speech; (2) speeded speech, twice the normal rate; (3) selective listening, tracking one speaker of many, as at a cocktail party; (4) reverberated or echoed speech, as in a hall with unfavorable acoustics; and (5) interrupted speech, as with a poor telephone connection.

SOURCE: From Bergman et al. (1976), reproduced by permission.

frail elders. Individual programming of the devices becomes increasingly difficult due to accompanying declines in vision and manipulation of very small objects. Technology will therefore be needed that provides for far more user-friendly methods to fine-tune hearing aids than are currently available.

BASIC FINDINGS FROM THE EXPERIMENTAL LITERATURE ON COGNITIVE AGING

Much of the literature on cognitive aging is cross sectional in nature and frequently includes convenience samples of young adults (often sophomore psychology students) that are compared with other community-dwelling older adults (often participants in adult education programs). The major findings from this literature regarding age differences in cognitive performance include memory, attention, and language.

Memory

Older adults are currently thought to be at a disadvantage in retrieving information from memory when the information to be retrieved is complex and when there are few cues or other environmental supports. Hence, age differences are far greater in recall than in recognition of information. The magnitude of age differences in memory is also thought to be far greater when a task involves effortful processing than when automatic processing is involved. Hence, greater age differences have been found for explicit than for implicit or automatized and overlearned memory (such as responses needed to drive an automobile). Older adults seem to have greater difficulty in integrating the context of information they are trying to remember. Moreover, working memory capacity (that is, the information that is immediately accessible) becomes reduced with increasing age. But there is little evidence for age differences in long-term storage. Memory deficits occurring with age include nonverbal tasks such as memory for spatial location, memory for faces, and memory for actions and activities. Studies of prospective memory (i.e., remembering something to be done in the future) suggest that older people do well in remembering simple and event-based tasks, but are at a disadvantage when tasks become complex or are time-based. In sum, it appears that age differences are known to increase in magnitude as a function of the processing requirements of a given task (Bäckman, Small, and Wahlin, 2001).

Attention

Another recent body of research has considered the role of attention in explaining age differences in other cognitive processes. Attentional processes are implicated whenever individuals engage in multitasking or time-sharing activities. Examples of the consequence of age-related attention deficits can be found in research on inhibition, reading comprehension (see below), and many everyday activities that may be affected by age-related deficits in the ability to attend simultaneously to multiple tasks (e.g., Schieber, 2003; West, 1999; Zacks and Hasher, 1997). On the other hand, attention deficits have not been found to underlie age differences in episodic memory that involve remembering items associated with a specific time or place (Nyberg, Nilsson, Olofsson, and Bäckman, 1997). Age-related differences in attention may also be implicated in executive functioning, the ability to put things together on the basis of several items of information. One example would be considering the price and utility of a computer system in making a purchase decision (cf. Kramer, Larish, Weber, and Bardell, 1999).

Although some of the most exciting research in this area is the exploration of neurological bases for attention processes, there are also many practical applications in areas such as aging and technology use (cf. Rogers and Fisk, 2001).

Language

Age-related differences in language behavior are closely related to the processes of encoding and retrieving verbal materials as discussed above. In addition, there are greater age differences in textual tasks that involve recent connections than in those that involve recollection of older connections. Language production is adversely affected in older adults under intense time pressure. Word-finding difficulty (the interesting tip-of-the-tongue phenomenon), however, seems to be more likely with infrequently used words. Significant age differences have also been found in planning what one intends to say and how to say it during language production. Older adults are therefore more likely to hesitate, have false starts, as well as to engage in repetitions. Age-linked deficits in story recall may be more of a general deficit in connection formation than in specific communication ability. Older adults tend to benefit from textual material that provides priming of associations because it contains learned semantically linked information (McKay and Abrams, 1996). On the other hand, certain aspects of language processing seem to be relatively age invariant. These include particularly lexical access and semantic memory, which are resistant to normal aging, even though they are affected by Alzheimer's disease (Kemper and Mitzner, 2001).

Recent research on language and aging has also included applications of basic research knowledge to the development of guidelines for consumer standards and for electronic communication (cf. Charness, Park, and Sabel, 2001; Park, Nisbett, and Hedden, 1999).

BASIC FINDINGS FROM THE DESCRIPTIVE LITERATURE ON AGE CHANGES IN INTELLECTUAL COMPETENCE

Included here are findings from two rather different traditions. The first originated early in the history of psychology when the research on mental testing in children was extended to normal adults and older adults. The second tradition, now represented by the field of neuropsychology, originated with the clinical interest in assessing cognitive impairment and in diagnosing various forms of dementia.

Normal Populations

Investigations of the course of intellectual competence over the adult life span in normal populations has been dominated by research either with the Wechsler Intelligence Scale or with ability batteries derived from the Thurstonian Primary Mental Ability framework (Schaie, 1996b; Schaie and Hofer, 2001). A primary distinction is often made between fluid abilities, thought to be innate, and crystallized abilities, which involve the utilization of culturally acquired knowledge (Cattell, 1963). Further distinctions have been introduced more recently between the mechanics (or basic processes) of intellectual competence and the pragmatics that involve cultural mediation (Baltes, Dittman-Kohli, and Dixon, 1984).

Most longitudinal studies have found that the adult life course of mental abilities is not uniform. The fluid abilities (sometimes defined as cognitive mechanics or primitives) tend to peak in early midlife and begin to decline by the early 60s. Crystallized abilities that represent abilities acquired in a given cultural context (particularly verbal abilities), by contrast, do not usually peak until the 50s are reached and begin to show significant decline only in the 70s and often show only minimal decline even in the 80s (Schaie, 1996a). But with advanced age, increasing convergence and steeper decline for both aspects of intellectual competence may occur, probably caused by the increasing decline of sensory and central nervous system functions (Baltes and Lindenberger, 1997; Baltes and Mayer, 1999). Figure 2-5 provides longitudinal data on six cognitive abilities illustrating differences in average decline patterns for the different abilities.

Cross-sectional snapshots, obtained at a particular time, may yield very different ability profiles because of the fact that consecutive population cohorts reach different asymptotes in midlife. For the six abilities whose age trajectories are shown in Figure 2-5, the cumulative magnitude

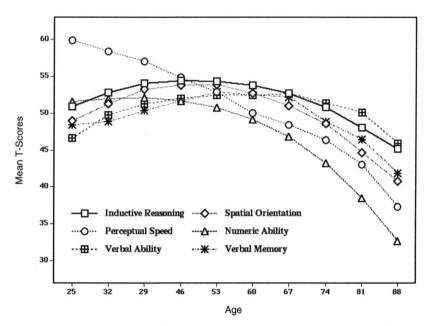

FIGURE 2-5 Longitudinal age changes from 25 to 88 years on six cognitive abilities. T-scores are standardized scores with a mean of 50 and a standard deviation of 10.
SOURCE: Schaie (1996a).

of the individual 7-year cohort differences are presented in Figure 2-6. For example, for the time frame shown there has been a positive linear cohort trend for inductive reasoning, the basic component of most problem-solving tasks, whereas there has been a negative trend in numeric skills. The magnitude of cohort differences in abilities over the past half-century has been comparable to the average age changes observed from young adulthood into the 70s (cf. Flynn, 1987). In the presence of positive cohort changes, older adults may appear to have declined markedly in comparison with their younger peers, even though they have not declined at all but simply attained a lower asymptote in young adulthood. Likewise, when there are negative cohort differences, older adults may compare favorably with their younger peers even when they are functioning below their earlier levels of performance (Schaie, 1996a; Schaie and Hofer, 2001).

Investigations of individual differences suggest that most persons have declined on some aspect of intellectual functioning from their own midlife peak as the 60s are reached. But specific patterns of decline may well depend on complex patterns of individual life experience. Most

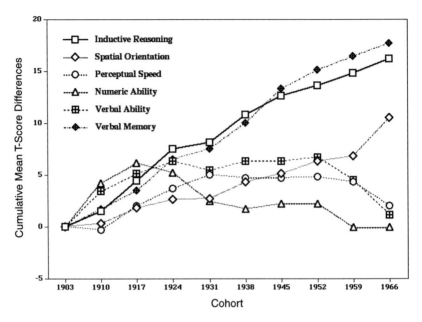

FIGURE 2-6 Cohort differences on six cognitive abilities for cohorts born from 1903 to 1966. T-scores are standardized scores with a mean of 50 and a standard deviation of 10.
SOURCE: Schaie (1996a).

healthy community-dwelling persons are able to maintain a high level of function until an advanced age (but see Baltes and Mayer, 1999, for the consequences of sensory dysfunctions). Because most tasks of daily living represent complex combinations of basic cognitive processes, many individuals can maintain their abilities above the minimally necessary threshold level for independent functioning by engaging in compensatory processes that may often be quite complex (cf. Baltes et al., 1984; Baltes and Mayer, 1999).

Neuropsychological Assessments of Normal and Cognitively Impaired Individuals

Measures used for neuropsychological assessment have also originated from the psychometric tradition (e.g., subtests from the Wechsler Memory Scales often form important components of neuropsychological assessment batteries). However, many measures designed for the identification of cognitive impairment and the diagnosis of the dementias are not particularly suitable for the study of cognitive aging because they were developed specifically to identify neuropathology. Hence, variability on these measures among cognitively unimpaired individuals may be quite limited, and such measures may therefore be less than ideal for the study of cognitive aging (cf. Lezak, 1995). This is unfortunate, for advances in prevention approaches to dementia may very well require the early detection of persons at excess risk for the eventual detection of dementia. This would require tests sensitive enough to detect small deviations from normal scores or subtle changes over time within individuals. Because of the age-related increase in the incidence of preclinical cognitive impairment, the detection of such individuals is of special interest to obtain better estimates for normal age changes.

Research is in progress in my laboratory to extend a neuropsychological battery into the primary mental ability space so as to facilitate the use of assessment instruments with wider ranges that are suitable for younger adults for the purpose of early detection of cognitive impairment (Schaie et al., in press).

DECISION MAKING AND PROBLEM SOLVING

An important extension of the research in cognitive psychology has been in the direction of going beyond the laboratory to the environmental context within which individuals solve problems of daily living and make consequential decisions. The decisions to be made are usually goal directed; in older adults, these decisions are related to instrumental activities of daily living and maintenance of independence (Schaie and Willis, 1999; Willis, 1996). Such decisions include management of one's medication regime and decisions about one's financial affairs. Antecedents of successful decision making in older adults have been identified as good physical health, adequate levels of functioning on basic intellectual skills, tolerance for ambiguity, as well as realistic beliefs about ways of knowing. Lessened tolerance of ambiguity in older adults has been noted to affect medical decision making in that older adults act more quickly to reduce ambiguous situations (Leventhal, Leventhal, Schaefer, and Easterling, 1993).

The problem-solving process involves task characteristics and knowledge systems. In older adults, task novelty can have a negative influence on effective problem solutions, as does task complexity and lack of task structure. Also of importance is the availability of declarative knowledge that is relevant to a particular decision. Older individuals tend to make critical decisions with less information than young or middle-aged adults (for an example of decision making and aging with a breast cancer scenario, see Meyer, Russo, and Talbot, 1995).

Decision making may also be affected by age-related processing styles. Youthful styles involve a bottom-up approach that involves intensive data gathering. Recourse must be had to formal integrated knowledge bases in order to compensate for a lack of personal experiences. The mature middle-aged style balances data gathering with the integration of accumulated experience. By contrast, the style of the older adult is to use acquired knowledge sometimes indiscriminately and inappropriately by applying heuristics that have worked well in the past (cf. Sinnot, 1989).

CAN COGNITIVE AGING BE SLOWED OR REVERSED?

Cognitive training programs have been developed in a number of laboratories (primarily in the United States and Germany). They have been applied in the laboratory, and more recently in cooperative multisite intervention trials (cf. Ball et al., 2002). Unlike training young children, where it can be assumed that new skills are conveyed, older adults most often have had access to the skills being trained, but have lost their proficiency through disuse. Information from longitudinal studies is therefore useful in distinguishing individuals who have declined from those who have remained stable. For those who have declined, the training objective involves remediation of loss. But for those who have remained stable, enhancement of previous levels of functioning is intended to compensate for possibly cohort-based disadvantages of older persons (cf. Willis, 2001).

Findings from cognitive intervention studies suggest that cognitive decline in old age, for many older adults, might be attributed to disuse rather than to the deterioration of the physiological or neural substrates of cognitive behavior. For example, a brief 5-hour training program for persons over age 65 resulted in average training gains of about 0.5 standard deviation on the abilities of spatial orientation and inductive reasoning. All study participants had been followed for 14 years prior to the intervention. Approximately half had remained stable and half had shown significant decline.

Of those participants for whom significant decrement could be documented over a 14-year period, roughly 40 percent were returned to the level at which they had functioned when first studied. Figure 2-7 shows findings by gender for the percentage of individuals who showed significant training gain, as well as the percentage whose performance was raised to the level they had achieved 14 years earlier (cf. Schaie, 1996a; Willis and Schaie, 1994).

The analyses of structural relationships among the ability measures prior to and after training further allow the conclusion that training does not result in qualitative changes in ability structures and is thus highly specific to the targeted abilities. A 7-year follow-up study further demonstrated that those subjects who showed significant decline at initial training retained a substantial advantage over untrained comparison groups

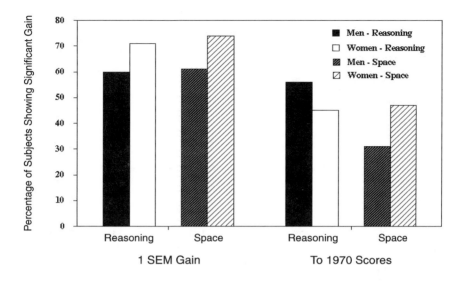

FIGURE 2-7 Percentage of study participants with significant training improvement of ±1 standard error of measurement (SEM) and with return to ability levels 14 years prior to the training intervention.
SOURCE: Schaie (1996a).

(Willis and Schaie, 1994). It should be noted, however, that although cognitive training may improve performance in older adults and may function to reduce effects of age decrement, such training will also be effective in enhancing the performance of young adults, so age differences tend to remain robust (cf. Baltes and Kliegl, 1992).

Many technologies that promise to compensate for age-related changes in behavioral efficiency will also require the increased utilization of cognitive skills that have become "rusty" through disuse. Cognitive training paradigms may therefore be helpful in enhancing the cognitive infrastructures required for the successful utilization of complex technology.

OTHER RELATED TOPICS IN COGNITIVE AGING

Research on cognitive aging in the past has been largely concerned with age-related aspects of the development of the basic processes of cognition. It should be recognized that the current focus in the study of cognitive aging is beginning to turn to the determination of how these basic processes operate within more complex domains. Of particular interest here are the study of wisdom and creativity (e.g., Baltes and Staudinger, 2000; Sternberg and Lubart, 2001), the application of basic cognitive processes to social cognition (e.g., Staudinger, 1998), and the development of software expert systems (e.g., Charness and Bosman, 1990). Although the extensive literature on these topics is beyond the scope of this chapter, it should be noted that this is the area of cognitive content where older adults often compare relatively well with the young whenever content is examined that was present in the life experience of older adults.

FUTURE DIRECTION

It is to be expected that much future research in cognitive aging will be directed toward detecting the neural substrates of cognitive processes over the adult life span. An essential element of such research, however, will be to attend to change over time within individuals, as much of what has been done thus far is largely limited to cross-sectional studies (Albert and Killiany, 2001). Similarly, we are just beginning to see longitudinal data emerging on the traditional measures of memory and executive functioning (cf. Bäckman et al., 2001).

To apply much of the basic knowledge on cognitive aging to everyday behavior and human factors considerations involved in the better utilization of modern technology (cf. Schaie and Charness, 2003), we still need to obtain a better understanding of the relationship between basic cognitive processes and everyday function. Similarly, further research will be needed to determine how interventions designed to enhance basic cognitive processes will express themselves in improving effective functioning on complex processes. And above all, far more attention needs to be paid to individual differences in adult cognitive development so that we can move beyond the naive notion that a single grand scheme can account for the behavior of all.

REFERENCES

Albert, M.S., and Killiany, R.J. (2001). Age-related cognitive change and brain-behavior relationships. In J.E. Birren and K.W. Schaie (Eds.), *Handbook of the psychology of aging* (5 ed., pp. 161-185). San Diego, CA: Academic Press.

Bäckman, L., Small, B.J., and Wahlin, A. (2001). Aging and memory: Cognitive and biological perspectives. In J.E. Birren and K.W. Schaie (Eds.), *Handbook of the psychology of aging* (5 ed., pp. 349-377). San Diego, CA: Academic Press.

Ball, K., Berch, D.B., Helmers, K.F., Jobe, J.B., Leveck, M.D., Marsiske, M., Morris, J.N., Rebok, G.W., Smith, D.M., Tennstedt, S.L., Unverzagt, F.W., and Willis, S.L. (2002). Effects of cognitive training interventions with older adults: A randomized controlled trial. *Journal of the American Medical Association, 288*(18), 2271-2281.

Baltes, P.B., and Kliegl, R. (1992). Further testing of limits of cognitive plasticity: Negative age differences in a mnemonic skill are robust. *Developmental Psychology, 28*(1), 121-125.

Baltes, P.B., and Lindenberger, U. (1997). Emergence of a powerful connection between sensory and cognitive functions across the adult life span: A new window to the study of cognitive aging? *Psychology and Aging, 12*(1), 12-21.

Baltes, P.B., and Mayer, K.U. (1999). *The Berlin Aging Study: Aging from 70 to 100*. Cambridge, England: Cambridge University Press.

Baltes, P.B., and Staudinger, U.M. (2000). Wisdom: A metaheuristic (pragmatic) to orchestrate mind and virtue toward excellence. *American Psychologist, 55*(1), 122-136.

Baltes, P.B., Dittman-Kohli, F., and Dixon, R.A. (1984). New perspectives on the development of intelligence in adulthood: Toward a duel process conception and a model of selective optimization with compensation. In P.B. Baltes and O.G. Brim Jr. (Eds.), *Lifespan development and behavior* (vol. 6, pp. 33-76). New York: Academic Press.

Bergman, M., Blumenfeld, V.G., Casardo, D., Dash, B., Levett, H., and Margulies, M.K. (1976). Age-related decrement in hearing for speech: Sampling and longitudinal studies. *Journal of Gerontology, 31*, 533-538.

Campbell, D.T., and Stanley, J.C. (1966). *Experimental and quasi-experimental designs for research in teaching*. Chicago: Rand McNally.

Cattell, R.B. (1963). Theory of fluid and crystallized intelligence: A critical experiment. *Journal of Educational Psychology, 54*, 1-22.

Cerella, J. (1990). Aging and information-processing rate. In J.E. Birren and K.W. Schaie (Eds.), *Handbook of the psychology of aging* (3rd ed., pp. 201-221). San Diego, CA: Academic Press.

Charness, N., and Bosman, E.A. (1990). Expertise and aging: Life in the lab. In T.M. Hess (Ed.), *Aging and cognition: Knowledge organization and utilization* (pp. 343-385). North Holland, Amsterdam: Elsevier Science.

Charness, N., Park, D.C., and Sabel, B.A. (2001). *Communication, technology and aging: Opportunities and challenges for the future*. New York: Springer-Verlag.

Flynn, J.R. (1987). Massive IQ gains in 14 nations: What IQ tests really measure. *Psychological Bulletin, 101*(2), 171-191.

Fozard, J.L. (2000). Sensory and cognitive changes with age. In K.W. Schaie and M. Pietrucha (Eds.), *Mobility and transportation in the elderly* (pp. 1-44). New York: Springer-Verlag.

Fozard, J.L., and Gordon-Salant, S. (2001). Changes in vision and hearing with aging. In J.E. Birren and K.W. Schaie (Eds.), *Handbook of the psychology of aging* (pp. 241-266). San Diego, CA: Academic Press.

Kemper, S., and Mitzner, T.L. (2001). Language production and comprehension. In J.E. Birren and K.W. Schaie (Eds.), *Handbook of the psychology of aging* (5th ed., pp. 378-398). San Diego, CA: Academic Press.

Ketcham, C.J., and Stelmach, G.E. (2004). Movement control in the older adult. In National Research Council, *Technology for adaptive aging* (pp. 64-92). Steering Committee for the Workshop on Technology for Adaptive Aging. R.W. Pew and S.B. Van Hemel (Eds.). Board on Behavioral, Cognitive, and Sensory Sciences. Division of Behavioral and Social Sciences and Education. Washington, DC: The National Academies Press.

Kramer, A.F., Larish, J.L., Weber, T.A., and Bardell, L. (1999). Training for executive control: Task coordination strategies and aging. In D. Gopher and A. Koriat (Eds.), *Attention and performance XVII: Cognitive regulation of performance: Interaction of theory and application* (pp. 617-652). Cambridge, MA: MIT Press.

Leventhal, E.A., Leventhal, H., Schaefer, P., and Easterling, D. (1993). Conservation of energy, uncertainty reduction, and swift utilization of medical care among the elderly. *Journal of Gerontology, 48*(2), 78-86.

Lezak, M.D. (1995). *Neuropsychological assessment* (3rd ed.). New York: Oxford University Press.

Madden, D.J. (2001). Speed and timing of behavioral processes. In J.E. Birren and K.W. Schaie (Eds.), *Handbook of the psychology of aging* (5th ed., pp. 288-312). San Diego, CA: Academic Press.

McKay, D.G., and Abrams, L. (1996). Language, memory, and aging: Distributed deficits and the structure of new-versus-old connections. In J.E. Birren and K.W. Schaie (Eds.), *Handbook of the psychology of aging* (4th ed., pp. 288-312). San Diego, CA: Academic Press.

Meyer, B.J.F., Russo, C., and Talbot, A. (1995). Discourse comprehension and problem solving: Decisions about the treatment of breast cancer by women across the life-span. *Psychology and Aging, 10,* 84-103.

National Center for Health Statistics. (1994). *Evaluation of national health interview survey diagnostic reporting.* (Vital and Health Statistics, Series 2 No. 120.) Hyattsville, MD: Centers for Disease Control and Prevention.

Nyberg, L., Nilsson, L.G., Olofsson, U., and Bäckman, L. (1997). Effects of division of attention during encoding and retrieval on age differences in episodic memory. *Experimental Aging Research, 23*(2), 137-143.

Park, D.C., Nisbett, R., and Hedden, T. (1999). Aging, culture, and cognition. *Journal of Gerontology: Psychological Sciences, 54B*(2), 75-84.

Rogers, W.A., and Fisk, A.D. (2001). *Human factors interventions for the health care of older adults.* Mahwah, NJ: Lawrence Erlbaum.

Rudinger, G., and Rietz, C. (2001). Structural equation modeling in longitudinal research on aging. In J.E. Birren and K.W. Schaie (Eds), *Handbook of the psychology of aging* (5th ed., pp. 29-52). San Diego, CA: Academic Press.

Salthouse, T.A. (1999). Theories of cognition. In V.L. Bengtson and K.W. Schaie (Eds.), *Handbook of theories of aging* (pp. 196-208). New York: Springer-Verlag.

Schaie, K.W. (1965). A general model for the study of developmental problems. *Psychological Bulletin, 64,* 92-107.

Schaie, K.W. (1989). Individual differences in rate of cognitive change in adulthood. In V.L. Bengtson, and K.W. Schaie (Eds.), *The course of later life: Research and reflections* (pp. 65-85). New York: Springer-Verlag.

Schaie, K.W. (1996a). *Intellectual development in adulthood: The Seattle Longitudinal Study.* New York: Cambridge University Press.

Schaie, K.W. (1996b). Intellectual functioning and aging. In J.E. Birren and K.W. Schaie (Eds.), *Handbook of the psychology of aging* (4th ed., pp. 266-286). San Diego, CA: Academic Press.

Schaie, K.W. (in press). *Developmental influences on adult intelligence: The Seattle Longitudinal Study.* New York: Oxford University Press.

Schaie, K.W., and Charness, N. (2003). *Influences of technolgical change on individual aging.* New York: Springer-Verlag.

Schaie, K.W., and Hofer, S.M. (2001). Longitudinal studies in research on aging. In J.E. Birren and K.W. Schaie (Eds.), *Handbook of the psychology of aging* (5th ed., pp. 55-77). San Diego, CA: Academic Press.

Schaie, K.W., and Willis, S.L. (1999). Theories of everyday competence. In V.L. Bengtson and K.W. Schaie (Eds.), *Handbook of theories of aging* (pp. 174-195). New York: Springer.

Schaie, K.W., and Willis, S.L. (2002). *Adult development and aging* (5th ed.). Upper Saddle River, NJ: Prentice-Hall.

Schaie, K.W., Caskie, G.I.L., Revell, A.J., Willis, S.L., Kaszniak, A.W., and Teri, L. (in press). Extending neuropsychological assessments into the primary mental ability space. *Aging, Neuropsychology and Cognition.*

Schieber, F. (2003). Human factors and aging: Identifying and compensating for age-related deficits in sensory and cognitive function. In K.W. Schaie and N. Charness (Eds.), *Influences of technological change on individual aging.* New York: Springer-Verlag.

Sinnot, J.D. (1989). A model for solution of ill-structured problems: Implications for every-day and abstract problem solving. In J.D. Sinnot (Ed.), *Everyday problem solving: Theory and applications* (pp. 72-99). New York: Praeger.

Staudinger, U.M. (1998). Social cognition and psychological approach to an art of life. In F. Blanchard-Fields and T.B. Hess (Eds.), *Social cognition, adult development and aging.* San Diego, CA: Academic Press.

Sternberg, R.J., and Lubart, T.I. (2001). Wisdom and creativity. In J.E. Birren and K.W. Schaie (Eds.), *Handbook of the psychology of aging* (5th ed., pp. 500-522). San Diego, CA: Academic Press.

West, R. (1999). Age differences in lapse of intention in the Stroop task. *Journals of Gerontology: Psychological Sciences, 54,* 34-43.

Willis, S.L. (1996). Everyday problem solving. In J.E. Birren and K.W. Schaie (Eds.), *Handbook of the psychology of aging* (4th ed., pp. 287-307). San Diego, CA: Academic Press.

Willis, S.L. (2001). Methodological issues in behavioral intervention research with the elderly. In J.E. Birren and K.W. Schaie (Eds.), *Handbook of the psychology of aging* (5th ed., pp. 78-108). San Diego, CA: Academic Press.

Willis, S.L., and Schaie, K.W. (1986). Training the elderly on the ability factors of spatial orientation and inductive reasoning. *Psychology and Aging, 1*(3), 239-247.

Willis, S.L., and Schaie, K.W. (1994). Cognitive training in the normal elderly. In F. Forette, Y. Christen, and F. Boller (Eds.), *Plasticite cerebrale et stimulation cognitive [Cerebral plasticity and cognitive stimulation]* (pp. 91-113). Paris, France: Fondation Nationale de Gerontologie.

Zacks, R., and Hasher, L. (1997). Cognitive gerontology and attentional inhibition. *Journal of Gerontology: Psychological Sciences, 52B,* 274-283.

3

Movement Control in the Older Adult

Caroline J. Ketcham and *George E. Stelmach*

INTRODUCTION

The control of movements is a complex interaction of cognitive and sensorimotor systems. Researchers in movement science aim to understand how an action is produced and what mechanisms are involved in regulating the movement. Motor control declines in older adults include changes in both the peripheral and the central nervous system, which lead to an array of behavioral decrements (Salthouse, 1985; Welford, 1977; Ketcham and Stelmach, 2002). It is well known that as adults age, the execution of movement becomes slow and more variable, and there is emerging evidence that the microstructure of the movement also changes. In this chapter we document most of the major changes that occur in the control and coordination of movement with respect to aging. In the studies reviewed, older adults are classified as over 60 years and are compared with young adults typically between 18 and 30 years of age in a cross-sectional manner (see Schaie, this volume, for a methodological description). Results reported are means derived from age-group comparisons and do not address individual differences.

The review begins with a discussion of processing speed defined by reaction time and presents differences between young and older adults on simple and complex tasks. The following topics include changes that occur in older adults related to the control of movement including: reduced movement speed, movement composition differences, increased variability, reduced force control, and coordination difficulties. Subsequently highlighted are some of the possible sensorimotor changes that may contribute to slower, more-variable movements and reduced strength observed in older adults. Changes in posture and balance are then discussed, as a stable base of support is necessary to execute precise motor skills as well as being important for mobility of older adults. Finally, an overview of motor learning research as well as a discussion of improvements in motor function with generalized and specific training programs are presented. As is apparent, changes in control and coordination of movement significantly affect the type of activities that older adults can efficiently perform and often determine whether they can live independently. Thus, those involved in enhancing the performance capabilities of these individuals need to have a good understanding of how the aging processes diminish motor performance.

RESPONSE INITIATION

Reaction time is defined as the time required to initiate a movement response following a visual, auditory, or other sensory signal and is thought to reflect the speed of transmission of the central nervous system (Stelmach and Goggin, 1988). Experiments are conducted to measure the time it takes to initiate a response when an imperative stimulus is presented. The imperative stimulus is usually visual, but may be auditory or tactile. Such reactions can be to a single stimulus, multiple stimuli, or may include incompatible responses. In a simple reaction-time task, where one stimulus is given and one response is required, it has been demonstrated that reaction time increases in range from 0.5 ms/yr (5 ms/decade) (Fozard, Vercryssen, Reynolds, Hancock, and Quilter, 1994) to 2 ms/decade (Gottsdanker, 1982). It has been widely shown in the research that the speed of processing information decreases (i.e., the time increases) with advanced age on the order of 26 percent (264 ms in the young—20 years old—versus 327 ms in older adults—60 years old) (Welford, 1984). Similar findings have been reported for auditory and tactile simple reaction times as well (Redfern, Muller, Jennings, and Furman, 2002; Walhovd and Fjell, 2001; Liu, 2001; Walker, Alicandri, Sedney, and Roberts, 1991). This approximately 50-ms increase in simple reaction times is consistent across studies that have examined such changes across the life span (Fozard et al., 1994) as well as those that compare groups of young and older adults on the same reaction-time tasks (Amrhein, Stelmach, and Goggin, 1991; Walker, Philbin, and Fisk, 1997; Stelmach and Goggin, 1988; Cerella, 1985; Cerella, Poon, and Williams, 1980; Bashore, Ridderinkhof, and van der Molen, 1997; Gottsdanker, 1982; Stelmach and Goggin, 1988). See Schaie (in this volume) for a similar discussion of response speed with respect to cognitive changes that occur with advanced age.

The slowing of processing speed in older adults is greater in tasks that require more complicated processing to initiate the appropriate response (Amrhein et al., 1991; Goggin and Stelmach, 1990; Larish and Stelmach, 1982; Stelmach, Goggin, and Garcia-Colera, 1987; Diggles-Buckles and Vercruyssen, 1990; Simon, 1967; Welford, 1977; Bashore et al., 1997; Cerella, 1985; Cerella et al., 1980; Fozard et al., 1994; Melis, Soetens, and van der Molen, 2002; Gottsdanker, 1982; Stelmach and Goggin, 1988). In a choice reaction-time task, subjects are required to select the appropriate response that corresponds to a specific stimulus. These reaction times are typically longer than in simple reaction-time tasks as they include an additional element of selecting the appropriate response. Older adults are 30-60 percent (50–500 ms) slower than young adults in reaction-time tasks with two to four choices (Amrhein et al., 1991; Simon, 1967; Welford, 1984; Jordan and Rabbitt, 1977; Stelmach and Goggin, 1988). Choice reaction time in older adults has been found to increase by 1.6 ms/yr and is amplified as the number of choices increases (Fozard et al., 1994). For example, in a two-, four-, and seven-choice reaction-time task, older adults were 39, 40, and 45 percent slower than young adults, respectively. Furthermore, older adults respond similarly to young adults: When the number of response choices increases, reaction time increases (Hick, 1952); however, the delays in responding are more substantial with multiple response choices.

Some researchers have sought to decompose reaction time into premotor and motor time. Premotor time is defined as the time from the presentation of the stimulus until the onset of muscle activity and is thought to reflect cognitive processes, whereas motor time is the time from muscle activation to the beginning of the movement and reflects efficiency of the motor system. These studies have shown that most of the response delays in older adults are accounted for in the premotor or cognitive period (Clarkson, 1978; Hart, 1980; Spirduso, 1995). Further studies have decomposed the premotor cognitive processes into the time it takes to detect, prepare, and initiate an appropriate response. The majority of these studies have shown that the time utilized for each of these elementary components is prolonged equally in older adults (Simon and Pouraghabagher, 1978; Gottsdanker, 1982; Stelmach and Goggin, 1988; Stelmach et al., 1987, 1988). Collectively, the literature on response speed documents delayed initiation of a response in older adults compared with young adults across an array of simple and complex tasks.

MOVEMENT CONTROL DECREMENTS

Movement Duration

Movement duration is defined as the time from the initiation of the movement to the termination of the movement (Birren, 1974; Salthouse,

1985). Movement time is increased in older adults for a variety of tasks including point-to-point movements (Amrhein et al., 1991; Cerella, 1985; Cooke, Brown, and Cunningham, 1989; Ketcham, Seidler, Van Gemmert, and Stelmach, 2002; Goggin and Meeuwsen, 1992), reaching and grasping movements (Carnahan, Vandervoort, and Swanson, 1998; Bennett and Castiello, 1994), handwriting (Amrhein and Theios, 1993; Dixon, Kurzman, and Friesen, 1993; Contreras-Vidal, Teulings, and Stelmach, 1998), and continuous movements (Greene and Williams, 1996; Pohl, Winstein, and Fisher, 1996; Wishart, Lee, Murdoch, and Hodges, 2000; Ketcham, Dounskaia, and Stelmach, 2001). Movement durations are on the order of 30-60 percent (50-90 ms) longer in older adults compared with young adults in tasks ranging from simple to complex (Welford, 1977); in extreme cases, slowing has been reported as great as 69 percent (421 ms compared with 132 ms in young adults) in a point-to-point movement (Stelmach et al., 1988). Although movement time is an important measure of how the motor system is performing, the effects observed vary greatly depending on the task.

One common approach to assessing movement slowing is to manipulate task difficulty (information to be processed) in a stepwise fashion. Fitts's law, a well-studied law in motor control research (Fitts, 1954), states that, as the difficulty of the movement increases, the speed of the movement decreases. A typical task would require the subject to move a hand as quickly as possible from a starting position to touch a target with a stylus when a "go" signal is given. The size of the target and the distance from the starting point to the target can be varied. The index of difficulty (ID) is greater for smaller targets and for longer movements. Research has shown that, in such tasks, older adults tend to move slower than young adults at all levels of difficulty but are differentially slower at higher levels of difficulty (Bashore, Osman, and Heffley, 1989; Goggin and Meeuwsen, 1992; Hines, 1979; Ketcham et al., 2002; Salthouse, 1988; Pohl et al., 1996; Walker et al., 1997; Brogmus, 1991; Fozard et al., 1994). For example, Ketcham and colleagues (2002) reported movement durations of a low ID to be 333 and 642 ms in young and older adults, respectively. At the higher ID, movement time of young adults was on average 717 ms compared with 1304 ms for older adults. Pohl and colleagues (1996) reported similar differences on a continuous movement task. Differences in movement times between young and older adults were amplified as task difficulty increased with an 80-ms time difference at the high ID compared with a 29-ms difference at the low ID. Task difficulty according to Fitts's law can be manipulated in two ways: by a change in either the target size or the distance between the start and the end of the movement. When target size and movement distance are manipulated separately, researchers have demonstrated that older compared with younger adults are more affected by increases in movement amplitude (a change from 9.6 to 19.2 cm resulted in a 108-ms increase in movement time for young adults versus 293 ms for older adults) but not by decreases in target size (Ketcham et al., 2002; Goggin and Meeuwsen, 1992). Some authors have speculated that these effects are caused by the reduced ability of older adults to produce and maintain forces across the entire spectrum of the movement (Ketcham et al., 2002; Galganski, Fuglevand, and Enoka, 1993; Darling, Cooke, and Brown, 1989), which may have real-world implications on a variety of precision aiming tasks.

Movement Components

Modern data-acquisition techniques make it possible to record and reconstruct movements in real time, which permit investigators to decompose a movement trajectory to gain information on how a movement is controlled and coordinated. Trajectory profiles are processed to yield velocity and acceleration profiles, which are further decomposed into acceleration and deceleration phases as well as parsed into movement substructures. Experiments that have employed these kinematic analyses have provided insights into how the movements produced by older adults differ from those of young adults (Slavin, Phillips, and Bradshaw, 1996). It has been shown that the velocity profiles of young adults are typically bell shaped, where the acceleration phase equals the deceleration phase. In studies that have examined trajectory profiles of young and older adults, it has been observed that for older adults the trajectories are asymmetrical with a longer deceleration phase (Ketcham et al., 2002; Bennett and Castiello, 1994; Brown, 1996; Cooke et al., 1989; Darling et al., 1989; Goggin and Stelmach, 1990; Marteniuk, MacKenzie, Jeannerod, Athenes, and Dugas, 1987; Pratt, Chasteen, and Abrams, 1994).

The deceleration phase has been suggested to contain the portion of movement that is under corrective control because there is sufficient time for sensory feedback to be processed and implemented into the control of the terminal phase of the movement. The deceleration phase in older adults is on the order of 20-40 percent longer than that of young adults (Brown, 1996; Cooke et al., 1989; Pratt et al., 1994; Bennett and Castiello, 1994; Morgan et al., 1994).

In addition to longer deceleration phases, older adults produce movements with 30-70 percent lower peak velocity compared with young adults (Ketcham et al., 2002; Bellgrove, Phillips, Bradshaw, and Gallucci, 1998; Cooke et al., 1989; Goggin and Meeuwsen, 1992; Pratt et al., 1994) (see Figure 3-1). Furthermore, when movement distance increases, older adults do not increase the velocity of their movements to the same degree as young adults (Ketcham et al., 2002; Gutman, Latash, Almeida,

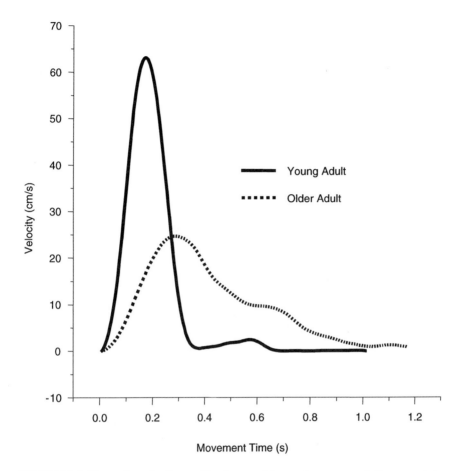

FIGURE 3-1 Example velocity profiles for an older and a young adult on a point-to-point aiming task.
SOURCE: Adapted from Ketcham et al. (2002, p. 56).

and Gottlieb, 1993). For example, Ketcham and colleagues (2002) found that the peak velocity of a shorter-distance movement was 15.9 cm/s in older adults and 29 cm/s in young adults. When movement distance was increased from 9.6 to 19.2 cm, the peak velocity of older adults was 27.6 cm/s whereas for young adults it was 48 cm/s.

Acceleration profiles can be partitioned into movement substructures (primary and secondary submovements) for a more in-depth analysis. The movement optimization model (Meyer, Abrams, Kornblum, Wright, and Smith, 1988) maintains that the primary submovement represents the portion of the movement under preplanned control where the limb is propelled to the target during the acceleration phase, whereas the secondary submovement represents the feedback-controlled portion of the movement. The closer to the target the primary submovement ends, the more efficient the motor system is thought to be (Meyer et al., 1988). Overall, research has demonstrated that older adults cover 10-70 percent less distance with their primary submovement compared with young adults, depending on the task (Bellgrove et al., 1998; Darling et al., 1989; Hsu, Huang, Tsuang, and Sun, 1997; Ketcham et al., 2002; Pratt et al., 1994; Walker et al., 1997; Romero, Van Gemmert, Adler, Bekkering, and Stelmach, 2003; Seidler-Dobrin, He, and Stelmach, 1998). Pratt and colleagues (1994) found that older adults covered 50 percent of the distance to the target with the primary submovement compared with young adults who traveled 70 percent of the distance (Figure 3-2). Because the primary submovement ends further from the movement end point, older adults need to make one or more adjustments with the secondary submovement to complete the movement accurately (Goggin and Meeuwsen, 1992; Hsu et al., 1997; Ketcham et al., 2002; Pohl et al., 1996; Pratt et al., 1994; Seidler-Dobrin and Stelmach, 1998; Walker et al., 1997).

Researchers have extended the use of substructure analysis to assess how young and older adults differ in improving their movements with practice. Pratt et al. (1994) and Seidler-Dobrin and Stelmach (1998) demonstrated that both groups improved their movement times with practice, but they did it quite differently. Older adults only slightly increased (50 to

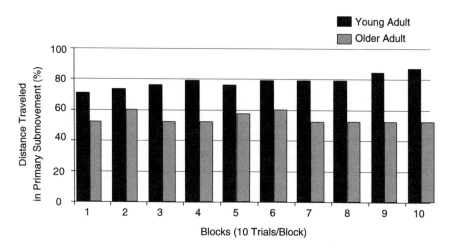

FIGURE 3-2 Percentage of distance traveled in the primary submovement for older and young adults in a point-to-point aiming task over 10 blocks of 10 trials. SOURCE: Adapted from Pratt et al. (1994, p. 360).

51 percent) the portion of the movement covered with the primary submovement with 100 trials of practice whereas young adults increased the distance covered from 67 to 75 percent. These data, along with other studies that have used kinematic and movement subparsing techniques, have shown that the initial phases of the movement are similar in young and older adults, with older adults producing movements with lower peak velocity outputs. Conversely, these methods have shown marked differences in the terminal phase of the movement, measured by the deceleration phase, proportion of the movement covered in the primary submovement, and the subsequent secondary submovements, suggesting that older adults need to make corrective adjustments to their movement as they approach the target.

Movement Variability

Movement variability refers to an individual's overall consistency of an executed task across trials. Increased variability may reflect decrements in the motor system in its ability to produce the same movement output repeatedly. There are two types of movement variability: variability of the end point and variability of the components of the movement trajectory.

Over a wide variety of tasks, researchers report higher variability in the trajectory and end-point position of movements of older adults compared with young adults overall and when performance is examined in a more detailed trial-by-trial basis in a rapid aiming task (Brown, 1996; Cooke et al., 1989; Greene and Williams, 1996; Seidler-Dobrin et al., 1998; Ketcham et al., 2002; Darling et al., 1989; Welford, 1984; Abrams, Pratt, and Chasteen, 1998; Warabi, Kase, and Kato, 1984; Tedeschi et al., 1989). Walker et al. (1997) have shown that older adults have higher variability of end-point of their first submovement compared with young adults. For both young and older adults, as acceleration increased, the variability of end-point position also increased—however, at a significantly greater rate for older adults. Pratt and colleagues (1994) documented that older adults had higher end-point variability than young adults. Both young and older adults showed decreased end-point variability after extended practice; however, older adults did not improve as much as young adults.

In addition to end-point analyses, researchers also have examined the variability of the movement trajectory using kinematic analysis techniques. Cooke and colleagues (1989) found that older adults were significantly more variable compared with young adults on measures including movement duration, peak velocity, and the acceleration/deceleration ratio. Furthermore, the variability of acceleration and deceleration increased differentially for older adults compared with young adults as the amplitude of the movement increased (Darling et al., 1989). Pratt et al. (1994) found that older adults showed higher variability in the distance traveled in the primary submovement that did not improve as much as young adults with extensive practice. It has been suggested that the irregularity of the amplitude and timing of muscle output in older adults is responsible for this overall increased variability in the trajectory of movements as well as variability of end-point position (Darling et al., 1989; Cooke et al., 1989; Brown, 1996; Goggin and Meeuwsen, 1992; Ketcham et al., 2002; Greene and Williams, 1996).

Variability of executed movements on a moment-to-moment basis has large implications for daily activities of older adults. For example, if the motor system is quite variable, it is difficult to know whether you may knock over a glass when you reach for it. If you know you will always undershoot the glass, then you can plan for, prepare for, and compensate for that decrement.

Speed and Accuracy

Movements made to functional targets have a known speed-accuracy relationship. As individuals attempt to move faster, there is a point where the response accuracy is compromised. Individuals, based on their ability, often have different speed-accuracy behavioral patterns. The literature has shown that the reaction time and movement time of older adults are slower than those of young adults (see "Response Initiation" and "Movement Duration" above). One common observation of those investigators who have made cross-sectional comparisons is that older adults have a bias for accuracy at the expense of speed (Salthouse, 1985). Older adults are often more conservative with respect to speed than young adults (Salthouse and Somberg, 1982; Ketcham et al., 2002; Walker et al., 1997; Goggin and Meeuwsen, 1992; Darling et al., 1989). The question arises as to whether such differences are caused by changes in the neurophysiological factors or by different cognitive strategies. Do older adults purposely slow down their movements to ensure that they are made with a high level of accuracy? Most of the studies have attributed the observed slowing in movement control to physiological factors with only a few examining directly whether the speed-accuracy trade-offs actually exist (Salthouse, 1985; Bashore et al., 1989). Salthouse (1985) cited two studies that examined age differences in the speed-accuracy trade-off by manipulating the instructions or incentives that the subjects received for emphasizing speed or accuracy, respectively. Salthouse (1985) further states that both of these studies reported that adults of different ages have specific speed-accuracy characteristics, which show slower response speed as target accuracy becomes more precise, with older adults having slower response speeds than young adults at the same level of precision. Thus, age differences in relation to speed production, with an accuracy component, do exist independently of the subject's emphasis on speed or accuracy. Therefore, in any study showing speed differences in cross-sectional age-group comparisons, the speed versus accuracy relationship should be determined. When an individual trades response speed for response accuracy, it is an example of the influence of cognitive processes on motor performance. Such cognitive strategies make it difficult to accurately determine the amount of change across age groups that is due to neurophysiological factors. This has significant implications for those who work with older adults. First, training programs should challenge older adults to move faster while maintaining accuracy. In addition, when assessing capabilities of older adults, it is important to give older adults more time to complete the task as they perform with accuracy levels similar to young adults when given enough time.

Force Control and Regulation

Force control is an elementary component of movement production because smooth and accurate movements require efficient modulation of force outputs. Changes in the regulation of force outputs lead to decrements in the initiation and control of movements. Older compared with young adults have decreased force outputs and inefficient force regulation making it difficult to initiate and execute movements quickly and accurately across a variety of tasks (Brown, 1996; Campbell, McComas, and Petito, 1973; Clamann, 1993; Cooke et al., 1989; Darling et al., 1989; Davies and White, 1983; Doherty, Vandervoort, and Brown, 1993; Galganski et al., 1993; Izquierdo, Aguado, Gonzalez, Lopez, and Hakkinen, 1999; Larsson and Karlsson, 1978; Milner-Brown, Stein, and Yemm, 1973; Milner, Cloutier, Leger, and Franklin, 1995; Roos, Rice, Connelly, and Vandervoort, 1999; Singh et al., 1999; Stelmach, Teasdale, Phillips, and Worringham, 1989). Stelmach and colleagues (1989), using an isometric task, demonstrated that older adults have a reduced range of force production and higher force output variability compared with young adults. In addition, their rate of force production was substantially slower, as it took 20 ms longer to achieve a force level 45 percent of their maximum (15 N). Ng and Kent-Braun (1999) documented similar findings with older adults. They reported 60-N lower peak force output in older adults compared with young adults and a 20-ms-longer time for force production.

It has been shown that older adults produce multiple bursts of force in tasks when they must achieve targeted force levels approaching maximum (Kinoshita and Francis, 1996; Brown, 1996; Galganski et al., 1993).

This is in contrast to young adults who produce a single burst to the targeted force level. Although these irregularities are small and occur over short periods, they do suggest a reason why control and coordination change with advanced age. Changes in force regulation and control have large implications for most functional tasks—for example, turning a door knob or picking up a glass of liquid. These changes may be a result of motor unit reorganization and muscle composition changes; see "Muscle Composition and Muscle Activation Patterns" below (Erim, Beg, Burke, and de Luca, 1999; Galganski et al., 1993; Hakkinen et al., 1996; Yue, Ranganathan, Siemionow, Liu, and Sahgal, 1999; Clamann, 1993; Davies and White, 1983; Milner-Brown et al., 1973).

Coordination

Coordination is the ability to control a number of movement segments or body parts in a refined manner resulting in a well-timed motor output. The ability to control multiple movement components at any one particular time becomes increasingly difficult with advanced age across a variety of movements including aiming, reaching and grasping, drawing, handwriting, and bimanual coordination tasks (Bennett and Castiello, 1994; Carnahan et al., 1998; Teulings and Stelmach, 1993; Greene and Williams, 1996; Swinnen et al., 1998; Wishart et al., 2000; Ketcham et al., 2001). For example in reach-to-grasp tasks, there are transport and grasp components that must be coordinated both spatially and temporally. Researchers have shown that older adults exhibit unstable temporal coupling between these components (Bennett and Castiello, 1994; Carnahan et al., 1998). Conversely, tasks such as drawing or handwriting that require subjects to control multiple joints in a linked segment have demonstrated that the joints involved require more regulation at fast movement speeds (Teulings and Stelmach, 1993; Ketcham et al., 2001). For example, Ketcham and colleagues (2001) found that in a cyclical drawing task older adults begin to distort their movements at 2.0 Hz (two cycles per second) compared with young adults who begin distortions at 2.5 Hz. It appeared that older adults were unable to accurately control the passive properties of linked segments, resulting in slower, more variable movements. Seidler and colleagues (2002) found that aiming movements away from the body, that required shoulder and elbow participation, became less smooth and decoupled as shoulder contribution increased (Figure 3-3). Furthermore, young adults tended to increase activity of opposing muscles as shoulder involvement increased, whereas older adults coactivated these muscles at high levels during single joint elbow movements and reduced coactivation as shoulder involvement increased.

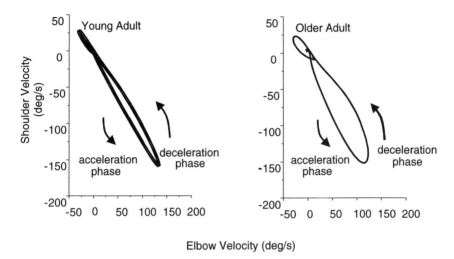

FIGURE 3-3 Coordination of shoulder and elbow joint rotations in a point-to-point aiming task for an example of a young and an older adult.

Bimanual coordination is also a widely researched topic in older adults. In these tasks subjects are asked to produce the same movement with left and right limbs. These movements are typically either in phase, where the two limbs move in the same anatomical direction (homologous muscles activated together), or antiphase, where the two limbs move in the same absolute direction (homologous muscles activated at a 180-degree offset or opposite of each other). In these experiments older adults tend to have difficulty maintaining the more complicated antiphase movements as movement speeds increase (Swinnen et al., 1998; Greene and Williams, 1996; Wishart et al., 2000). Older adults were less accurate at movement speeds of 1.5 and 2.0 Hz compared with young adults, with absolute errors on the order of 20 degrees of relative phase offset. Overall, it has been shown that older adults have increased difficulty controlling and regulating multiple segments to produce smooth motor outputs. Coordination is a part of most tasks of daily living and therefore it is essential to understand breakdowns in control and regulation.

SENSORIMOTOR DECLINES WITH AGE

There are a variety of neurophysiological changes that occur with aging that affect how movements are controlled and regulated in older adults. In this section we focus on declines in proprioception, changes that occur in the composition and activation patterns of muscle, and changes in flexibility. Although we acknowledge that there are important changes that occur in other anatomical and physiological components, they are beyond the scope of this chapter.

Proprioception

Proprioception is a term used to denote the sense of how body segments are oriented in relation to each other. It depends on receptors in the joints and muscles. Research has shown that older adults have decreased proprioceptive capabilities, which includes joint and muscular sensitivity (Levin and Benton, 1973; Ferrell, Crighton, and Sturrock, 1992; Hurley, Rees, and Newham, 1998; Kaplan, Nixon, Reitz, Rindfleish, and Tucker, 1985; Pai, Rymer, Chang, and Sharma, 1997; Skinner, Barrack, and Cook, 1984; Lord, Rogers, Howland, and Fitzpatrick, 1999). To produce smoothly controlled and regulated movements, the central nervous system must be able to accurately identify movement onsets and determine the exact location of the limb at any given time. A reduced capability to detect the position of the limb has large implications for movement control, and therefore it is important to identify age differences in proprioception. Investigators test proprioceptive capabilities by having individuals reproduce joint positions or recognize joint displacements. Smaller errors reflect better proprioceptive acuity. Research has shown that errors in determining joint positions are approximately three times greater in older adults than in young adults (Petrella, Lattanzio, and Nelson, 1997; Kaplan et al., 1985; Ferrell et al., 1992). Petrella and colleagues (1997) assessed the capability to reproduce joint angles in the knee and found that older adults had errors of ±1.2 degrees compared with young subjects who had errors of only ±0.4 degrees. Skinner and colleagues (1984) have suggested, by comparing subjects across age, that for each additional year the ability to detect changes in joint positions decreases by approximately 0.06 degrees.

In paradigms where subjects are asked to match one limb posture with that of the contralateral limb, errors in older adults are on the order of two times greater than those of young adults (Kaplan et al., 1985; Stelmach and Sirica, 1986; Stelmach and Worringham, 1985). Kaplan et al. (1985) found matching errors of ±4 degrees for young adults and ±7 degrees for older adults. The largest errors in both groups were found for the largest joint angles, with the older adults tending to underestimate the joint angle. The reduced ability in older adults to accurately detect movement or localize a body segment position makes it difficult to produce rapid, well-coordinated movements. This has major functional implications for older adults in a variety of tasks of daily living, from sitting in a chair to reaching for an object.

Muscle Composition and Muscle Activation Patterns

The loss of muscle mass in older adults leads to overall decreases in magnitude of force production (Doherty et al., 1993; Lexell, 1993; Metter et al., 1999; Roos et al., 1997, 1999). It has been shown that the number and the size of muscle fibers decrease in older adults, with the most substantial decrease occurring in fast-twitch fibers, which can be activated quickly for large force outputs, but are unable to sustain force output for long periods of time (Yamada, Masuda, and Okada, 2002). It has been estimated that type II (fast-twitch) muscle fibers decrease by approximately 40 percent in older adults, whereas slow-twitch muscle fibers stay relatively stable across the life span (Aniansson, Hedberg, Henning, and Grimby, 1986; Lexell, 1993; Singh et al., 1999; Yamada et al., 2002). In addition to changes in fiber composition, it has also been shown that there is a reorganization of existing motor units (Doherty et al., 1993; Campbell et al., 1973; Yamada et al., 2002). The existing motor units are reorganized to include more muscle fibers per innervation and subsequently change the way force outputs are achieved. Activation of muscle is more bursty and less smooth than in young adults, resulting in force outputs of large incremental steps (Brown, 1972; McComas, Fawcett, Campbell, and Sica, 1971; Roos et al., 1997, 1999). Moreover, the contractile speed of muscles in older adults is slower than in young adults, which also influences the ability to ramp forces in any given muscle (Davies and White, 1983; Larsson, Li, and Frontera, 1997; Ng and Kent-Braun, 1999; Roos et al., 1997).

For most movements, the underlying muscle activation patterns are organized in a triphasic pattern consisting of two bursts of agonist muscle activity separated by a single burst of antagonistic muscle activity (Berardelli et al., 1996). This triphasic pattern of muscle activity produces a smooth trajectory of a body segment from one position to another, with the first agonist burst initiating the movement, overcoming inertial forces; then the subsequent two bursts decelerate or brake the movement of the limb to the desired position (Berardelli et al., 1996; Brown, 1996; Buneo, Soechting, and Flanders, 1994; Darling et al., 1989). Research has found that older adults do not tightly couple the triphasic agonist-antagonist-agonist activation pattern as young adults do. The timing of the triphasic muscle activity is highly variable, without a clear alternating pattern of agonist-antagonist activation. The antagonist burst is not well defined and occurs abnormally early (Darling et al., 1989). Consequently, older adults often produce movements that have prolonged deceleration patterns or periods of braking of the movement (Berardelli et al., 1996; Brown, 1996; Seidler-Dobrin et al., 1998; Darling et al., 1989).

Joint Characteristics and Flexibility Changes

Movement can be restricted by changes in joint characteristics, including tight ligaments, tendons, and muscle; decreased amounts of cartilage; and thicker consistency or decreased amounts of synovial fluid. With advanced age, the length of muscles around the joints is reduced as a result of lower flexibility of joint structures (Nonaka et al., 2002; Wachtel, Maroudas, and Schneiderman, 1995). The deterioration of these structures is thought to result from changes in the hydration and microstructure of collagen within the joint (Bailey and Mansell, 1997; Wachtel et al., 1995). In addition, the loss of cartilage surface and the chemical characteristic changes of this surface lead to osteoarthritic changes common in older adults (Laver-Rubich and Silbermann, 1985; Beaupre, Stevens, and Carter, 2000; Bernick and Cailliet, 1982). The prevalence of joint diseases such as osteoarthritis is extremely high in older adults, on the order of 80 percent of adults over the age of 65 years (Spirduso, 1995; Reginster, 2002). However, even without diseases of the joints, older adults show substantial loss in the range of motion of their joints due to the anatomical changes in joint structures (Bloem, Allum, Carpenter, Verschuuren, and Honegger, 2002; Ronsky, Nigg, and Fisher, 1995; Nonaka et al., 2002).

Range of movement of a joint refers to the excursion a segment can make before being impeded by bone, tight ligaments and tendons, or muscles. Changes in joint characteristics, muscle composition, and activation characteristics as well as higher levels of disuse in older adults (Raab, Agre, McAdam, and Smith, 1988; Bassey, 1998) lead to overall decreases in flexibility in older adults (Shepard, Berridge, and Montelpare, 1990; Spirduso, 1995). Spirduso (1995) cites a study by Kuo (1990), which tested 3,562 Japanese subjects of ages 25-80 years on trunk flexibility. He reported decreases in range of motion on the order of 20 percent in women and 40 percent in men 55 years and older compared with 25-30-year-old subjects. Decreases in range of motion have been largely reported in the lower limbs, primarily in the hip, knee, and ankle joints of men (Ronsky et al., 1995; Nonaka et al., 2002; Bell and Hoshizaki, 1981; Gehlsen and Whaley, 1990). Decreased flexibility has implications for tasks of daily living as it often determines whether a task, like putting on socks or stockings, safely pulling out into traffic, picking up a dropped object, can be successfully completed (Gehlsen and Whaley, 1990; Nonaka et al., 2002; Shepard et al., 1990; Spirduso, 1995).

CHANGES IN POSTURE AND BALANCE

Most skilled movement involves posture in some manner because there needs to be a stable base of support to perform motor skills such as pointing, reaching, and grasping. The ability to stabilize posture is important not only for upright stance, but also when performing a variety of upper-extremity movements. Balance and posture control is assessed to understand motor decrements that contribute to instability. Postural stability is commonly measured during quiet stance or following platform perturbations. Older adults have been shown to have deficits during both quiet stance and perturbation-induced sway balance tests (Maki, Holliday, and Fernie, 1990). Older adults exhibited increased sway range (18 percent), sway variability (16 percent), and sway velocity (43 percent) compared with young adults when standing with eyes open (Teasdale, Stelmach, and Breunig, 1991a). Larger variability in postural sway in the absence of vision in older adults is well documented (Woollacott, 1993; Whipple, Wolfson, Derby, Singh, and Tobin, 1993; Peterka and Black, 1990). Older adults had considerable trouble maintaining balance when the eyes were closed (Whipple et al., 1993; Stelmach and Worringham, 1985). Research has also reported that postural sway range and velocity increased when vision was occluded. When vision was occluded and proprioception disturbed, sway substantially increased (65 percent compared with young adults) (Hay, Bard, Fleury, and Teasdale, 1996; Woollacott, 1993; Schieppati, Grasso, Siliotto, and Nardone, 1993; Sheldon, 1963; Teasdale et al., 1991a). Collins and colleagues (1995) studied postural control mechanisms during quiet stance over a 30-s period. They compared early and late sway stability and found that older adults were substantially more unstable than young adult controls in the first 200 ms of the trial when sensory feedback was not available; they became increasingly stable after 200 ms, similar to young adult controls, when sensory feedback had sufficient time to be processed and implemented into control (Collins et al., 1995). Therefore, during quiet stance, disturbances in incoming information greatly affect postural stability in older adults whereas young adults can quickly and effectively recover from such disturbances.

To further test the capability to recover from perturbation, researchers disturb the support surface while a participant is standing. When platform perturbations are introduced that destabilize the body, older adults take longer to initiate corrective or protective actions than young adults. These delays greatly increase the risk of falling as the time period to prevent destabilization is quite short (Tinetti, Speechley, and Ginter, 1988; Stelmach and Worringham, 1985). Furthermore, older adults become unstable even with small perturbations that typically require moderate corrective actions (Maki et al., 1990; Woollacott, Moore, and Hu, 1993; Hu and Woollacott, 1994). Other types of studies found that the combination of visual occlusion and compliant surface conditions resulted in increased variability, velocity, range, and dispersion of postural sway

(Teasdale et al., 1991a, 1991b; Hu and Woollacott, 1994; Maki et al., 1990; Redfern, Moore, and Yarsky, 1997). Overall, data on balance and postural stability in older adults document that older adults show declines in the ability to maintain and recover from disturbances to their upright stance. These decrements result in an increased risk for falls and greatly influence functional tasks of daily living.

SKILL LEARNING

The ability of older adults to learn new skills and relearn previously learned skills is an important area of motor behavior research. Overall, it has been shown that older adults are able to relearn old skills and learn novel skills, but at a much slower rate than young adults (Spirduso, 1995; Murrell, 1970; Salthouse, 1984). Skilled abilities such as coordination, balance, associative learning, and handwriting all improve with extended practice, although not always to the level of young adults (Czaja and Sharit, 1998; Harrington and Haaland, 1992; Lazarus and Haynes, 1997; Strayer and Kramer, 1994; Judge, King, Whipple, Clive, and Wolfson, 1995; Dixon et al., 1993; Woollacott, 1993). Older adults require more time to practice a skill before improvements are shown. For example, Judge and colleagues (1995) found that older adults were able to improve their balance, measured by postural sway range and recovery, when vision and proprioception were distorted but required substantial practice. Similar improvements were found for recovery of balance with a postural perturbation task after substantial practice (Woollacott, 1993). Improvements with practice have also been documented with speed of handwriting. Dixon et al. (1993) found that older adults were almost two times slower than young adults prior to practice, but they improved to being just as fast as the young adults after extensive practice. Although these data document the ability of older adults to relearn a skill, research examining the ability to learn novel tasks will better address the question of motor learning in older adults.

Novel tasks have been studied to assess how older adults are able to learn a new skill. For example, Seidler-Dobrin and Stelmach (1998) and Pratt et al. (1994) had participants perform an aiming task with accuracy requirements. Both of these studies found that, with extensive practice, overall performance (measured by movement time) improved. However, older adults did not improve the distance traveled in the primary submovement, or ballistic phase (see "Movement Components" above) of the movement, whereas young participants did. Others have reported similar overall improvements, but no specific improvements in variables that measure the fundamental components of movement (Cerella et al., 1980; Seidler-Dobrin et al., 1998; Brown, 1996; Darling et al., 1989; Murrell, 1970).

Another example of skill aquisition on a novel task was done by Etnier and Landers (1998), who demonstrated on a mirror star-tracing task that older adults learned at a much slower rate than young adults as measured by time on target. Furthermore, they showed that older adults who had more practice also had better retention. Overall, these data suggest that older subjects are able to learn and improve new skills. Furthermore, the data suggest that improvements may occur in different ways than in young adults, which has implications for motor performance in older adults.

There is some evidence that cognitive strategies, specifically having older adults verbalize a sequence of content-specific cues, improve the speed of learning in older adults (Greenwood, Meeuswsen, and French, 1993; Proteau, Charest, and Chaput, 1994). These strategies help speed up the learning process, make learning more enjoyable, and therefore result in lower attrition rates of older adults in tasks that are novel. In addition there are some studies that show that exercise improves the cognitive abilities (i.e., executive functions) of older adults and subsequently their ability to learn a task (Churchill et al., 2002; Fillit et al., 2002). Churchill et al. (2002) found that executive functions of older adults were maintained or enhanced in individuals with higher levels of fitness. Knowledge about improvements in cognition and movement with exercise has important implications for rehabilitation and training programs for older adults.

TRAINING PROGRAMS

Although there are several studies that have documented age-related decrements in older adults, few have demonstrated how interventions or lifestyle can maintain abilities or even reverse changes observed with advanced age. There is evidence that maintaining an active lifestyle preserves motor functions (Spirduso, 1975; Spirduso and Clifford, 1978; Raab et al., 1988; Fatouros et al., 2002; Gehlsen and Whaley, 1990; Girouard and Hurley, 1995; Drowatzky and Drowatzky, 1999; Morey et al., 1999). Spirduso (1975) and Spirduso and Clifford (1978) performed a study in which they compared active and sedentary young and older adults on reaction and movement time skills. They also addressed whether specificity of skill or overall general fitness influenced reaction and movement time performance by testing an active group, subjects who were either runners or racquet sport players. Spirduso and Clifford also found that older active adults had faster reaction times and movement times than sedentary men of the same age regardless of whether they were runners or racquet sport players. Although these studies have been criticized for not having adequate controls, which may lead to different outcomes in the magnitude of differences, they nevertheless suggest that older adults who maintain an active lifestyle show positive effects of exercise on the production of movement.

Exercise training (both aerobic and strength) has also been shown to have general beneficial effects on strength and flexibility in older adults. It has been found that exercise training slows the adverse affects of aging even in those who start exercising as late as 80 years of age (Cress et al., 1999). Several studies have shown that light resistance training, stretching, and moderate aerobic exercise have a beneficial effect on strength, balance, flexibility, coordination, and range of motion in older adults (Raab et al., 1988; Fatouros et al., 2002; Gehlsen and Whaley, 1990; Girouard and Hurley, 1995; Drowatzky and Drowatzky, 1999; Morey et al., 1999).

Strength training has been shown to have a specific impact on muscle composition and subsequent motor function. One of the major decrements in older adults is the change in composition of muscle. The decrease in muscle fibers, particularly type II muscle fibers (fast twitch), is largely associated with the lack of use. If the level of exercise training is maintained, the loss of muscle fibers is slowed or does not occur (Rogers and Evans, 1993; Frischknecht, 1998; Fielding, 1995). Weight training increases the number of type II fibers by 20 percent (Drowatzky and Drowatzky, 1999).

It has also been shown that strength training increases maximum torque in plantar flexion movements in the feet, which are important for balance and mobility (Blanpied and Smidt, 1993). Increases in muscle mass and range of motion have been shown to reduce the risk of detrimental falls (Allander, Bjornsson, Olafsson, Sigfusson, and Thorsteinsson, 1974; Hortobagyi and DeVita, 1999; Pendergast, Fisher, and Calkins, 1993). Similar improvements have been found in dynamic balancing of older athletes with increased muscle mass and range of motion (Raty, Impivaara, and Karppi, 2002). Overall, the research shows that maintaining physical activity, including strength and flexibility training, slows the effects of aging on the motor system and may prevent some irreversible injuries or declines.

Other data show more specific improvements in cognitive and motor function with specialized training. Kramer, Hahn, and Gopher (1999) have shown very specific benefits from training over several sessions on a dual-task paradigm. They showed that older adults, compared with young adults, have large time costs, measured by reaction time, when performing tasks that require switching of attention from one task to another. However, with modest practice, older adults were able to reduce the costs of switching between tasks. These improvements were maintained over a 2-month period. These data show that highly specialized training can improve a very specific kind of performance.

Similar specialized training benefits have been shown with balance training interventions, particularly multifactor training (Daubney and Culham, 1999; Hu and Woollacott, 1994; Tang and Woollacott, 1996). Multifactor balance training requires several modalities of sensory information to be processed and integrated simultaneously. A review conducted by Tang and Woollacott (1996) found that multifactor balance training targeted to specific subsystems, working on individual needs, showed the most improvements in balance and postural responses. Training on a set of specific defined deficits in individuals resulted in improvements in stability and recovery from postural disturbances. Shumway-Cooke and colleagues (1997) have demonstrated that balance training programs that include tasks that involve multiple processes increase the attentional demands associated with balance control and become more like real-world experiences in which a person must respond to multiple inputs. Tasks such as maintaining balance while performing rhythmic movements between limbs increase the postural response resources available to individuals and subsequently improve compensatory strategies (Tang and Woollacott, 1998).

Rose and Clark (2000) have reported that a biofeedback-based balance intervention improves balance control in older adults as measured by postural sway. Individuals who participated in biofeedback balance training were able to make quicker corrections to perturbations and able to recover from larger sway dispersions, suggesting more control of their center of gravity. Proprioception and gait training has also been observed to be beneficial to older adults to maintain balance (Gauchard, Jeandel, Tessier, and Perrin, 1999; Galindo-Ciocon, Ciocon, and Galindo, 1995).

Overall, most available data that measure defined motor performance variables suggest that the benefits of intervention training are relatively specific. It needs to be determined whether more generalized intervention strategies such as exercise produce specific improvements in motor function such as speed, accuracy, coordination, and balance control.

Another area that has begun to emerge, but needs to become the forefront of the field, is how technology can assist movement control and accuracy. There have been few studies that have shown the benefits of devices that improve the speed and accuracy of movements, as well as coordination and balance, in older adults. Maki and colleagues (1999) performed a study in which enhanced sensory inserts (raised edge around perimeter of foot) were put in the soles of subjects' shoes. They found that this intervention improved the efficiency of stabilizing reactions elicited by unpredictable postural perturbations. This device targets improving balance control by enhancing sensation in the soles of individuals' feet so that postural disturbances can be recognized and corrected before a detrimental outcome occurs. The results may be important in the design of assistive technologies to reduce instability and risk of falling in older adults. Technological advances in devices that assist older adults should target improving parameters of movement performance that have the largest impact on the skills of daily living. It is important for future technological advancements for older adults to incorporate and capitalize on the intact ability of older adults, while compensating for declines. This will lead to improvements in performance with training as well as help older adults maintain skills in which they are proficient.

REFERENCES

Abrams, R.A., Pratt, J., and Chasteen, A.L. (1998). Aging and movement: Variability of force pulses for saccadic eye movements. *Psychology and Aging, 13*(3), 387-395.

Allander, E., Bjornsson, O.J., Olafsson, O., Sigfusson, N., and Thorsteinsson, J. (1974). Normal range of joint movements in shoulder, hip, wrist and thumb with special reference to side: A comparison between two populations. *International Journal of Epidemiology, 3*(3), 253-261.

Amrhein, P.C., and Theios, J. (1993). The time it takes elderly and young individuals to draw pictures and write words. *Psychology and Aging, 8*(2), 197-206.

Amrhein, P.C., Stelmach, G.E., and Goggin, N.L. (1991). Age differences in the maintenance and restructuring of movement preparation. *Psychology and Aging, 6*(3), 451-466.

Aniansson, A., Hedberg, M., Henning, G.B., and Grimby, G. (1986). Muscle morphology, enzymatic activity, and muscle strength in elderly men: A follow-up study. *Muscle and Nerve, 9*(7), 585-591.

Bailey, A.J., and Mansell, J.P. (1997). Do subchondral bone changes exacerbate or precede articular cartilage destruction in osteoarthritis of the elderly? [Review]. *Gerontology, 43*(5), 296-304.

Bashore, T.R., Osman, A., and Heffley, E.F. (1989). Mental slowing in elderly persons: A cognitive psychophysiological analysis. *Psychology and Aging, 4*(2), 235-244.

Bashore, T.R., Ridderinkhof, K.R., and van der Molen, M.W. (1997). The decline of cognitive processing speed in old age. *Current Directions in Psychological Science, 6*(6), 163-169.

Bassey, E.J. (1998). Longitudinal changes in selected physical capabilities: Muscle strength, flexibility and body size. *Age and Ageing, 27*(Suppl 3), 12-16.

Beaupre, G.S., Stevens, S.S., and Carter, D.R. (2000). Mechanobiology in the development, maintenance, and degeneration of articular cartilage. [Comment]. *Journal of Rehabilitation Research and Development, 37*(2), 145-151.

Bell, R.D., and Hoshizaki, T.B. (1981). Relationships of age and sex with range of motion of seventeen joint actions in humans. *Journal Canadien Des Sciences Appliquees Au Sport, 6*(4), 202-206.

Bellgrove, M.A., Phillips, J.G., Bradshaw, J.L., and Gallucci, R.M. (1998). Response (re-) programming in aging: A kinematic analysis. *Journals of Gerontology Series A: Biological Sciences and Medical Sciences, 53*(A3), M222-M227.

Bennett, K.M., and Castiello, U. (1994). Reach to grasp: Changes with age. *Journal of Gerontology, 49*(B1), P1-P7.

Berardelli, A., Hallett, M., Rothwell, J.C., Agostino, R., Manfredi, M., Thompson, P.D., and Marsden, C.D. (1996). Single-joint rapid arm movements in normal subjects and in patients with motor disorders. *Brain, 119*, 661-674.

Bernick, S., and Cailliet, R. (1982). Vertebral end-plate changes with aging of human vertebrae. *Spine, 7*(2), 97-102.

Birren, J.E. (1974). Translations in gerontology: From lab to life. Psychophysiology and speed of response. *American Psychologist, 29*(11), 808-815.

Blanpied, P., and Smidt, G.L. (1993). The difference in stiffness of the active plantarflexors between young and elderly human females. *Journal of Gerontology, 48*(2), M58-M63.

Bloem, B.R., Allum, J.H., Carpenter, M.G., Verschuuren, J.J., and Honegger, F. (2002). Triggering of balance corrections and compensatory strategies in a patient with total leg proprioceptive loss. *Experimental Brain Research, 142*(1), 91-107.

Brogmus, G.E. (1991). Effects of age and sex on speed and accuracy of hand movements and the refinements they suggest for Fitts' law. Paper presented at the Human Factors Society 35th Annual Meeting, September 2-6, San Francisco, CA.

Brown, S.H. (1996). Control of simple arm movements in the elderly. In A.-M. Ferrandez and N. Teasdale (Eds.), *Changes in sensory motor behavior in aging. Advances in psychology* (Vol. 114, pp. 27-52). North Holland, Amsterdam: Elsevier Science.

Brown, W.F. (1972). A method for estimating the number of motor units in thenar muscles and the changes in motor unit count with ageing. *Journal of Neurology, Neurosurgery and Psychiatry, 35*(6), 845-852.

Buneo, C.A., Soechting, J.F., and Flanders, M. (1994). Muscle activation patterns for reaching: The representation of distance and time. *Journal of Neurophysiology, 71*(4), 1546-1558.

Campbell, M.J., McComas, A.J., and Petito, F. (1973). Physiological changes in ageing muscles. *Journal of Neurology, Neurosurgery and Psychiatry, 36*(2), 174-182.

Carnahan, H., Vandervoort, A.A., and Swanson, L.R. (1998). The influence of aging and target motion on the control of prehension. *Experimental Aging Research, 24*(3), 289-306.

Cerella, J. (1985). Information processing rates in the elderly. *Psychological Bulletin, 98*(1), 67-83.

Cerella, J., Poon, L.W., and Williams, D.M. (1980). Age and the complexity hypothesis. In L. Poon (Ed.), *Aging in the 1980's: Psychological issues.* Washington, DC: American Psychological Association.

Churchill, J.D., Galvez, R., Colcombe, S., Swain, R.A., Kramer, A.F., and Greenough, W.T. (2002). Exercise, experience and the aging brain. *Neurobiology of Aging, 23*(5), 941-955.

Clamann, H.P. (1993). Motor unit recruitment and the gradation of muscle force. *Physical Therapy, 73*(12), 830-483.

Clarkson, P.M. (1978). The effect of age and activity level on simple and choice fractionated response time. *European Journal of Applied Physiology, 40,* 17-25.

Collins, J.J., DeLuca, C.J., Burrows, A., and Lipsitz, L.A. (1995). Age-related changes in open-loop and closed-loop postural control mechanisms. *Experimental Brain Research, 104,* 480-492.

Contreras-Vidal, J.L., Teulings, H.L., and Stelmach, G.E. (1998). Elderly subjects are impaired in spatial coordination in fine motor control. *Acta Psychologica, 100*(1-2), 25-35.

Cooke, J.D., Brown, S.H., and Cunningham, D.A. (1989). Kinematics of arm movements in elderly humans. *Neurobiology of Aging, 10*(2), 159-65.

Cress, M.E., Buchner, D.M., Questad, K.A., Esselman, P.C., deLateur, B.J., and Schwartz, R.S. (1999). Exercise: Effects on physical functional performance in independent older adults. *Journals of Gerontology Series A: Biological Sciences and Medical Sciences, 54*(5), M242-248.

Czaja, S.J., and Sharit, J. (1998). Ability-performance relationships as a function of age and task experience for a data entry task. *Journal of Experimental Psychology: Applied, 4*(4), 332-351.

Darling, W.G., Cooke, J.D., and Brown, S.H. (1989). Control of simple arm movements in elderly humans. *Neurobiology of Aging, 10*(2), 149-157.

Daubney, M.E., and Culham, E.G. (1999). Lower-extremity muscle force and balance perfor-
   mance in adults aged 65 years and older. *Physical Therapy, 79*(12), 1177-1185.
Davies, C.T., and White, M.J. (1983). Contractile properties of elderly human triceps surae.
   Gerontology, 29(1), 19-25.
Diggles-Buckles, V., and Vercruyssen, M. (1990). Age-related slowing, S-R compatibility,
   and stages of information processing. Paper presented at the Human Factors Society
   34th Annual Meeting, October 8-12, Orlando, FL.
Dixon, R.A., Kurzman, D., and Friesen, I.C. (1993). Handwriting performance in younger
   and older adults: Age, familiarity, and practice effects. *Psychology and Aging, 8*(3), 360-
   370.
Doherty, T.J., Vandervoort, A.A., and Brown, W.F. (1993). Effects of ageing on the motor
   unit: A brief review. *Canadian Journal of Applied Physiology, 18*(4), 331-358.
Drowatzky, K.L., and Drowatzky, J.N. (1999). Physical training programs for the elderly.
   Clinical Kinesiology, 53(3), 52-62.
Erim, Z., Beg, M.F., Burke, D.T., and de Luca, C.J. (1999). Effects of aging on motor-unit
   control properties. *Journal of Neurophysiology, 82*(5), 2081-2091.
Etnier, J.L., and Landers, D.M. (1998). Motor performance and motor learning as a function
   of age and fitness. *Research Quarterly for Exercise and Sport, 69*(2), 136-146.
Fatouros, I.G., Taxildaris, K., Tokmakidis, S.P., Kalapotharakos, V., Aggelousis, N.,
   Athanasopoulos, S., Zeeris, I., and Katrabasas, I. (2002). The effects of strength training, cardiovascular training and their combination on flexibility of inactive older
   adults. *International Journal of Sports Medicine, 23*(2), 112-119.
Ferrell, W.R., Crighton, A., and Sturrock, R.D. (1992). Age-dependent changes in position
   sense in human proximal interphalangeal joints. *NeuroReport, 3*(3), 259-261.
Fielding, R.A. (1995). The role of progressive resistance training and nutrition in the preser-
   vation of lean body mass in the elderly. *Journal of the American College of Nutrition, 14*
   (6), 587-594.
Fillit, H.M., Butler, R.N., O'Connell, A.W., Albert, M.S., Birren, J.E., Cotman, C.W.,
   Greenough, W.T., Gold, P.E., Kramer, A.F., Kuller, L.H., Perls, T.T., Sahagan, B.G., and
   Tully, T. (2002). Achieving and maintaining cognitive vitality with aging. *Mayo Clinic
   Proceeds, 77*(7), 681-696.
Fitts, P.M. (1954). The information capacity of the human motor system in controlling the
   amplitude of movement. *Journal of Experimental Psychology, 47*, 381-391.
Fozard, J.L., Vercryssen, M., Reynolds, S.L., Hancock, P.A., and Quilter, R.E. (1994). Age
   differences and changes in reaction time: The Baltimore Longitudinal Study of Aging.
   Journal of Gerontology, 49(4), P179-189.
Frischknecht, R. (1998). Effect of training on muscle strength and motor function in the
   elderly. *Reproduction, Nutrition, Development, 38*(2), 167-174.
Galganski, M.E., Fuglevand, A.J., and Enoka, R.M. (1993). Reduced control of motor output
   in a human hand muscle of elderly subjects during submaximal contractions. *Journal of
   Neurophysiology, 69*(6), 2108-2115.
Galindo-Ciocon, D.J., Ciocon, J.O., and Galindo, D.J. (1995). Gait training and falls in the
   elderly. *Journal of Gerontological Nursing, 21*(6), 10-17.
Gauchard, G.C., Jeandel, C., Tessier, A., and Perrin, P.P. (1999). Beneficial effect of proprio-
   ceptive physical activities on balance control in elderly human subjects. *Neuroscience
   Letters, 273*(2), 81-84.
Gehlsen, G.M., and Whaley, M.H. (1990). Falls in the elderly: Part II, Balance, strength, and
   flexibility. *Archives of Physical Medicine and Rehabilitation, 71*(10), 739-741.
Girouard, C.K., and Hurley, B.F. (1995). Does strength training inhibit gains in range of
   motion from flexibility training in older adults? *Medicine and Science in Sports and Exercise, 27*(10), 1444-1449.

Goggin, N.L., and Meeuwsen, H.J. (1992). Age-related differences in the control of spatial aiming movements. *Research Quarterly for Exercise and Sport, 63*(4), 366-372.

Goggin, N.L., and Stelmach, G.E. (1990). Age-related differences in a kinematic analysis of precued movements. *Canadian Journal on Aging, 9*(4), 371-385.

Gottsdanker, R. (1982). Age and simple reaction time. *Journal of Gerontology, 37*(3), 342-348.

Greene, L.S., and Williams, H.G. (1996). Aging and coordination from the dynamic pattern perspective. In A. Ferrandez and N. Teasdale (Eds.), *Changes in sensory motor behavior in aging* (Vol. 114, pp. 89-131). North Holland, Amsterdam: Elsevier Science.

Greenwood, M., Meeuswsen, H., and French, R. (1993). Effects of cognitive learning strategies, verbal reinforcement, and gender on the performance of closed motor skills in older adults. *Activities, Adaptation and Aging, 17*(3), 39-53.

Gutman, S.R., Latash, M.L., Almeida, G.L., and Gottlieb, G.L. (1993). Kinematic description of variability of fast movements: Analytical and experimental approaches. *Biological Cybernetics, 69*(5-6), 485-492.

Hakkinen, K., Kraemer, W.J., Kallinen, M., Linnamo, V., Pastinen, U. M., and Newton, R.U. (1996). Bilateral and unilateral neuromuscular function and muscle cross-sectional area in middle-aged and elderly men and women. *Journals of Gerontology Series A: Biological Sciences and Medical Sciences, 51*(1), B21-29.

Harrington, D.L., and Haaland, K.Y. (1992). Skill learning in the elderly: Diminished implicit and explicit memory for a motor response. *Psychology and Aging, 7*(3), 425-434.

Hart, B.A. (1980). *Fractionated reflex and response times in women by activity level and age.* Unpublished doctoral dissertation. University of Massachusetts, Amherst.

Hay, L., Bard, C., Fleury, M., and Teasdale, N. (1996). Availability of visual and proprioceptive afferent messages and postural control in elderly adults. *Experimental Brain Research, 108*(1), 129-139.

Hick, W. (1952). On the rate of gain of information. *Quarterly Journal of Experimental Psychology, 4*, 11-26.

Hines, T. (1979). Information feedback, reaction time and error rates in young and old subjects. *Experimental Aging Research, 5*(3), 207-215.

Hortobagyi, T., and DeVita, P. (1999). Altered movement strategy increases lower extremity stiffness during stepping down in the aged. *Journals of Gerontology: Biological Sciences and Medical Sciences, 54*(2), B63-70.

Hsu, S.H., Huang, C.C., Tsuang, Y.H., and Sun, J.S. (1997). Age differences in remote pointing performance. *Perceptual and Motor Skills, 85*(2), 515-527.

Hu, M.H., and Woollacott, M.H. (1994). Multisensory training of standing balance in older adults: II. Kinematic and electromyographic postural responses. *Journal of Gerontology, 49*(2), M62-M71.

Hurley, M.V., Rees, J., and Newham, D.J. (1998). Quadriceps function, proprioceptive acuity and functional performance in healthy young, middle-aged and elderly subjects. *Age and Ageing, 27*(1), 55-62.

Izquierdo, M., Aguado, X., Gonzalez, R., Lopez, J.L., and Hakkinen, K. (1999). Maximal and explosive force production capacity and balance performance in men of different ages. *European Journal of Applied Physiology and Occupational Physiology, 79*(3), 260-267.

Jordan, T.C., and Rabbitt, P.M. (1977). Response times to stimuli of increasing complexity as a function of ageing. *British Journal of Psychology, 68*(2), 189-201.

Judge, J.O., King, M.B., Whipple, R., Clive, J., and Wolfson, L.I. (1995). Dynamic balance in older persons: Effects of reduced visual and proprioceptive input. *Journal of Gerontology, 50A*(5), M263-M270.

Kaplan, F.S., Nixon, J.E., Reitz, M., Rindfleish, L., and Tucker, J. (1985). Age-related changes in proprioception and sensation of joint position. *Acta Orthopaedica Scandinavica, 56*(1), 72-74.

Ketcham, C.J., and Stelmach, G.E. (2002). Motor control of older adults. In D.J. Ekerdt, R.A. Applebaum, K.C. Holden, S.G. Post, K. Rockwood, R. Schulz, R.L. Sprott, and P. Uhlenberg (Eds.), *Encyclopedia of aging.* New York: Macmillan Reference USA.

Ketcham, C.J., Dounskaia, N., and Stelmach, G.E. (2001). Older adults demonstrate trajectory distortions in multijoint coordination. *Society for Neuroscience Abstracts, 27*(Program number 834.1).

Ketcham, C.J., Seidler, R.D., Van Gemmert, A.W., and Stelmach, G.E. (2002). Age-related kinematic differences as influenced by task difficulty, target size, and movement amplitude. *Journals of Gerontology: Psychological Sciences and Social Sciences, 57*(1), P54-64.

Kinoshita, H., and Francis, P.R. (1996). A comparison of prehension force control in young and elderly individuals. *European Journal of Applied Physiology and Occupational Physiology, 74*(5), 450-460.

Kramer, A.F., Hahn, S., and Gopher, D. (1999). Task coordination and aging: Explorations of executive control processes in the task switching paradigm. *Acta Psychologica, 101*(2-3), 339-378.

Kuo, G.H. (1990). Physical fitness of the people in Taipei including the aged. In M. Kaneko (Ed.), *Fitness for the aged, disabled, and industrial worker* (pp. 21-24). Champaign, IL: Human Kinetics.

Larish, D.D., and Stelmach, G.E. (1982). Preprogramming, programming, and reprogramming of aimed hand movements as a function of age. *Journal of Motor Behavior, 14*(4), 322-340.

Larsson, L., and Karlsson, J. (1978). Isometric and dynamic endurance as a function of age and skeletal muscle characteristics. *Acta Physiologica Scandinavica, 104*(2), 129-136.

Larsson, L., Li, X., and Frontera, W.R. (1997). Effects of aging on shortening velocity and myosin isoform composition in single human skeletal muscle cells. *American Journal of Physiology, 272*(Cell Physiology 41), C638-C649.

Laver-Rubich, Z., and Silbermann, M. (1985). Cartilage surface charge: A possible determinant in aging and osteoarthritic processes. *Arthritis and Rheumatism, 28*(6), 660-670.

Lazarus, J.C., and Haynes, J.M. (1997). Isometric pinch force control and learning in older adults. *Experimental Aging Research, 23,* 179-200.

Levin, H.S., and Benton, A.L. (1973). Age effects in proprioceptive feedback performance. *Gerontologia Clinica, 15*(3), 161-169.

Lexell, J. (1993). What is the cause of the ageing atrophy? Assessment of the fiber type composition in whole human muscles. In G.E. Stelmach and V. Homberg (Eds.), *Sensorimotor impairment in the elderly* (pp. 143-153). North Holland, Amsterdam: Elsevier Science.

Lord, S.R., Rogers, M.W., Howland, A., and Fitzpatrick, R. (1999). Lateral stability, sensorimotor function and falls in older people. *Journal of the American Geriatrics Society, 47*(9), 1077-1081.

Liu, Y.C. (2001). Comparative study of effects of auditory, visual and multimodality displays on drivers' performance in advanced traveler information systems. *Ergonomics, 44*(4), 425-442.

Maki, B.E., Holliday, P.J., and Fernie, G.R. (1990). Aging and postural control: A comparison of spontaneous and induced sway balance tests. *Journal of the American Geriatrics Society, 38,* 1-9.

Maki, B.E., Perry, S.D., Norrie, R.G., and McIlroy, W.E. (1999). Effect of facilitation of sensation from plantar foot-surface boundaries on postural stabilization in young and older adults. *Journals of Gerontology Series A: Biological Sciences and Medical Sciences, 54*(6), M281-M287.

Marteniuk, R.G., MacKenzie, C.L., Jeannerod, M., Athenes, S., and Dugas, C. (1987). Constraints on human arm movement trajectories. *Canadian Journal of Psychology, 41*(3), 365-378.

McComas, A.J., Fawcett, P.R., Campbell, M.J., and Sica, R.E. (1971) Electrophysiological estimation of the number of motor units within a human muscle. *Journal of Neurology, Neurosurgery and Psychiatry, 34*(2), 121-131.

Melis, A., Soetens, E., and van der Molen, M.W. (2002). Process-specific slowing with advancing age: Evidence derived from the analysis of sequential effects. *Brain and Cognition, 49*, 420-435.

Metter, E.J., Lynch, N., Conwit, R., Lindle, R., Tobin, J., and Hurley, B. (1999). Muscle quality and age: Cross-sectional and longitudinal comparisons. *Journals of Gerontology Series A: Biological Sciences and Medical Sciences, 54*(5), B207-B218.

Meyer, D.E., Abrams, R.A., Kornblum, S., Wright, C.E., and Smith, J.E.K. (1988). Optimality in human motor performance: Ideal control of rapid aimed movements. *Psychological Review, 95*(3), 340-370.

Milner, T.E., Cloutier, C., Leger, A.B., and Franklin, D.W. (1995). Inability to activate muscles maximally during cocontraction and the effect on joint stiffness. *Experimental Brain Research, 107*(2), 293-305.

Milner-Brown, H.S., Stein, R.B., and Yemm, R. (1973). The contractile properties of human motor units during voluntary isometric contractions. *Journal of Physiology, 228*(2), 285-306.

Morey, M.C., Schenkman, M., Studenski, S.A., Chandler, J.M., Crowley, G.M., Sullivan, R.J., Jr, Pieper, C.F., Doyle, M.E., Higginbotham, M.B., Horner, R.D., MacAller, H., Puglisi, C.M., Morris, K.G., and Weinberger, M. (1999). Spinal-flexibility-plus-aerobic versus aerobic-only training: Effect of a randomized clinical trial on function in at-risk older adults. *Journals of Gerontology Series A: Biological Sciences and Medical Sciences, 54*(7), M335-M342.

Morgan, M., Phillips, J.G., Bradshaw, J.L., Mittingley, J.B., Iasek, R., and Bradshaw, J.A. (1994). Age-related motor slowness: Simply strategic? *Journal of Gerontology, 49*(3), M133-M139.

Murrell, F.H. (1970). The effect of extensive practice on age differences in reation time. *Journal of Gerontology, 25*, 268-274.

Ng, A.V., and Kent-Braun, J.A. (1999). Slowed muscle contractile properties are not associated with a decreased EMG/force relationship in older humans. *Journals of Gerontology Series A: Biological Sciences and Medical Sciences, 54*(10), B452-B458.

Nonaka, H., Mita, K., Watakabe, M., Akataki, K., Suzuki, N., Okuwa, T., and Yabe, K. (2002). Age-related changes in the interactive mobility of the hip and knee joints: A geometrical analysis. *Gait and Posture, 15*(3), 236-243.

Pai, Y.C., Rymer, W.Z., Chang, R.W., and Sharma, L. (1997). Effect of age and osteoarthritis on knee proprioception. *Arthritis and Rheumatism, 40*(12), 2260-2265.

Pendergast, D.R., Fisher, N.M., and Calkins, E. (1993). Cardiovascular, neuromuscular, and metabolic alteration with age leading to fraility. *Journal of Gerontology, 48*, 61-67.

Peterka, R.J., and Black, F.O. (1990). Age-related changes in human posture control sensory organization tests. *Journal of Vestibular Research, 1*, 73-85.

Petrella, R.J., Lattanzio, P.J., and Nelson, M.G. (1997). Effect of age and activity on knee joint proprioception. *American Journal of Physical Medicine and Rehabilitation, 76*(3), 235-241.

Pohl, P.S., Winstein, C.J., and Fisher, B.E. (1996). The locus of age-related movement slowing: Sensory processing in continuous goal-directed aiming. *Journals of Gerontology Series B: Psychological Sciences and Social Sciences, 51*(2), P94-P102.

Pratt, J., Chasteen, A.L., and Abrams, R.A. (1994). Rapid aimed limb movements: Age differences and practice effects in component submovements. *Psychology and Aging, 9*(2), 325-334.

Proteau, L., Charest, I., and Chaput, S. (1994). Differential roles with aging of visual and proprioceptive afferent information for fine motor control. *Journal of Gerontology, 49B*(3), P100-P107.

Raab, D.M., Agre, J.C., McAdam, M., and Smith, E.L. (1988). Light resistance and stretching exercise in elderly women: Effect upon flexibility. *Archives of Physical Medicine and Rehabilitation, 69*(4), 268-272.

Raty, H.P., Impivaara, O., and Karppi, S.L. (2002). Dynamic balance in former elite male athletes and in community control subjects. *Scandinavian Journal of Medicine and Science in Sports, 12*(2), 111-116.

Redfern, M.S., Moore, P.L., and Yarsky, C.M. (1997). The influence of flooring on standing balance among older persons. *Human Factors, 39*(3), 445-455.

Redfern, M.S., Muller, M.L., Jennings, J.R., and Furman, J.M. (2002). Attentional dynamics in postural control during perturbations in young and older adults. *Journals of Gerontology: Biological Sciences and Medical Sciences, 57*(8), B298-B303.

Reginster, J.Y. (2002). The prevalence and burden of arthritis. *Rheumatology, 41 Supp*(1), 3-6.

Rogers, M.A., and Evans, W.J. (1993). Changes in skeletal muscle with aging: Effects of exercise training. *Exercise and Sport Sciences Reviews, 21*, 65-102.

Romero, D.H., Van Gemmert, A.W.A., Adler, C.H., Bekkering, H., and Stelmach, G.E. (2003). Time delays prior to movement alter the drawing kinematics of elderly adults. *Human Movement Science, 22*(2), 207-220.

Ronsky, J.L., Nigg, B.M., and Fisher, V. (1995). Correlation between physical activity and the gait characteristics and ankle joint flexibility of the elderly. *Clinical Biomechanics, 10*(1), 41-49.

Roos, M.R., Rice, C.L., and Vandervoort, A.A. (1997). Age-related changes in motor unit function. *Muscle and Nerve, 20*(6), 679-690.

Roos, M.R., Rice, C.L., Connelly, D.M., and Vandervoort, A.A. (1999). Quadriceps muscle strength, contractile properties, and motor unit firing rates in young and old men. *Muscle and Nerve, 22*(8), 1094-1103.

Rose, D.J., and Clark, S. (2000). Can the control of bodily orientation be significantly improved in a group of older adults with a history of falls? *Journal of the American Geriatrics Society, 48*(3), 275-282.

Salthouse, T.A. (1984). Effects of age and skill in typing. *Journal of Experimental Psychology: General, 113*, 345-371.

Salthouse, T.A. (1985). Speed of behavior and its implications for cognition. In J.E. Birren and K.W. Schaie (Eds.), *Handbook of the psychology of aging* (2nd ed., pp. 400-426). New York: Van Nostrand Reinhold.

Salthouse, T.A. (1988). Cognitive aspects of motor functioning. *Annals of the New York Academy of Sciences, 515*, 33-41.

Salthouse, T.A., and Somberg, B.L. (1982). Isolating the age deficit in speeded performance. *Journal of Gerontology, 37*, 59-63.

Schaie, K.W. (2004). Cognitive aging. In National Research Council, *Technology for adaptive aging* (pp. 43-63). Steering Committee for the Workshop on Technology for Adaptive Aging. R.W. Pew and S.B. Van Hemel (Eds.). Board on Behavioral, Cognitive, and Sensory Sciences. Division of Behavioral and Social Sciences and Education. Washington, DC: The National Academies Press.

Schieppati, M., Grasso, M., Siliotto, R., and Nardone, A. (1993). Effect of age, chronic diseases and Parkinsonism on postural control. In G.E. Stelmach and V. Homberg (Eds.), *Sensorimotor impairments in the elderly* (pp. 355-373). Dordrecht, Amsterdam: Kluwer Academic.

Seidler, R.D., Alberts, J.L., and Stelmach, G.E. (2002). Changes in multi-joint performance with age. *Motor Control*, 6(1), 19-31.

Seidler-Dobrin, R.D., and Stelmach, G.E. (1998). Persistence in visual feedback control by the elderly. *Experimental Brain Research*, 119(4), 467-474.

Seidler-Dobrin, R.D., He, J., and Stelmach, G.E. (1998). Coactivation to reduce variability in the elderly. *Motor Control*, 2(4), 314-330.

Sheldon, J.H. (1963). The effect of age on the control of sway. *Gerontology Clinical*, 5, 129-138.

Shepard, R.J., Berridge, M., and Montelpare, W. (1990). On the generality of the "sit and reach" test: An analysis of flexibility data for an aging population. *Research Quarterly Exercise and Sport*, 61(4), 326-330.

Shumway-Cook, A., Woollacott, M., Kerns, K.A., and Baldwin, M. (1997). The effects of two types of cognitive tasks on postural stability in older adults with and without a history of falls. *Journals of Gerontology Series A: Biological Sciences & Medical Sciences*, 52(4), M232-M240.

Simon, J.R. (1967). Choice reaction time as a function of auditory S-R correspondence, age and sex. *Ergonomics*, 10(6), 559-564.

Simon, J.R., and Pouraghabagher, A.R. (1978). The effect of aging on the stages of processing in a choice reation time task. *Journal of Gerontology*, 33(4), 553-561.

Singh, M.A., Ding, W., Manfredi, T.J., Solares, G.S., O'Neill, E.F., Clements, K.M., Ryan, N.D., Kehayias, J.J., Fielding, R.A., and Evans, W.J. (1999). Insulin-like growth factor I in skeletal muscle after weight-lifting exercise in frail elders. *American Journal of Physiology*, 277(Endocrinology and Metabolism 40), E135-E143.

Skinner, H.B., Barrack, R.L., and Cook, S.D. (1984). Age-related decline in proprioception. *Clinical Orthopaedics and Related Research*, 184, 208-211.

Slavin, M.J., Phillips, J.G., and Bradshaw, J.L. (1996). Visual cues in the handwriting of older adults: A kinematic analysis. *Psychology and Aging*, 11(3), 521-526.

Spirduso, W.W. (1975). Reaction and movement time as a function of age and physical activity level. *Journal of Gerontology*, 30(4), 435-440.

Spirduso, W.W. (1995). *Physical dimensions of aging*. Champaign, IL: Human Kinetics.

Spirduso, W.W., and Clifford, P. (1978). Replication of age and physical activity effects on reaction time and movement time. *Journal of Gerontology*, 33(1), 26-30.

Stelmach, G.E., and Goggin, N.L. (1988). Psychomotor decline with age. *Physical Activity and Aging*, 22, 6-17.

Stelmach, G.E., and Sirica, A. (1986). Aging and proprioception. *Age*, 9, 99-103.

Stelmach, G.E., and Worringham, C.J. (1985). Sensorimotor deficits related to postural stability: Implications for falling in the elderly [Review]. *Clinics in Geriatric Medicine*, 1(3), 679-694.

Stelmach, G.E., Goggin, N.L., and Amrhein, P.C. (1988). Aging and the restructuring of precued movements. *Psychology and Aging*, 3(2), 151-157.

Stelmach, G.E., Goggin, N.L., and Garcia-Colera, A. (1987). Movement specification time with age. *Experimental Aging Research*, 13(1-2), 39-46.

Stelmach, G.E., Teasdale, N., Phillips, J., and Worringham, C.J. (1989). Force production characteristics in Parkinson's disease. *Experimental Brain Research*, 76(1), 165-172.

Strayer, D.L., and Kramer, A.F. (1994). Aging and skill acquisition: Learning-performance distinctions. *Psychology and Aging*, 9(4), 589-605.

Swinnen, S.P., Verschueren, S.M.P., Bogaerts, H., Dounskaia, N., Lee, T.D., Stelmach, G.E., and Serrien, D.J. (1998). Age-related deficits in motor learning and differences in feedback processing during the production of a bimanual corrdination pattern. *Cognitive Neuropsychology*, 15(5), 439-466.

Tang, P.F., and Woollacott, M.H. (1996). Balance control in older adults: Training effects on balance control and the integration of balance control into walking. In A.-M. Ferrandez and N. Teasdale (Eds.), *Changes in sensory motor behavior in aging* (Vol. 114, pp. 339-367). North Holland, Amsterdam: Elsevier Science.

Tang, P.F., and Woollacott, M.H. (1998). Inefficient postural response to unexpected slips during walking in older adults. *Journal of Gerontology, 53A*(6), M471-M480.

Teasdale, N., Stelmach, G.E., and Breunig, A. (1991a). Postural sway characteristics of the elderly under normal and altered visual and support surface conditions. *Journal of Gerontology, 46A*(6), B238-B244.

Teasdale, N., Stelmach, G.E., Breunig, A., and Meeuwsen, H.J. (1991b). Age differences in visual sensory integration. *Experimental Brain Reseach, 85*, 691-696.

Tedeschi, G., Di Costanzo, A., Allocca, S., Quattrone, A., Casucci, G., Russo, L., and Bonavita, V. (1989). Age-dependent changes in visually guided saccadic eye movements. *Functional Neurology, 4*(4), 363-367.

Teulings, H.L., and Stelmach, G.E. (1993). Signal-to-noise ratio of handwriting size, force, and time: Cues to early markers of Parkinson's disease. In G.E. Stelmach and V. Homberg (Eds.), *Sensorimotor impairment in the elderly* (pp. 311-327). Dordrecht, Amsterdam: Kluver Academic.

Tinetti, M.E., Speechley, M., and Ginter, S.F. (1988). Risk factors for falls among elderly persons living in the community. *New England Journal of Medicine, 319*, 1701-1707.

Wachtel, E., Maroudas, A., and Schneiderman, R. (1995). Age-related changes in collagen packing of human articular cartilage. *Biochimica and Biophysica Acta, 1243*(2), 239-243.

Walhovd, K.B., and Fjell, A.M. (2001). Two- and three-stimuli auditory oddball ERP tasks and neuropsychological measures in aging. *Neuroreport, 12*(14), 3149-3153.

Walker, J., Alicandri, E., Sedney, C., and Roberts, K. (1991). In-vehicle navigation devices: Effects on the safety of driver performance. In *Vehicle navigation and information systems conference proceedings* (pp. 499-525). Warrendale, PA: Society of Automotive Engineers.

Walker, N., Philbin, D.A., and Fisk, A.D. (1997). Age-related differences in movement control: Adjusting submovement structure to optimize performance. *Journals of Gerontology Series B: Psychological Sciences and Social Sciences, 52*(1), P40-P52.

Warabi, T., Kase, M., and Kato, T. (1984). Effect of aging on the accuracy of visually guided saccadic eye movement. *Annals of Neurology, 16*(4), 449-454.

Welford, A.T. (1977). Motor performance. In J.E. Birren and K.W. Schaie (Eds.), *Handbook for the psychology of aging*. New York: Van Nostrand Reinhold.

Welford, A.T. (1984). Between bodily changes and performance: Some possible reasons for slowing with age. *Experimental Aging Research, 10*(2), 73-88.

Whipple, R., Wolfson, L., Derby, C., Singh, D., and Tobin, J. (1993). Altered sensory function and balance in older persons. *The Journal of Gerontology, 48*(SI), 71-76.

Wishart, L.R., Lee, T.D., Murdoch, J.E., and Hodges, N.J. (2000). Effects of aging on automatic and effortful processes in bimanual coordination. *Journal of Gerontology, 53B*(2), P85-P94.

Woollacott, M.H. (1993). Age-related changes in posture and movement. *Journal of Gerontology, 48*(SI), 56-60.

Woollacott, M.H., Moore, S., and Hu, M.H. (1993). Improvements in balance in the elderly through training in sensory organization abilities. In G.E. Stelmach and V. Homberg (Eds.), *Sensorimotor impairment in the elderly* (pp. 377-392). Dordrecht, Amsterdam: Kluver Academic.

Yamada, H., Masuda, T., and Okada, M. (2002). Age-related EMG variables during maximum voluntary contraction. *Perceptual and Motor Skills, 95*(1), 10-14.

Yue, G.H., Ranganathan, V.K., Siemionow, V., Liu, J.Z., and Sahgal, V. (1999). Older adults exhibit a reduced ability to fully activate their biceps brachii muscle. *Journals of Gerontology Series A: Biological Sciences and Medical Sciences, 54*(5), M249-M253.

4

Methodological Issues in the Assessment of Technology Use for Older Adults

Christopher Hertzog and *Leah Light*

Principles of social research are abstractions that are made concrete and manifest through the decisions made by researchers. The research tools we use must be flexibly adapted to the complex problem of understanding how our population is embedded in and responds to a rapidly changing historical context. No context is more complex, it seems, than the flux and rapid progression that is technology use in modern Western societies. The start of the twenty-first century has been characterized by mind-numbing changes in the way in which we engage the world, from the advent of the microcomputer through development of mobile communications technology. Yet the evolution of technology is merely one aspect of the problem. Historical trends in technology encompass individuals who are more or less knowledgeable, more or less skilled, and more or less avoidant of learning how to engage technological innovation. Individual differences in existing knowledge and skill provide a background that strongly influences adaptation to new technologies (Czaja, Sharit, Charness, Fisk, and Rogers, 2003). Moreover, the normative and non-normative changes that accompany aging create a situation in which individuals with changing physical, social, and cognitive resources (the "gains and losses" associated with adult development) (Baltes, 1993) must adapt to new technologies while simultaneously adjusting to and compensating for various negative effects of aging so as to achieve "successful aging" (Rowe and Kahn, 1987).

Understanding the impact of technology on older adults thus requires empirical approaches that can gauge changes on numerous dimensions, including physiological, behavioral, cognitive, and social psychological outcomes. Given the law of unintended consequences, not all effects of the introduction of new technologies are likely to be planned or even anticipated when the technology is designed. Furthermore, research on human factors and aging strongly indicates that technology designers often do not consider the information processing limitations of humans, let alone their existing behavioral repertoire of skills, their attitudes, and their preferences regarding how to achieve goals (Czaja, 2001). Thus, there is a critical need for effective and reliable methods for judging the efficacy of technological interventions for improving the functioning of older persons, for assisting them in performing tasks necessary for everyday living, for enhancing their capacity to engage in desired behaviors, and for generally improving their quality of life.

Fortunately, the means for accomplishing these tasks are, by and large, available. Social scientists have engaged the generic problem of effective methods for program evaluation in a variety of domains, including education and clinical psychology (e.g., Zigler and Styfco, 2001). The pioneering efforts of scientists such as Donald T. Campbell (Bickman, 2000; Campbell and Stanley, 1966; Cook and Campbell, 1979) in the latter half of the twentieth century have produced well-established principles for conducting experimental and quasi-experimental evaluations of social trends and interventions that are intended to modify them (e.g., Berk and Rossi, 1999; Boruch, 1997; Shadish, Cook, and Leviton, 1995). The seminal study by Campbell and Stanley (1966) also had a strong influence on thinking about how to approach problems of research on aging (Nesselroade and Labouvie, 1985; Schaie, 1977). The dominant approach has been to emphasize quantitative methods for evaluating program impact, but there has also been renewed attention to and appreciation of the benefits of qualitative approaches for certain questions and problems (e.g., Patton, 2001).

A hallmark of modern approaches to program evaluation is an appreciation of the critical role that measurement quality plays in generating valid research conclusions (e.g., Campbell and Russo, 2001). Arguably, selection or development of sensitive and valid measurement techniques is the most important aspect of successful evaluation research. Finally, our sampling methods (for example, ones that achieve representativeness to a target population) have evolved considerably over the past 50 years and are widely employed in sociology, demography, and other disciplines (for an introduction, see Babbie, 2003). These issues are of course highly relevant to research on aging (Alwin and Campbell, 2001; Lawton and Herzog, 1989).

Generally speaking, research design can be viewed as a process of making compromises regarding what and when one measures so as to answer a research question (Cronbach, 1986; Hertzog and Dixon, 1996; Nesselroade, 1988). Design is the art of compromise because not all variables can be measured easily, and not all confounding variables can be directly controlled to rule out competing interpretations of the data. The practical realities of research necessitate exchanging the optimal for the feasible. Our belief is that theory-guided research is to be preferred when possible (Mead, Batsakes, Fisk, and Mykityshyn, 1999), but theory-guided evaluation may not always be possible or even desirable (e.g., Creswell, 1994). Nonetheless, explicit statements of the research questions, and explorations of what one is and is not attempting to accomplish, are critical first steps if we are to make valid decisions about design issues. Our goal in this chapter is not to provide a compendium of "dos" and don'ts" or a series of checklists for translational research, but rather to provide a *vade mecum*, or tour guide, for those embarking on such endeavors. We do not treat important practical issues associated with designing and implementing research in field settings (but see Ball, Wadley, and Roenker, 2003); instead we focus on an illustration of principles of research design that are generically relevant to applied research. We hope that consideration of issues involved in the assessment of the impact of technologies on the lives of older adults will help researchers to make thoughtful design decisions that maximize the usefulness of the evaluations they undertake.

We begin our discussion with an overview of some issues that apply quite universally to the design of studies to evaluate the impact of technological interventions on adaptive functioning in older adults. We then review in more detail some fundamental measurement issues as well as basic features of experimental and quasi-experimental intervention designs, ending with a short discussion of the social significance of research outcomes.

BASIC ISSUES IN EVALUATING
TECHNOLOGICAL INTERVENTIONS

What Are the Research Questions?

It is important for social scientists to appreciate that the nature of the research question is often different in evaluation research than in research focused on identifying basic mechanisms. Experimental psychologists (like ourselves) are oriented toward isolating causal mechanisms through achieving experimental control over independent variables. The research questions they ask are about structure, mechanism, and process. Evaluation research often dictates a different kind of research question concerning the *functional impact* of existing or new conditions on the broader population (or specific subpopulations). Consider, for example, the disparity between research questions focusing on understanding age changes in perception and the potential impact of such changes on cognitive performance. An experimental psychologist might ask whether age-related impairments in perception have a detrimental impact on comprehending presented information. Designing research on this topic might focus on manipulating stimulus parameters (e.g., background noise, illumination, glare) to determine the conditions in which perceptual deficits do or do not impact comprehension (e.g., Schneider and Pichora-Fuller, 2000; Wingfield and Stine-Morrow, 2000). The research question might dictate describing the relationship between manipulated perceptual deficit and comprehension outcomes. A practical outcome for comprehension researchers might be guidelines for stimulus characteristics in experiments that eliminate or at least minimize the influence of perceptual limitations on comprehension task performance. A researcher interested in the functional impact of perceptual limitations in typical environments would, in contrast, not want to remove the influences of perceptual limitations, except as the target of an intervention design. Instead, that researcher would first design a study that focused on observing or simulating conditions that constrain perception in common everyday environments and ask questions such as, "What proportion of the population is adversely affected by these kinds of conditions? What is the nature of the functional impact? What can be done to mitigate this functional impact?"

Gerontologists have long recognized that phenomena identified in the laboratory do not necessarily translate directly into improved lives for older adults (Birren, 1974; Czaja and Sharit, 2003; Schonfeld, 1974), although well-designed simulations of everyday tasks in the laboratory may well predict actual performance (e.g., Angell, Young, Hankey, and Dingus, 2002). Translating laboratory research into statements about functional impact on everyday life requires an understanding of the similarity and differences between the laboratory setting and the ecological setting, accounting for the vagaries of human behavior. People develop practical knowledge about how to achieve goals in everyday life that is difficult to "control" in the laboratory. In everyday life, for example, adults can change the requirements of a task by adjusting their strategic approach to the task. Remembering to take medications on schedule requires effective memory processes, unless the adult who is memory impaired obtains assistance from a care provider, family, or friends. Remembering to take medications may be as much a function of social support as it is an ecological test of intact memory functioning (see Park and Kidder, 1996).

Ultimately, understanding the functional impact of technology requires *both* an understanding of underlying mechanisms *and* an understanding of normal environmental contexts (e.g., ranges of variation in perceptual conditions, characteristics of persons in the populations) that affect this impact.

Such an assessment is likely to involve simultaneous consideration of many design features and outcome variables. For example, the ultimate standards for usability of a hearing aid for older adults are (a) whether it improves auditory discrimination in all or most of the contexts in which adults who are hearing impaired find themselves (rather than just in the tightly controlled conditions of an audiometric examination), (b) whether it improves not only hearing but also more-complex behaviors that rely on hearing (e.g., social interaction), (c) whether it has been designed to take into account problems in small motor control that might make fine adjustments of its settings difficult for the user, and (d) whether it is unobtrusive enough to permit use without stigmatization (Kemper and Lacal, this volume; Pichora-Fuller and Carson, 2001).

What Are the Populations (or Subpopulations) of Interest?

Any intervention or evaluation study must consider carefully the issue of the target groups of interest for the intervention. Research design needs to carefully consider rival explanations for observed outcomes—often referred to as internal validity threats (Berk and Rossi, 1999; Campbell and Stanley, 1966; Schaie, 1988)—so as to ensure a valid assessment of intervention effects, controlling for potentially confounded variables that could mimic the pattern of expected treatment benefits. Arguably, however, just as much attention needs to be given to matters of external validity—that is, designing studies with an eye to generalizing results of a specific study to different target populations, settings, and time periods (Cook and Campbell, 1979; Hultsch and Hickey, 1978). This is especially the case in technological interventions, which are often designed for compensatory or prosthetic support. Full understanding of the range of attributes in the target group to receive an intervention is critical to ensure that individuals have sufficient cognitive ability or comprehension skills to understand directions or training regimens. Furthermore, careful preliminary research on need and potential benefit may be critical for tailoring the intervention itself.

Older populations are a special case in point. They are characterized by heterogeneity, relative to younger populations (e.g., Nelson and Dannefer, 1992; Hultsch, Hertzog, Dixon, and Small, 1998). Some older adults function at extraordinarily high levels. Others are afflicted with physical and psychological burdens, including chronic diseases such as arthritis, frailty, or depression. Many lack the economic resources to be able to take full advantage of technological innovations that carry some financial costs for implementation and maintenance.

Some products or assistive technologies are designed explicitly for use by people who have disabilities or specific medical conditions. For example, assistive listening devices are intended for people who have hearing difficulties, and blood glucose monitors are intended for people who have diabetes. However, everyone in our society, including those with functional limitations, needs to access a wide spectrum of technologies during the course of the day, at home, at work, and while carrying out the usual round of daily activities in the community. Most technological devices are designed for those in the 20-50-year age range (Kroemer, 1997). In considering the aging population, however, it is necessary to take into account the fact that aging, and a number of pathological conditions encountered with greater frequency during aging, lead to manifestations of a range of problems. Conditions that affect technology use may be associated with chronological age in a linear or in a quadratic fashion and will vary in severity and incidence, making it difficult to determine "the average person" who is the potential technology user. Vanderheiden (1997) suggests that many designers aim for usability by the upper 95 percent of the population. However, that 95 percent figure applies to each dimension that may lead to limitations in usability—e.g., poor vision, poor hearing, arthritis, learning disabilities. Although many such limitations are independent of each other, a given individual, especially an older individual, may have several. Taking a simple case in which the probabilities of each disability are independent and constant in magnitude, say 10 percent, if a product requires that a person lie in the upper 90 percent of each distribution, the percentage of individuals who can actually use the product will be much less than 90 percent.

Also, because relationships between individual abilities and performance may be nonlinear, there may be threshold effects in which a minimum level of memory, or reasoning, or physical mobility may be required. For example, those who score below a minimum level of performance may be unable to benefit from audiological rehabilitation programs in which complex new skills must be acquired (Pichora-Fuller and Carson, 2001). Some products or devices may be relatively costly and not subsidized by medical insurance—e.g., computers. It is critical, then, that any intervention study consider carefully the targeted recipients, their likelihood to benefit from the intervention, and any unanticipated costs or burdens that may be imposed by the intervention.

Attention to the issue of subpopulation selection also has critical importance for thinking about the nature of the intervention design. Often, interventions are cast in the traditional experimental framework and rely on analysis of variance approaches to identify average treatment benefit. Under these circumstances, individual differences are treated only as error variance. However, research in several domains, including human abilities, cognitive aging, and educational psychology, points to the fact that treatments or interventions may be differentially effective for individuals varying along some dimension (in analysis of variance terms, these are person by treatment interactions) (Baltes, Reese, and Nesselroade, 1988; Cook and Campbell, 1979; Cronbach and Snow, 1977).

Individuals differ in terms of the background skills, knowledge, beliefs, and behaviors that are relevant to shaping intervention effectiveness. For example, health beliefs play a great role in determining whether older adults will comply with physician instructions (Leventhal, Rabin, Leventhal, and Burns, 2001), and style of personal organization may be an important determinant of whether individuals successfully adhere to medication regimens (Brown and Park, 2003; Park and Kidder, 1996). In cognitive task environments, the particular strategies people select for approaching a task can have a profound impact on novice and skilled performance of older adults (Hertzog, 1985; 1996; Rogers, 2000; Touron and Hertzog, in press).

In the domain of technological intervention, individuals vary widely in past experience regarding computers, VCRs, ATMs, and other devices, and their attitudes toward technology, self-efficacy beliefs in technology use, and general ability may have important influences on their willingness to use and effectiveness in using complex technical devices (Czaja, 2001). For example, some window interfaces may work better for novices than for expert mouse users whereas other interfaces may work better for experts than for novices (Tombaugh, Lickorish, and Wright, 1987).

Evaluators of the usability of heads-up devices for detecting objects on the road ahead may focus on individuals who are familiar with a specific make of automobile or may test individuals new to both the type of auto used in the assessment and to the display device. Choice between these user groups will impact the conclusions that can be drawn.

Therefore, a critical issue for researchers is to determine whether an evaluation design needs to be able to detect interactions of person differences with the target outcome variables. If so, more-complicated statistical analyses are needed for designs that have identified the relevant variables, measured the relevant covariates, and have sampled enough individuals to be able to have the power to detect possible interactions between characteristics of persons and the benefit they derive from intervention. A prior question for the researcher is whether such heterogeneity should be explicitly evaluated, with a larger sample, or whether people will be deliberately selected for homogeneity on particular variables, arguing that a particular target group or groups is the right starting point for evaluating a technical intervention (see Schaie, 1973).

What Are the Outcome (Dependent) Variables of Interest?

Choice of dependent variables will necessarily depend on the research question at hand. In early stages of design and redesign of technology, the focus is likely to be on issues of usability and safety, rather than on costs and benefits of technology. Once implemented, the dependent variables of interest may shift more toward issues of costs and benefits. Costs and benefits can be assessed at a number of levels, but the nature of these must first be defined. They may be construed narrowly or broadly; as affecting the individual using the technology; as affecting others with whom the user interacts at home, in the workplace, and in the community; or as affecting society more broadly. They may be defined very specifically with regard to the task at hand. For example, the benefit of a telephone reminder system may be assessed quite simply by comparing rates of keeping appointments with healthcare providers or in terms of cost-benefit analyses that take into account the costs of missed appointments and the cost of implementing the reminder system.

The impact of a new technology in the workplace can be evaluated in terms of increased efficiency assessed by speed or accuracy of output (or some measure of efficiency that takes both into account), in terms of quality of interpersonal relationships among users of the technology, in terms of increased sense of well-being or efficacy on the part of the user, or in terms of increases or decreases in stress associated with performing particular tasks after introduction of the technology. The use of ATMs may produce benefits for both users and banks in terms of time saved for transactions, but there may be potential costs in terms of frustration in learning to use the ATM and in loss of personal contact with bank employees. Telemedicine may bring diagnostic and health maintenance services to those without transportation or who live far from specialized medical facilities, but there may be costs if the accuracy of the instrumentation is not high or if there are differences in the nature of information provided by patients to healthcare providers via telecommunication devices and in face-to-face interactions. Learning data entry or other computer skills may bring the opportunity of employment both in the work place and from the home (telecommuting) to older adults, providing enhancements in income during retirement. Maintaining the presence of older adults in the work force can have benefits at the individual level in terms of increased income and sense of self-worth, as well as effects at a societal level that may vary depending on the state of the economy and the need for workers in particular job categories. Use of the computer or telecommunication devices as adjuncts to psychotherapy for caregivers of patients with dementia can reduce the perceived burden of caregiving, provide information about support groups and other services, and allow for extended communication with family members. Below we discuss in more detail issues associated with the choice of specific measures for assessing outcomes.

Is Event or Time Sampling Needed?

Another critical design issue is whether individuals must be followed over time to evaluate treatment efficacy. Sometimes long-term retention of a newly acquired skill is a crucial issue, and a follow-up to training after an extended lag is needed to fully evaluate training effectiveness. For example, a critical test of a memory intervention may not be whether individuals' memory performance is better immediately after training, but whether trained skills and memory performance improvements are maintained over days, months, or years (Neely and Bäckman, 1993). Furthermore, the nature of technology use can be conceptualized as the development of skilled behavioral repertoires over time. Hence, one may need to evaluate changes in behavior over the course of training in order to understand how skills develop over time, as well as the relevance of other variables as mediators or moderators of training effectiveness at various stages after the introduction of some technology (Kanfer and Ackerman, 1989).

The literature suggests that older adults can often acquire new skills, but that they do so more slowly at best, and are sometimes differentially susceptible to influences that can impede skill acquisition (Charness and Bosman, 1992; Kausler, 1994; Touron and Hertzog, in press). Nevertheless, assessment of skills or attitudes at a single point in time may not provide results that generalize to real-world settings, where skills are often acquired over long periods of time in intermittent, dispersed learning contexts. Assessment of change over time becomes critical for understanding how much or what kind of training produces optimal use of new technology.

Event sampling may be important for other questions. Event sampling here refers to collecting data when (or if) a specific event or state change occurs. For example, individuals may be maintained in a research panel but may be transferred to a different protocol contingent on specific events (e.g., progression of pathology to a functional level requiring new forms of technological support). Alternatively, data may be sampled according to the onset of specific events encountered by participants (e.g., elevation of blood pressure or blood glucose, a social encounter).

Time sampling may also be an important method for establishing preintervention equivalence when a randomized experiment is not feasible. Introduction of time or event sampling in the design can improve the ability of the design to address critical research questions, but it is almost always accompanied by an increase in the complexity of the design and the resulting data analyses.

MEASUREMENT ISSUES IN ASSESSMENT AND EVALUATION

Here we consider some general issues associated with common methods of measurement in the social sciences used in field and laboratory settings that are relevant to assessing the impact of technology for older adults.

Reliability and Validity

Any method used to decide whether outcomes are meaningful must involve measures that are reliable or consistent. Reliability is often operationalized as stable or consistent individual differences in item responses, either in terms of test-retest correlations, correlations of alternate forms, or measures of internal consistency in responses to sets of relatively homogeneous items (Guion, 2002). More generally, it is the ratio of consistent to total variance. Reliability, by standard accounts, is necessary but not sufficient for establishing construct validity—a variable can repeatedly and consistently measure something(s) other than the construct of interest. However, developmental methodologists have repeatedly shown that stable individual differences are not necessarily the critical measure of consistency; labile measures of psychological states (e.g., mood or affect) often show good reliability within an occasion, but little between-person correlation across different times (Hertzog and Nesselroade, 1987, in press; Nesselroade, 1991). To establish reliability and validity of a given variable, it is critical to consider whether the construct is static or dynamic and the conditions that would give rise to static or dynamic sources of measurement error.

Generically, the most important issue facing any research is ensuring the construct validity of target measures, that is, whether a measure actually taps the construct of interest as conceptualized in a research question (Cronbach and Meehl, 1955; Guion, 2002). This issue can be framed as one of considering the (potentially) multiple sources of variance that affect responses on questionnaires, surveys, or psychological tasks. Variables with higher ratios of construct-relevant variance to total variance, or in regression terms, higher validity coefficients, are of course preferred to variables with low validity coefficients. However, given that we cannot directly observe many important psychological constructs, the problem of comparing validity coefficients is not at all transparent.

What is needed is research that establishes what Cronbach and Meehl (1955) termed a nomological net, that is, a pattern of relationships among variables that is consistent with theoretical arguments about how a construct should relate to other constructs. Measures should show good convergent validity with other measures of the same construct, provided that the same facets of the construct are being measured. At the same time, they should diverge from measures of related but distinct constructs (discriminant validity—Campbell and Fiske, 1959; see Campbell and Russo, 2001). They should also show differential patterns of predictive validity to related or cognate constructs.

In practice, addressing issues of construct validity often involves the use of complex multivariate statistics, such as confirmatory factor analysis and structural equation models (Hertzog, 1996; McArdle and Prescott, 1994; Schaie and Hertzog, 1985). These approaches can be used to estimate construct-related or method-related sources of variance (Widaman, 1985) and can be used to test hypotheses about construct relations in ways that adjust for measurement properties of the variables (e.g., Hertzog and Bleckley, 2001).

One important lesson that can be learned from validation research is that testing models of nomological nets cannot be separated from asking substantive questions about the possible implications of different theories from data. One does not create valid measures in a first step and then do substantive research on validated measures in a second step. Instead, the process of addressing substantive questions inevitably involves also collecting information on the validity of measurement assumptions and decisions and the behavior of variables.

The extent to which these considerations play a role in evaluating societal impact varies from domain to domain and research question to research question. Measures must always be reliable and valid, but validity may be easier to assess in some situations than in others. Face validity (what a scale seems to measure) of measures may be relatively transparent in many problems. Face validity is also often useful for promoting participant satisfaction and compliance (Babbie, 2003). If one wants to know whether use of infrared devices for detecting objects in the dark reduces nighttime accidents in older adults, archival records of accidents would be appropriate sources of evidence; and the operationalization of the measure and its relationship to the construct of interest is straightforward. If one wants to know whether changing the features on a mouse improves the ability to click on a small window on the screen, this too has a straightforward dependent measure with a straightforward interpretation. On the other hand, face validity can reduce construct validity if people react to the apparent goal of the measure by altering their responses (as in the case of emitting socially desirable responses).

Evaluating construct validity can be complex. Consider the case of caregiving and the Resources for Enhancing Alzheimer's Caregivers' Health (REACH) study. Gitlin et al. (2003) discuss two outcome measures. One was the Center for Epidemiological Studies—Depression

Scale (CES-D) (Radloff, 1977). The other was the Revised Memory and Behavior Problem Checklist (RMBPC) (Teri et al., 1992). Respondents were asked at baseline and 6 months later if their care recipients manifested each of a list of problem behaviors and, if so, how bothered or upset the caregivers were by each. Both the CES-D and the RMBPC are reliable measures that are widely used in studies of caregiving. In the Miami sample (and at other sites in this large multisite project), treatment had no effect on degree of change in RMBPC but there was an overall (although fairly small) effect of treatment over control on CES-D for some subsamples. Both the RMBPC and the CES-D might be considered to be measures of the impact of caregiving, but their precise relationship to each other depends on theories of the effects of stressors on perceptions of caregiver burden and the relationship between perception of burden and outcomes such as depression. Interpretation of what it means for one of these variables to show a treatment effect whereas the other does not also requires a theory of their relationship to each other and to other constructs.

A construct that illustrates the import of defining terms is the notion of quality of life. This term has been used to refer to a number of related but not necessarily identical concepts, including life satisfaction assessed either globally or in a particular domain, sense of well-being, social and emotional functioning, health, and social-material conditions (e.g., employment, income, housing), all highly relevant for assessing the impact of assistive technologies on everyday life (Gladis, Gosch, Dishuk, and Crits-Christoph, 1999; Namba and Kuwano, 1999). Instruments used to measure quality of life typically involve self-report, and there is a debate in the field as to whether there is a need for more putatively objective measures such as reports by clinicians or significant others. Gladis et al. note that the best way to operationalize the construct of quality of life may be different at different points in the life span for patients with dementia.

Quality of life is obviously a multifarious concept, and, as noted by Czaja and Schulz (2003), different facets of quality of life may be more appropriate outcome measures depending on the issue under study. Caregiver burden, ability to perform activities of daily living and instrumental activities of daily living, depressive symptoms, and enjoyment of leisure activities may all represent quality of life.

Measurement Equivalence

Research with older adults, as well as research on special subpopulations needing or benefiting from technology, often involves comparisons between subpopulations on variables of interest (e.g., background knowledge about computers, attitudes toward technology). In addition, subgroups are often compared on correlations between two or more measures. Quantitative comparison of means, correlations, regression coefficients, and other test statistics between groups assumes that the variables being analyzed have equivalent measurement properties. That is, one cannot merely assume that the variable is reliable and valid in all the groups; one needs to also assume that the variable is equivalently scaled in different subpopulations (Baltes et al., 1988; Labouvie, 1980). Otherwise, quantitative comparisons of the variables are, strictly speaking, problematic. Use of comparative statistical techniques such as confirmatory factor analysis or item-response theory to evaluate scaling in different groups may be required.

Research has suggested, for example, that older and younger adults respond similarly to some but not all affect rating items (Hertzog, Van Alstine, Usala, Hultsch, and Dixon, 1990; Liang, 1985; Maitland, Dixon, Hultsch, and Hertzog, 2001); likewise, ethnic subgroups can differ in responses to such items (e.g., Miller, Markides, and Black, 1997). To take another example, it is often found that young and older adults give very similar subjective health ratings, but the number of medical conditions reported increases with age; this strongly suggests that young and older adults have different bases for assigning scale values on indices of subjective health. Some data also suggest that older adults differ from younger adults in responses to certain types of telephone-administered surveys (Herzog and Kulka, 1989). Special attention needs to be placed on ensuring that sensory and perceptual difficulties do not dilute the validity of older adults' responses on questionnaires, interviews, and cognitive tasks (e.g., Schneider and Pichora-Fuller, 2000).

Measurement of Change

If the goal of the research is to assess change over time, a methodological issue that must be addressed is whether measures can be repeatedly administered without altering the validity of the instruments (see also the notion of response shift as in Schwartz and Sprangers, 1999). Some cognitive tests, for example, may be inappropriate for repeated multiple administrations because of reactive effects of testing or practice effects, memory for item solutions, etc. If an aim of the study is to measure intraindividual variability by repeated measurement (Nesselroade, 1991), then development of multiple equivalent or parallel forms is needed (e.g., Hertzog, Dixon, and Hultsch, 1992).

Some measures are also subject to contrast- and adaptation-level effects that occur over time. In a famous study, Brickman, Coates, and Janoff-Bulmer (1978) found that lottery winners did not differ in rated happiness from controls and that paraplegics were not as miserable as intuition might predict, presumably because of adaptation to changed lifestyle or reassessment of earlier states. Concerns about adaptation or response shift effects are endemic to research in which self-reports are obtained, especially in the area of health evaluation, and have been observed (for example) in assessment of the effectiveness of hearing aids (Joore, Potjewijd, Timmerman, and Anteunis, 2002). Finding similar subjective health ratings in young and older groups may well be an example of such adaptation-level phenomena.

Another issue is whether the measures have been designed to be sensitive to change. Given that measures are often validated by seeking stable individual differences in responses, there can be some concern that a carefully validated measure might inadvertently emphasize (or diffentially weight) stable versus labile components of variance (Roberts and Del Vecchio, 2000).

The goal of evaluating individual differences in intervention effects requires an analysis of stability and change within a population of persons experiencing an intervention effect. Mean change (the average intervention effect, relative to an appropriate baseline comparison) can be contrasted with stability of individual differences within the intervention group, which reflects variation in the impact of the intervention on outcome measures (Campbell and Reichardt, 1991). Statistical estimation of the relative effect of variables predicting differential benefit may profit considerably from more-complicated models or methods for estimating change over time (e.g., Collins and Sayer, 2001; McArdle and Bell, 2000; see Hertzog and Nesselroade, in press, for a conceptually oriented review of these techniques).

Personalized Assessment

Another measurement issue is whether one should use the same variable to measure a hypothetical construct for every individual. For example, assume one wishes to evaluate individuals' current technical competence with using a computer. It may be better to observe the ways in which different people actually use the computer and to evaluate competence in the context of success with frequently used software, as opposed to evaluating performance on a standard, uniform software program. In this sense, the construct of effective computer use is personalized to assess what individuals actually do and how effectively they do it. There are potential problems of equivalence of scaling across alternative methods, and almost certainly qualitative coding would be needed in some cases rather than development of quantitative conversions across different task types. Nevertheless, consideration of the potential benefits of tailored, personalized assessment could be crucial for measurement regarding some kinds of technology.

Self-Reports

Many measures assess personal characteristics of individuals by asking them to respond with what we can consider self-reports in individual or group interviews (including focus groups), questionnaires, or surveys (for more detailed discussion of these approaches, see Beith, 2002; Nielsen, 1997; and Salvendy and Carayon, 1997). Use of self-report measures requires attention to a number of methodological issues that we discuss in some detail because of their centrality to valid measurement.

"Objective" Versus Subjective Assessment

It is unfortunately easy to design interview and survey questions using implicit but erroneous assumptions of universal and rapid accessibility of target information. For example, one cannot assume that self-reports are inevitably a mirror into objective status. A large body of research shows that subjective health status, as measured by symptom checklists, ratings of functional health, or other methods (e.g., Liang, 1986), often correlates poorly with assessments of physical health by physicians (Pinquart, 2001). This does not imply that the self-reports are necessarily invalid; in fact, subjective health assessments may have better predictive validity for later development of morbidity and mortality than certain kinds of physician assessments.

A large body of literature also shows that self-reported memory complaints are not necessarily a proxy for objective memory problems, as measured by performance on standardized memory tests (e.g., Rabbit, Maylor, and McInnes, 1995). Memory complaints are often more correlated with feelings of depression than they are with actual memory problems. Hertzog, Park, Morrell, and Martin (2000) demonstrated that self-reports of problems with medication adherence had good predictive validity for later medication adherence problems, but that a standardized questionnaire for measuring memory complaints did not predict these problems.

The explanation of the difference appears to involve the fact that the subjective measures of adherence problems were done in the context of reporting medication regimens, and individuals were asked about problems taking the medications as they showed the interviewer the bottle of medication and the instructions on the bottle. As in the cognitive interview (see Jobe and Mingay, 1991), this approach may have created a rich retrieval context for episodes of memory failures. Furthermore, asking about specific behaviors rather than general classes of problems (e.g., "How often do you forget information you read in a newspaper?") may increase the validity of self-reports.

The separation of objective and subjective status variables is not surprising, given that individuals' beliefs about themselves and others are complex, multiply determined, and grounded in social contexts of personal experience and of self-reports. Nevertheless, scientists should not assume that self-report measures are inevitably useful substitutes for measures of background status variables or actual outcomes. A similar concern arises for evaluating the implications of attitudes toward technology for possible use of technology. Social psychologists have known for some time that there is a fundamental distinction between intentions and behavior. Asking individuals about their attitudes toward an assistive device, about their willingness to try to use such a device, or whether they would be likely to use an assistive device in the future are not equivalent to measuring the frequency of actual use. The self-reports of attitudes or intentions may have very little predictive value for actual behavior.

Context Effects

Crafting questionnaires is a highly skilled activity and there may be complicating factors when the sample includes older participants. To continue with the healthcare example introduced above, there is abundant evidence that responses to retrospective questions about personal behavior (e.g., medical healthcare visits over the past year) change as a function of the way in which the questions are asked, suggesting that individuals can respond on the basis of different sources of information (Jobe and Mingay, 1991). For example, the accuracy of retrospective estimates of the frequency of doctor visits increases when individuals are provided with a series of questions that establish a retrieval context for specific episodes of illness and treatment. Otherwise, individuals can base responses on some schema-based aspects of self-beliefs (e.g., "I'm a healthy individual, I didn't go to the doctor last year").

The content of prior questions can influence answers given to later ones in other ways. If asked about satisfaction with life in general, respondents who have just been queried about satisfaction with marriage are likely to include information about marriage in assessing overall satisfaction and may respond more positively if their response to the marriage question has been positive (Schwarz, Strack, and Mai, 1991). Primacy and recency effects may also occur. That is, particular items may be endorsed at higher rates depending on their position in a list, perhaps because list position is associated with cognitive resources necessary to evaluate the items. Such effects may be exacerbated by oral rather than visual presentation (e.g., Schwarz, Hippler, and Noelle-Neumann, 1992). Because older adults may have reduced resources that affect their ability to keep in mind either prior questions or lists of response alternatives, question order effects are expected to be smaller than for young adults, whereas response order effects are expected to be larger in older adults. Knauper (1999) reviews evidence that this is indeed the case.

Even seemingly innocuous questions have the potential to affect responses to other questions. Take for example the role of filter questions in surveys (Martin and Harlow, 1992). Filter questions can be used to determine knowledge without directly asking for a self-report. So one might be asked, "Do you happen to remember anything special that your U. S. representative has done for your district or for the people in your district while he has been in Congress? (IF YES): What was that?" Such questions are difficult to answer, and failure to answer them correctly can lead to attributions about level of knowledge in some domain and to negative feelings about failure to answer correctly (e.g., embarrassment, disappointment, lack of self-efficacy). Failure to answer filter questions may also lead to distraction and reduction of effort in answering subsequent questions, leading to different patterns of correlations between responses to questions in related and unrelated domains. Whether such effects would be exacerbated in older groups is an interesting question in the context of technology use.

The Social Context of Self-Report

Interviews have been thought of as social exchanges with fairly circumscribed roles for the participants. The interviewer seeks information and the respondent provides it. The assumption is that the interviewer poses a question, the respondent divines the intent of the question and provides a full and unconditional response. Current theorizing has led to a much more complex view of the interview process in which the beliefs, attitudes, and expectations of both interviewer and respondent are critical determinants of how questions are interpreted and answered (e.g., Kwong See and Ryan, 1999; Merton, Fiske, and Kendall, 1990; Saris, 1991). A number of these issues are important for interviewing older adults. Interviewers may hold stereotyped views about cognition in old age, including views about reduced memory and language comprehension and they may, consequently, adopt an interview style believed to be more helpful to older adults (cf. Kwong See and Ryan, 1999; Belli, Weiss, and Lepkowski, 1999). Interviewers are expected to read questions exactly as written, to probe inadequate answers in a nondirective way, to record answers without distortion, and to be nonjudgmental about the content of answers (cf. Fowler and Mangione, 1990), but there is a fair amount of latitude inasmuch as respondents may not be responsive in choosing among alternatives that are provided, or may give responses that are internally inconsistent, or may ask for repetition or clarification (e.g., Schechter, Beatty, and Willis, 1999).

Deviations from exact wording by interviewers may affect accuracy of responses for retrospective questions, but it is possible that interviewer tailoring occurs more often for older adults and that the form of such tailoring is differentially effective (or costly) for older adults than for young adults. Belli et al. (1999) report that older adults "are more likely to engage in verbal comments such as interruptions, expressions of uncertainty, and uncodable responses" and that "interviewers are more likely to engage in verbal behaviors that are discrepant from the ideals of standardized interviewing with older respondents, perhaps as attempts to tailor their communication to meet the perceived challenges that they face (p. 323)." Interviewers tend to produce more significant changes in question reading, more probing, and more feedback for responses with older participants. Belli et al. suggest that these may constitute a form of "elderspeak"[1] in the interview situation. To the extent that the interviewer, in deviating from the standard script for an interview, manages to convey negative impressions about aging, the self-efficacy of older adults about encounters with technology could affect their responses.

In carrying out laboratory experiments on cognitive aging, it is our experience that young and older adults construe the interaction between experimenter and participant in different ways. Young adults tend to be quite task oriented and may be participating to fulfill a course requirement or to earn small sums of money. Older adults are often interested in the scientific aspects of the work and view the experimental session as an opportunity for a social interaction. The extent to which such differences may impact the interview process is unknown.

In focus groups, small numbers of people are brought together to discuss a particular topic or topics under the guidance of a trained moderator (Morgan, 1998). Focus groups are useful for exploration and discovery when relatively little is known in advance about an issue or a group (e.g., Rogers, Meyer, Walker, and Fisk, 1998). In focus groups, unlike surveys, there is considerable flexibility in how questions are asked and how participants shape their responses and direct the flow of the conversation. The format permits participants to interact and to develop ideas in a dynamic way as they respond to each other's ideas. It is the role of the moderator to make sure that the group stays on target and to ask follow-up questions to generate more information on relevant topics.

Focus groups are often used as the first stage in needs assessments or in the development of surveys or interventions. They generate opinions, rather than behavior, and, like other forms of verbal report, are not necessarily predictive of how people will in fact behave. Focus groups are

---

[1]See Chapter 5, this volume, for a definition and discussion of elderspeak.

potentially subject to the kinds of interviewer bias effects discussed above. They are also subject to problems of group dynamics associated with perceptions of rank or personality differences (Beith, 2002). For example, one could imagine that mixed groups of novice and expert users of web browsers might be dominated by experts, with novice users less willing to speak at all, much less to describe difficulties with particular aspects of software or hardware. There are alternative approaches. Instead of communicating verbally, participants can type in responses to questions and view their own responses and those of other group members anonymously presented on a screen. Or people can provide responses on paper that are compiled and returned to participants within groups or posted on bulletin boards where participants or researchers can sort them into categories based on similar responses.

Think-Aloud Strategies

There are several strategies for obtaining verbal reports from users of technological devices (Nielsen, 1997). Plausible applications are easy to envision. For example, people can be asked to verbalize their thoughts as they use the web to search for information needed to answer questions (e.g., Mead et al., 1999). Thinking aloud may provide a window on the user's view of the application or device and may permit identification of the nature of specific areas of difficulty in conceptualizing procedures. Nonetheless, thinking-aloud strategies may not always be appropriate or easy to use (Nielsen, 1997). For example, the act of thinking aloud may change people's strategies for better or worse. Thinking aloud also slows people down, so performance measures may not be comparable to those obtained under "normal" conditions. Thinking aloud may also be viewed as a form of divided attention—one reports on the task as it is being performed and the performance and the report must be coordinated, something that might prove difficult for older adults. Certain types of task may also not lend themselves well to this approach. Imagine thinking aloud while trying to evaluate information from heads-up devices that show obstacles ahead on the highway and simultaneously steering a vehicle. Verbalization may also prove more difficult for experts who have automatized certain procedural aspects of a task than for novices who are aware of each step they take.

Observational Evaluation Strategies

Given that people may not be good observers of their own behavior and may not be able to describe in detail how they behave in interacting with technological devices, observational techniques in which people are monitored and perhaps recorded while actually engaged in using technology can be informative not only about the level of performance that is achieved but also about aspects of the technology that are problematic or stressful. For example, Fernie (1997) describes a procedure for assessing the usability of a four-wheeled walker. A video system tracked the movement of light-reflective markers on a participant standing on a large platform that could move unpredictably in one dimension or another. Electrodes applied to the skin measured electrical activity of the muscles, and there were load cells on the walker to measure the force applied to brake handles and force plates to measure components of floor contact.

Videotapes of users may also reveal musculoskeletal discomfort— e.g., rubbing one's neck or fidgeting (Salvendy and Carayon, 1997). Czaja and Sharit (1993) monitored physiological indicators of stress while young and older adults engaged in three simulated real-world computer tasks (data entry, file modification, inventory management) and found that older adults showed increased arousal on a number of measures of respiratory function and also took longer to return to baseline on these measures than younger adults.

Keeping track of the sequence of actions performed while engaging in a task may reveal how efficient a user is, rather than just whether some task was completed successfully. For example, Czaja, Sharit, Ownby, Roth, and Nair (2001) assessed navigational efficiency for problems solved successfully in a complex information search and retrieval task. An on-line technique that may hold promise for elucidating problems in use of the Internet is eye movement tracking. Noting where people look as they search for information may be informative about optimal placement of information on a screen.

EXPERIMENTAL AND QUASI-EXPERIMENTAL
DESIGN PRINCIPLES

Is a Randomized Experiment Possible?

One of the major considerations for evaluation research design is whether a randomized experiment is even possible (Boruch, 1997). A randomized experiment consists of a design with manipulated independent variables that have persons assigned at random to levels of the independent variable. For example, a researcher interested in evaluating a new technique for training data management might assign people at random to participate in either the new training protocol or a no-training or the current training control condition. All other things being equal, randomized experiments afford the greatest control of unwanted research confounds and are in general to be preferred to other approximate techniques for evaluating effectiveness (Cook and Campbell, 1979). However, randomized experiments are frequently difficult to conduct. Random assignment of persons within an organization to preferred and nonpreferred treatment conditions could lead to imitation of treatments (where individuals in the control group give themselves the intervention without experimenter awareness), resentful demoralization (where persons learn they are in the control group and are not receiving the treatment, with derivative consequences for enthusiasm and morale), and other problems. Interventions that are not under the researchers' control (e.g., introduction of a technology in the wider society) are not well suited for true experiments, unless screening on variables such as prior exposure to the technology is considered adequate, given the research questions. Furthermore, randomized experiments may not be warranted in some circumstances. For example, if the randomization would require withholding of effective treatment (such as a hearing aid) from a control group of individuals for which it had been recommended, this would be inappropriate on ethical grounds (e.g., Tesch-Römer, 1997).

Random assignment is irrelevant if the goal of the evaluation is to determine which aspects of a design seem to work and which cause usability problems for specific technologies within a particular organizational setting (e.g., Ellis and Kurniawan, 2000). In such circumstances, of course, the same kinds of issues about generalizability would arise as in other types of case studies—similarity of individuals, settings, and, here, technologies across groups to which extension is desired (see Yin, 2002, for a discussion of case study methodologies). In some cases, the goal is not only to develop particular technologies (e.g., the Nursebot, a robotic device capable, among other things, of tracking the whereabouts of people, guiding them through their environments, and reminding them of events or actions to be carried out), but also to develop them in ways that permit tailoring to the needs of individual users (e.g., Pineau, Montemerlo, Pollack, Roy, and Thurn, 2003). Here too, assessment is likely to be carried out at the individual level and considerations of random assignment are not at issue.

Randomized Experiments

The true (or randomized) experiment is generally considered an ideal in evaluation research, but one that may not be feasible due to practical constraints (Cook and Campbell, 1979). Figure 4-1 shows a typical intervention design, the pretest and posttest with randomized treatment and control groups. The design can be generalized to include multiple treatment conditions, or a factorial arrangement of treatment variables, following generic experimental design principles. It can also be extended to

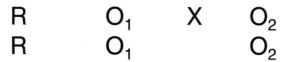

FIGURE 4-1 Standard representation of a randomized pretest-posttest design (see Campbell and Stanley, 1966). Individuals are randomly assigned (denoted by R) to one of two groups—the experimental group and the control group. After pretest (O_1), the experimental group (first row) receives the intervention (denoted as X); the control group does not. Both groups are then given the posttest (O_2). The design predicts equivalent pretest scores on all dependent variables (due to random assignment) but better performance at posttest (after the intervention) for the experimental group.

provide additional posttests to examine maintenance of intervention benefits over time. The central idea is that random assignment of persons to treatment conditions has the long-run expectation of equating groups on any and all individual differences characteristics. Therefore, any group differences in pretest scores should behave as if those differences reflect variation in random samples drawn from the larger population. The critical hypothesis is that the treatment group will improve more than the control group. Assuming an interval-scaled quantitative dependent variable, one would predict a reliable treatment X time (pretest-posttest) interaction.

The randomized design controls for a wide variety of potential confounded variables (Cook and Campbell, 1979) that are rival explanations for results that seem to indicate a treatment effect, including selection effects (differences in people chosen to be in the treatment and control groups). There are several advantages of the pretest-posttest feature of the design (over and above a posttest-only design). Repeated assessment typically produces a test of experimental effects that has greater statistical power (Cohen, 1988). The design's hypothesized interaction effect (i.e., people in the treatment group should improve more than people in the control group) has fewer plausible rival hypotheses, generically, than a simple treatment versus control group comparison.

In general, designing a study to generate a specific pattern of results if the intervention is effective is the best way to guard against rival explanations of the results. For example, extending the design to include multiple posttests generates a more subtle hypothesis about treatment benefit and its maintenance over time (Figure 4-2). Perhaps most importantly, individual differences in degree of treatment benefit (indexed by the difference between pretest and posttest scores) can be measured and correlated with other variables in a pretest-posttest design. Thus, it becomes possible to test whether people's characteristics, such as age, gender, back-

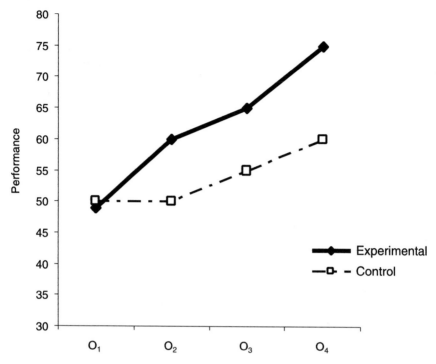

FIGURE 4-2 Hypothetical results from a multiple posttest design (in this case, O_1 is the pretest, O_2-O_4 are the posttests). Note that, although the control group shows increases in performance from O_2 through O_4 (perhaps for unknown reasons), the experimental group shows the same increases, so the benefit of the intervention between O_1 and O_2 (manifested by the experimental group's increase at O_2, relative to the control group) is maintained over time.

ground knowledge, and attitudes, are systematically correlated with the magnitude of the intervention effect. This pattern can also be indirectly evaluated by comparing regression equations between control and treatment groups, examining whether predictors of treatment group performance differ from predictors of control group performance. Nevertheless, testing the hypothesis is more straightforward if estimates of experimental benefits are available for all individuals.

Often it is the case that evaluation requires sampling larger units and then assigning treatment conditions to persons within those units. For example, if one were interested in the benefits of technology in assisted living settings, one might find it necessary to provide technological innovations to all persons in a particular setting. This approach may achieve more cooperation from residents and staff and it avoids potential confounds such as resentful demoralization in the control group denied the benefits of the new technology. A randomized experiment can still be achieved in such contexts if a sampling frame of the larger units is pre-defined, and then units are randomly assigned to treatment or control conditions. This establishes a hierarchical data structure, and optimal estimates of treatment effects can be obtained through application of mixed model procedures that allow for multilevel analysis (e.g., Bryk and Raudenbush, 1987; Willett, Singer, and Martin, 1998).

Quasi-Experimental (Nonequivalent Group) Designs

Sometimes random assignment, even of larger sampling units, is simply not feasible. Under these conditions researchers can attempt to approximate the experimental method by administering interventions to intact groups. For example (continuing the assisted living example), if one has a limited number of assisted living units willing to participate, random assignment is not likely to produce approximate equivalence. Under these conditions researchers might try to approximate the randomized block design approach by first assessing resident and staff characteristics (e.g., location, socioeconomic status, nature of activity programs, size, resident/staff ratios) that might have an impact on the delivery and benefit of the technological intervention. Then they would purposively assign pairs of maximally similar units to receive the treatment or control condition in a manner that would preserve comparability between the units. In this case, of course, selection confounds are a primary concern, given the researchers' deliberate selection of units to receive treatments. Statistical analysis of differences in pretest scores and other individual attributes becomes an important part of assessing whether the treatment and control groups are maximally similar on relevant variables prior to introduction of the treatment.

In such quasi-experimental contexts, experiments that can effectively employ within-subjects administration of treatment conditions are even more beneficial than when truly randomized experiments are feasible. One still benefits from the statistical power of repeated measures analyses (assuming the dependent variables are positively correlated across the different cells), and each person effectively serves as his or her own control. When a limited number of sampling units are contemplated, the problem becomes more interwoven with generalizability of estimated treatment effects to other contexts.

Principles of quasi-experimental design can also be applied to comparisons of self-selected populations (e.g., those who do and do not opt to use certain kinds of technologies). Here, the problem becomes one of achieving statistical control on nuisance variables, as well as statistical evaluation of differences in persons experiencing the different conditions. In limited cases, matching of persons in quasi-experimental groups might be considered, but matching can be problematic when there are multiple characteristics that should be considered and when the persons to be matched differ in the aggregate (perhaps for unknown reasons) in the values of matching variables.

Generically a more valid approach that achieves statistical control is to collect large samples and use regression analysis to evaluate the consequences of technology use and the interactions of person characteristics with those consequences. Given this goal, and the need to control for static individual differences variables that are correlated with the outcomes measures of interest, repeated assessment of persons as they use the technology or become introduced to the technology becomes a valuable design feature. Longitudinal designs, in effect, become a more powerful means of evaluating changes in outcomes as a function of exposure to technology.

Time Series and Interrupted Time Series

In cases in which there is no opportunity for experimental or quasi-experimental manipulation of variables, observational designs can often be strengthened by conducting multivariate time-series observations on the critical variables of interest (Cook and Campbell, 1979; McCleary, 2000). This approach can sometimes produce better evidence for the linkage of technical changes with changes in outcome variables. Statistical models are available for time-series designs that allow for estimates of change in variables adjusting for regular temporal influences (autocorrelation) in the time series.

Intensive intraindividual assessment designs can also be helpful in evaluating coherence of variability in a person or set of persons. For example, if older adults' subjective well-being is thought to be influenced by degree of e-mail contact with family and peers, intensive repeated assessment of well-being and communication patterns can establish whether there is covariation within persons of these variables (e.g., Molenaar, 1994; Nesselroade, 1991).

An important generalization of time-series principles for quasi-experimental designs is the interrupted time-series design (see Figure 4-3). Here, the idea is that one establishes time-related trends on relevant variables prior to introduction of the new technology and then observes whether this interruption produces qualitative change in the shape of the temporal function, or quantitative change in level, slope of change, or variability over time.

This type of design is recommended when it is not generically feasible to assign persons to different treatments and when a discrete inter-

$$O_1 \ O_2 \ O_3 \ O_4 \ O_5 \ \ X \ \ O_6 \ O_7 \ O_8 \ O_9 \ O_{10}$$

FIGURE 4-3 Standard representation of an interrupted time-series design in a single group (see Campbell and Stanley, 1966). In this case, individuals are measured at five points in time prior to the intervention and then five points in time after the intervention. The hypothesis is that the intervention will result in a different curve than would have been observed in the absence of the intervention. In practice, a larger number of observation points would often be necessary to determine that the curves before and after the intervention are discontinuous (McCleary, 2000). The design can be strengthened by adding randomized or quasi-experimental groups that do not receive the intervention.

vention event (possibly not under control of the experimenter) is scheduled sufficiently far in advance to enable the researcher to collect adequate baseline data on the time series before it is interrupted. An audiologic rehabilitation program described by Pichora-Fuller and Carson (2001) exemplifies this approach. In the first phase of the project, the measures of interest were administered on two occasions separated by 6 months, permitting assessment of change over time without intervention. The program was then implemented and the same measures were administered twice more, also at 6-month intervals, permitting assessment of change after the intervention. Comparison of change scores before and after the intervention helps to rule out the alternative explanation that the observed gains after the intervention were due simply to the presence of the researchers at the residential facility at which the program was introduced.

A critical problem for time-series designs is accounting for autocorrelation and distinguishing seasonal or temporal cycles from effects of societal interventions (McCleary, 2000). Descriptive time-series analysis often produces apparently interpretable patterns of flux that can be attributed to multiple, time-varying causes. For this reason, there may be so many rival explanations for the trends that definitive statements about causes of change are not possible. In contrast, the judicious introduction and removal of treatments in the context of time-series observations should produce lawful displacements from temporal flux that covary with the treatment's manipulations, provided that the intervention is effective (see Cook and Campbell, 1979; McCleary, 2000).

CONSIDERING THE IMPLICATIONS OF RESEARCH RESULTS

Within the community of physical and mental healthcare providers, issues of clinical significance are increasingly under evaluation (see e.g.,

Czaja and Schulz, 2003; Schulz et al., 2002). Czaja and Schulz (2003, p. 231) define clinical significance as "the practical importance of the effect of an intervention (treatment) or the extent to which the intervention makes a real difference to the individual or society. For the individual, clinical significance is obviously important. A treatment should effect a change on some outcome that is important to the life of an individual." In formulating policy within social agencies, both private and public, the goal is to have evidence-based interventions. We believe that the framework in which Czaja and Schulz (2003) cast issues of clinical significance can be usefully extended to issues of evaluating the impact of technology. Following their exposition, we discuss (a) defining what is meant by a significant outcome and selection of measures to index these outcomes and (b) social significance.

Defining Significant Outcomes

Issues of "significance" are sometimes defined in terms of statistical significance, but because statistical significance is a function of sample size as well as the heterogeneity of the group or groups being assessed, the reliability of the measures involved, and other factors, some statisticians prefer to think instead in terms of effect sizes such as r^2 or d. Deciding on the magnitude of an effect that is considered large or important, however, is a subject of some debate. For example, Cohen (1988) proposes that, for the t-test, ds of 0.20, 0.50, and 0.80 be considered small, medium, and large effect sizes. Rosenthal (1995) has noted that very small effect sizes may translate into important differences in terms of number of persons who benefit from medical treatments. Kazdin (1999) has also suggested that clinically significant outcomes can occur when change is large, small, or indeed absent!

What counts as a meaningful change in outcome measures will vary from domain to domain. Consider the case of CES-D as an outcome measure in the REACH study discussed above (Gitlin et al., 2003). In the Miami sample, one group of caregivers received an intervention called the Family-Based Structural Multisystem In-Home Intervention (FSMII) and another received the FSMII and a Computer Telephony Integration System (CTIS). The CTIS included use of a screen phone with text display screens and enhanced functions that allow both voice and text to be sent. The expectation was that this would facilitate communication in therapy sessions, increase access to support from family members and others, and provide access to medication and nutrition information and linkages to formal resources as well as some caregiver respite activities. A minimal support control group was also included. The group with CTIS showed a greater improvement in CES-D scores from baseline over a 6-month period than did the control group (Gitlin et al., 2003). The control group showed a small change from 18.34 to 17.73, whereas the CTIS group showed a decline from 16.08 to 13.88. There are different ways of evaluating the importance of this effect. A CES-D score of 16 is treated as the cutoff for persons to be at risk for major depression. So one way to look at this is that the CTIS group moved out of the at-risk category. Another way to evaluate the outcome would be to ask whether the CTIS group mean at 6 months looks more like some normative group than it did at baseline. This of course presumes that there is an appropriate comparison group. Other approaches are also possible (e.g., Jacobson, Roberts, Berns, and McGlinchey, 1999). Note, however, that in absolute terms the change of the CTIS group was 2.20 points whereas that of the control group was 0.61 points. The change here, although significant, may not make what Kazdin (1999, p. 332) refers to as "a real (e.g., genuine, palpable, practical, noticeable) difference in everyday life to the clients or to others with whom the clients interact." Here we could ask whether the CTIS led to perceived reductions in stress that were important to the caregiver's sense of quality of life or increased the ability to provide care so that the care recipient remained at home or lived longer. Similar issues presumably arise when one considers the effects of assistive devices. One can ask whether the use of particular walkers leads to a significant decrease in number of falls at home, fewer visits to healthcare providers, greater independence, reductions in difficulty performing activities of daily living and instrumental activities of daily living—and of course all of the interpretive issues described above would apply. In the case of hearing aids, one can ask what it means to be able to report back correctly one more word or sentence in noise. And so on. In some cases, it is likely to be very difficult to quantify the outcomes. For example, older adults use the Internet to get information about health and to plan travel. What is the appropriate measure here for determining the effect that these uses have?

Social Significance of Outcomes

Here the issue is the extent to which an intervention generates outcomes that are important to or have an impact on society. Social significance can be defined fairly simply in some cases. For example, in the case of caregiving, Czaja and Schulz (2003) point to measures of residential care, placement, patient longevity, patient functional status, service utilization, impact on employment, and cost-effectiveness. Some of these, of course, are also highly relevant for evaluating the result of providing assistive devices to those who need them. Other measures will vary from application to application. There might be costs associated with use of computers in interventions with caregivers—users might come to expect a higher level of accessibility to expert medical personnel, leading to additional issues of how to compensate healthcare providers for their time. Searching the Internet for medical information could lead to better informed physician-patient interactions but also to costs in terms of problems in understanding technical material available on the web and increases in self-medication or susceptibility to the consequences of faulty information sources (and scams). Providing state-of-the-art assistive devices such as artificial limbs might improve mobility and perceived quality of life, but such devices may be costly. Each of these examples suggests the need for definition of terms and selection of measures that are sensitive to the particular kinds of costs and benefits that are anticipated when a technology is implemented or discovered afterwards. How this might be accomplished is, regretfully, beyond the scope of this chapter.

CONCLUSIONS

We have attempted to identify the critical issues for researchers who are designing research to evaluate the impact of technological change on older adults. Our purpose in raising a number of difficult issues is not to imply that valid research in this area is impossible. To the contrary, we believe that inoculating researchers with information about challenges to good research in this domain is the best method of fostering quality research outcomes and sound scientific and policy inferences based on them. Indeed, the other chapters in this volume are a testament to the fact that high-quality scientific research about aging is abundant and is having a major impact on how we understand the aging process, older adults, and the impact of technology on them. Older populations present special problems for the researcher, as do the goals of evaluating older adults' current practices and formulating effective interventions that enhance older adults' functioning. We hope this chapter will raise awareness about the issues that must be tackled to ensure that our society responds to the challenges of enhancing the quality of life of older adults through technological innovation. If we have raised readers' consciousness about the importance of actually *evaluating* impact and benefit of technology, rather than presuming it, then we have accomplished one of our major goals.

REFERENCES

Alwin, D.F., and Campbell, R.T. (2001). Quantitative approaches: Longitudinal methods in the study of human development and aging. In R.H. Binstock and L.K. George (Eds.), *Handbook of aging and the social sciences* (pp. 22-43). San Diego, CA: Academic Press.

Angell, L.S., Young, R.A., Hankey, J.M., and Dingus, T.A. (2002). *An evaluation of alternative methods for assessing driver workload in the early development of in-vehicle information systems.* (Report No. SAE 2002-01-1981). Warrendale, PA: Society of Automotive Engineers.

Babbie, E.J. (2003). *The practice of social research* (10th ed.). Belmont, CA: Wadsworth.

Ball, K., Wadley, V., and Roenker, D. (2003). Obstacles to implementing research outcomes in community settings. *Gerontologist, 43*(1), 29-36.

Baltes, P.B. (1993). The aging mind: Potential and limits. *Gerontologist, 33,* 580-594.

Baltes, P.B., Reese, H.W., and Nesselroade, J.R. (1988). *Life-span developmental psychology: Introduction to research methods.* Mahwah, NJ: Lawrence Erlbaum.

Beith, B.H. (2002). Needs and requirements in health care for the older adults: Challenges and opportunities for the new millennium. In W.A. Rogers and A.D. Fisk (Eds.), *Human factors interventions for the health care of older adults* (pp. 13-30). Mahwah, NJ: Lawrence Erlbaum.

Belli, R.F., Weiss, P.S., and Lepkowski, J.M. (1999). Dynamics of survey interviewing and the quality of survey reports: Age comparisons. In N. Schwarz, D.C. Park, B. Knauper, and S. Sudman (Eds.), *Cognition, aging, and self-reports* (pp. 303-325). Philadelphia, PA: Psychology Press.

Berk, R.A., and Rossi, P.H. (1999). *Thinking about program evaluation* (2nd ed.). Thousand Oaks, CA: Sage.

Bickman, L. (2000). *Research design: Donald Campbell's legacy.* Thousand Oaks, CA: Sage.

Birren, J.E. (1974). Translations in gerontology from lab to life: Psychophysiology and the speed of response. *American Psychologist, 29,* 808-815.

Boruch, R.F. (1997). *Randomized experiments for planning and evaluation.* Thousand Oaks, CA: Sage.

Brickman, P., Coates, D., and Janoff-Bulmer, R. (1978). Lottery winners and accident victims: Is happiness relative? *Journal of Personality and Social Psychology, 36,* 917-927.

Brown, S.A., and Park, D.C. (2003). Theoretical models of cognitive aging and implications for translational research in medicine. *Gerontologist, 43*(1), 57-67.

Bryk, A.S., and Raudenbush, S.W. (1987). Application of hierarchical linear models to assessing change. *Psychological Bulletin, 101,* 147-158.

Campbell, D.T., and Fiske, D.W. (1959). Convergent and discriminant validation by the multitrait-multimethod matrix. *Psychological Bulletin, 56,* 81-105.

Campbell, D.T., and Reichardt, C.S. (1991). Problems in assuming the comparability of pretest and posttest in autoregressive and growth models. In R.E. Snow and D.E. Wiley (Eds.), *Improving inquiry in social science* (pp. 201-219). Mahwah, NJ: Lawrence Erlbaum.

Campbell, D.T., and Russo, M.J. (2001). *Social measurement.* Thousand Oaks, CA: Sage.

Campbell, D.T., and Stanley, J.C. (1966). *Experimental and quasi-experimental designs for research in teaching.* Chicago: Rand McNally.

Charness, N., and Bosman, E. (1992). Human factors and age. In F.I.M. Craik and T.A. Salthouse (Eds.), *Handbook of Aging and Cognition* (pp. 495-552). Mahwah, NJ: Lawrence Erlbaum.

Cohen, J. (1988). *Statistical power analysis for the behavioral sciences* (2nd ed.). Mahwah, NJ: Lawrence Erlbaum.

Collins, L.M., and Sayer, A.G. (2001). *New methods for the analysis of change.* Washington, DC: American Psychological Association.

Cook, T.D., and Campbell, D.T. (1979). *Quasi-experimentation: Design and analysis issues for field settings.* Chicago: Rand McNally.

Creswell, J.W. (1994). *Research design: Qualitative and quantitative approaches.* Thousand Oaks, CA: Sage.

Cronbach, L.J. (1986). Social inquiry by and for Earthlings. In D.W. Fiske and R.A. Shweder (Eds.), *Metatheory in social science: Pluralisms and subjectivities* (pp. 83-107). Chicago: University of Chicago Press.

Cronbach, L.J., and Meehl, P.E. (1955). Construct validity in psychological tests. *Psychological Bulletin, 52,* 281-302.

Cronbach, L.J., and Snow, R.E. (1977). *Aptitudes and instructional methods: A handbook for research on aptitude-treatment interactions.* New York: Irvington.

Czaja, S.J. (2001). Technology change and the older worker. In J. Birren and K.W. Schaie (Eds.), *Handbook of psychology and aging* (5th ed., pp. 547-568). San Diego, CA: Academic Press.

Czaja, S.J., and Schulz, R. (2003). Does the treatment make a real difference: The measurement of clinical significance. *Alzheimer's Care Quarterly, 4,* 229-240.

Czaja, S.J., and Sharit, J. (1993). Stress reactions to computer-interactive tasks as a function of task structure and individual differences. *International Journal of Human-Computer Interaction, 5,* 1-22.

Czaja, S.J., and Sharit, J. (2003). Practically relevant research: Capturing real world tasks, environments, and outcomes. *Gerontologist, 43,* 9-18.

Czaja, S.J., Sharit, J., Charness, N., Fisk, A.D., and Rogers, W.A. (2003). Factors predicting the use of technology: Findings from the center for research and education on aging and technology enhancement (CREATE). Unpublished manuscript.

Czaja, S.J., Sharit, J., Ownby, R., Roth, D.L., and Nair, S. (2001). Examining age differences in performance of a complex information search and retrieval task. *Psychology and Aging, 16*(4), 564-579.

Ellis, R.D., and Kurniawan, S.H. (2000). Increasing the usability of online information for older users: A case study in participatory design. *International Journal of Human-Computer Interaction, 12*(2), 263-276.

Fernie, G. (1997). Assistive devices. In A.D. Fisk and W.A. Rogers (Eds.), *Handbook of human factors and the older adult* (pp. 289-310). San Diego, CA: Academic Press.

Fowler, F.J., Jr., and Mangione, T.W. (1990). *Standardized survey interviewing: Minimizing interviewer-related error.* Thousand Oaks, CA: Sage.

Gitlin, L.N., Belle, S.H., Burgio, L.D., Czaja, S.J., Mahoney, D., Gallagher-Thompson, D., Burns, R., Hauck, W.W., Zhang, S., Schulz, R., and Ory, M.G. (2003). Effect of multi-component interventions on caregiver burden and depression: The REACH multisite initiative at 6-month follow-up. *Psychology and Aging, 18*(3), 361-374.

Gladis M.M., Gosch E.A., Dishuk N.M., and Crits-Christoph P. (1999). Quality of life: Expanding the scope of clinical significance. *Journal of Consulting and Clinical Psychology, 67*(3), 320-331.

Guion, R.M. (2002). Validity and reliability. In S.G. Rogelberg (Ed.), *Handbook of research methods in industrial and organizational psychology* (pp. 57-76). Malden, MA: Blackwell.

Hertzog, C. (1985). An individual differences perspective: Implications for cognitive research in gerontology. *Research on Aging, 7,* 7-45.

Hertzog, C. (1996). Research design in studies of aging and cognition. In J.E. Birren and K.W. Schaie (Eds.), *Handbook of the psychology of aging* (4th ed., pp. 24-37). New York: Academic Press.

Hertzog, C., and Bleckley, M.K. (2001). Age differences in the structure of intelligence: Influences of information processing speed. *Intelligence, 29,* 191-217.

Hertzog, C., and Dixon, R.A. (1996). Methodological issues in research on cognition and aging. In F. Blanchard-Fields and T. Hess (Eds.), *Perspectives on cognitive changes in adult development and aging* (pp. 66-121). New York: McGraw-Hill.

Hertzog, C., and Nesselroade, J.R. (1987). Beyond autoregressive models: Some implications of the trait-state distinction for the structural modeling of developmental change. *Child Development, 58,* 93-109.

Hertzog, C., and Nesselroade, J.R. (in press). Assessing psychological change in adulthood: An overview of methodological issues. *Psychology and Aging.*

Hertzog, C., Dixon, R.A., and Hultsch, D.F. (1992). Intraindividual change in text recall of the elderly. *Brain and Language, 42*(3), 248-269.

Hertzog, C., Park, D.C., Morrell, R.W., and Martin, M. (2000). Ask and ye shall receive: Behavioral specificity in the accuracy of subjective memory complaints. *Applied Cognitive Psychology, 14,* 257-275.

Hertzog, C., Van Alstine, J., Usala, P.D., Hultsch, D.F., and Dixon, R.A. (1990). Measurement properties of the Center for Epidemiological Studies Depression Scale (CES-D) in older populations. *Psychological Assessment, 2,* 64-72.

Herzog, A.R., and Kulka, R.A. (1989). Telephone and mail surveys with older populations: A methodological overview. In M.P. Lawton and A.R. Herzog (Eds.), *Special research methods for gerontology* (pp. 63-89). New York: Baywood.

Hultsch, D.F., and Hickey, T. (1978). External validity in the study of human development: Theoretical and methodological issues. *Human Development, 21*(2), 76-91.

Hultsch, D.F., Hertzog, C., Dixon, R.A., and Small, B.J. (1998). *Memory change in the aged.* New York: Cambridge University Press.

Jacobson, N.S., Roberts, L.J., Berns, S.B., and McGlinchey, J.B. (1999). Methods for defining and determining the clinical significance of treatment effects: Description, application, and alternatives. *Journal of Consulting and Clinical Psychology, 67*(3), 300-307.

Jobe, J.B., and Mingay, D.J. (1991). Cognition and survey measurement: History and overview. *Applied Cognitive Psychology, 5,* 175-192.

Joore, M.A., Potjewijd, J., Timmerman, A.A., and Anteunis, L.J. (2002). Response shift in the measurement of quality of life in hearing impaired adults after hearing aid fitting. *Quality of Life Research, 11*(4), 299-307.

Kanfer, R., and Ackerman, P.L. (1989). Motivation and cognitive abilities: An integrative aptitude-treatment interaction approach to skill acquistion. *Journal of Applied Psychology, 74,* 657-690.

Kausler, D.H. (1994). *Learning and memory in normal aging.* New York: Academic Press.

Kazdin, A.E. (1999). The meanings and measurement of clinical significance. *Journal of Consulting and Clinical Psychology, 67,* 332-339.

Knauper, B. (1999). Age differences in queston and response order effects. In N. Schwarz, D.C. Park, B. Knauper, and S. Sudman (Eds.), *Cognition, aging, and self-reports* (pp. 341-363). Philadelphia, PA: Psychology Press.

Kroemer, K.H.E. (1997). Anthropometry and biomechanics. In A.D. Fisk and W.A. Rogers (Eds.), *Handbook of human factors and the older adult* (pp. 87-124). San Diego, CA: Academic Press.

Kwong See, S.T., and Ryan, E.B. (1999). Intergenerational communication: The survey interview as a social exchange. In N. Schwarz, D.C. Park, B. Knauper, and S. Sudman (Eds.), *Cognition, aging, and self-reports* (pp. 245-262). Philadelphia, PA: Psychology Press.

Labouvie, E.W. (1980). Identity versus equivalence of psychological measures and constructs. In L.W. Poon (Ed.), *Aging in the 1980's: Selected contemporary issues in the psychology of aging* (pp. 493-502). Washington, DC: American Psychological Association.

Lawton, M.P., and Herzog, A.R. (1989). *Special research methods for gerontology.* New York: Baywood Press.

Leventhal, H., Rabin, C., Leventhal, E.A., and Burns, E. (2001). Health risk behaviors and aging. In J.E. Birren and K.W. Schaie (Eds.), *Handbook of the psychology of aging* (5 ed., pp. 186-214). San Diego, CA: Academic Press.

Liang, J. (1985). A structural integration of the Affect Balance Scale and the Life Satisfaction Index A. *Journal of Gerontology, 40*(5), 552-561.

Liang, J. (1986). Self-reported physical health among aged adults. *Journal of Gerontology, 41,* 248-260.

Maitland, S.B., Dixon, R.A., Hultsch, D.F., and Hertzog, C. (2001). Well-being as a moving target: Measurement equivalence of the Bradburn Affect Balance Scale. *Journals of Gerontology Series B: Psychological Sciences and Social Sciences, 56*(2), 69-77.

Martin, L.L., and Harlow, T.F. (1992). Basking and brooding: The motivating effects of filter questions in surveys. In N. Schwarz and S. Sudman (Eds.), *Context effects in social and psychological research* (pp. 81-95). New York: Springer-Verlag.

McArdle, J.J., and Bell, R.Q. (2000). An introduction to latent growth models for developmental data analysis. In T.D. Little, K.U. Schnabel, and J. Baumert (Eds.), *Modeling longitudinal and multilevel data: Practical issues, applied approaches, and specific examples* (pp. 69-107). Mahwah, NJ: Lawrence Erlbaum.

McArdle, R.D., and Prescott, C.A. (1994). Age-based construct validation using structural equation modeling. *Experimental Aging Research, 18,* 87-116.

McCleary, R.D. (2000). Evolution of the time-series experiment. In L. Bickman (Ed.), *Research design: Donald Campbell's legacy* (Vol. 2, pp. 215-234). Thousand Oaks, CA: Sage.

Mead, S.E., Batsakes, P., Fisk, A.D., and Mykityshyn, A. (1999). Applications of cognitive theory to training and design solutions for age-related computer use. *International Journal of Behavioral Development, 23*(3), 533-573.

Merton, R.K., Fiske, M., and Kendall, P.A. (1990). *The focused interview: A manual of problems and procedures* (2nd ed.). New York: Free Press.

Miller, T.Q., Markides, K.S., and Black, S.A. (1997). The factor structure of the CES-D in two surveys of elderly Mexican-Americans. *Journal of Gerontology: Social Sciences, 52,* S259-S269.

Molenaar, P.C.M. (1994). Dynamic latent variable models in developmental psychology. In A. von Eye and C.C. Clogg (Eds.), *Latent variables analysis: Applications for developmental research* (pp. 155-180). Thousand Oaks, CA: Sage.

Morgan, D.L. (1998). *The focus group guidebook: Focus group kit 1.* Thousand Oaks, CA: Sage.

Namba, S., and Kuwano, S. (1999). Human engineering for quality of life. In P.A. Hancock (Ed.), *Human performance and ergonomics* (pp. 69-86). San Diego, CA: Academic Press.

Neely, A.S., and Bäckman, L. (1993). Long-term maintenance of gains from memory training in older adults: Two 3-year follow-up studies. *Journal of Gerontology: Psychological Sciences, 48*(5), P233-P237.

Nelson, E.A., and Dannefer, D. (1992). Aged heterogeneity: Fact or fiction? The fate of diversity in gerontological research. *Gerontologist, 32*(1), 17-23.

Nesselroade, J.R. (1988). Sampling and generalizability: Adult development and aging issues examined within the general methodological framework of selection. In K.W. Schaie, R.T. Campbell, W. Meredith, and S.C. Rawlings (Eds.), *Methodological issues in aging research* (pp. 13-42). New York: Springer-Verlag.

Nesselroade, J.R. (1991). The warp and woof of the developmental fabric. In R.M. Downs, L.S. Liben, and D.S. Palermo (Eds.), *Visions of development, the environment, and aesthetics: The legacy of Joachim F. Wohlwill* (pp. 213-240). Mahwah, NJ: Lawrence Erlbaum.

Nesselroade, J.R., and Labouvie, E.W. (1985). Experimental design in research on aging. In J.E. Birren and K.W. Schaie (Eds.), *Handbook of the psychology of aging* (2nd ed., pp. 35-60). New York: Van Nostrand Reinhold.

Nielsen, J. (1997). Usability testing. In G. Salvendy (Ed.), *Handbook of human factors and ergonomics* (2nd ed., pp. 1543-1568). New York: John Wiley and Sons.

Park, D.C., and Kidder, D.P. (1996). Prospective memory and medication adherence. In M. Brandimonte and G.O. Einstein (Eds.), *Prospective memory: Theory and applications* (pp. 369-390). Mahwah, NJ: Lawrence Erlbaum.

Patton, M.Q. (2001). *Qualitative research and evaluation methods.* Thousand Oaks, CA: Sage.

Pichora-Fuller, M.K., and Carson, A.J. (2001). Hearing health and the listening experiences of older communicators. In M.L. Hummert and J.F. Nussbaum (Eds.), *Aging, communication, and health: Linking research and practice for successful aging* (pp. 43-74). Mahwah, NJ: Lawrence Erlbaum.

Pineau, J., Montemerlo, M., Pollack, M., Roy, N., and Thurn, S. (2003). Towards robotic assistants in nursing homes: Challenges and results. *Robotics and Autonomous Systems, 42*, 271-281.

Pinquart, M. (2001). Correlates of subjective health in older adults: A meta-analysis. *Psychology and Aging, 16*, 414-426.

Rabbit, P., Maylor, E., and McInnes, L. (1995). What goods can self-assessment questionnaires deliver for cognitive gerontology? *Applied Cognitive Psychology, 9*, S127-S152.

Radloff, L.S. (1977). The CES-D Scale: A self-report depression scale for research in the general population. *Applied Psychological Measurement, 1*, 385-401.

Roberts, B.W., and Del Vecchio, W.F. (2000). The rank-order consistency of personality traits from childhood to old age: A quantitative review of longitudinal studies. *Psychological Bulletin, 126*, 3-25.

Rogers, W.A. (2000). Attention and aging. In D. Park and N. Schwarz (Eds.), *Cognitive aging: A primer*. Philadelphia, PA: Psychology Press.

Rogers, W.A., Meyer, B., Walker, N., and Fisk, A.D. (1998). Functional limitations to daily living tasks in the aged: A focus group analysis. *Human Factors, 40*(1), 111-125.

Rosenthal, R. (1995). Methodology. In A. Tesser (Ed.), *Advanced social psychology* (pp. 17-49). New York: McGraw-Hill.

Rowe, J.W., and Kahn, R.L. (1987). Human aging: Usual and successful. *Science, 237*, 143-149.

Salvendy, G., and Carayon, P. (1997). Data collection and evaluation of outcome measures. In G. Salvendy (Ed.), *Handbook of human factors and ergonomics* (2nd ed., pp. 1451-1470). New York: John Wiley and Sons.

Saris, W.E. (1991). *Computer-assisted interviewing*. Thousand Oaks, CA: Sage.

Schaie, K.W. (1973). Methodological problems in descriptive developmental research on adulthood and aging. In J.R. Nesselroade and H.W. Reese (Eds.), *Life-span developmental psychology: Methodological issues* (pp. 253-280). New York: Academic Press.

Schaie, K.W. (1977). Quasi-experimental designs in the psychology of aging. In J.E. Birren and K.W. Schaie (Eds.), *Handbook of the psychology of aging* (pp. 39-58). New York: Van Nostrand Reinhold.

Schaie, K.W. (1988). Internal validity threats in studies of adult cognitive development. In M.L. Howe and C.J. Brainerd (Eds.), *Cognitive development in adulthood: Progress in cognitive developmental research* (pp. 241-272). New York: Springer-Verlag.

Schaie, K.W., and Hertzog, C. (1985). Measurement in the psychology of adulthood and aging. In J.E. Birren and K.W. Schaie (Eds.), *Handbook of the psychology of aging* (2nd ed., pp. 61-92). New York: Van Nostrand Reinhold.

Schechter, S., Beatty, P., and Willis, G.B. (1999). Asking survey respondents about health status: Judgement and response issues. In N. Schwarz, D.C. Park, B. Knauper, and S. Sudman (Eds.), *Cognition, aging, and self-reports* (pp. 265-283). Philadelphia, PA: Psychology Press.

Schneider, B.A., and Pichora-Fuller, M.K. (2000). Implications of perceptual deterioration for cognitive aging research. In F.I.M. Craik and T.A. Salthouse (Eds.), *The handbook of aging and cognition* (2nd ed., pp. 155-219). Mahwah, NJ: Lawrence Erlbaum.

Schonfeld, D. (1974). Translations in gerontology from lab to life: Utilizing information. *American Psychologist, 29*, 796-801.

Schulz, R., O'Brien, A., Czaja, S., Ory, M., Norris, R., Martire, L.M., Belle, S.H., Burgio, L., Gitlin, L., Coon, D., Burns, R., Gallagher-Thompson, D., and Stevens, A. (2002). Dementia caregiver intervention research: In search of clinical significance. *The Gerontologist, 42*(5), 589-602.

Schwartz, C.E., and Sprangers, M.A.G. (1999). Methodological approaches for assessing response shift in longitudinal health-related quality-of-life research. *Social Science and Medicine, 48,* 1531-1548.

Schwarz, N., Hippler, H.-J., and Noelle-Neumann, E. (1992). A cognitive model of response-order effects in survey measurement. In N. Schwarz and S. Sudman (Eds.), *Context effects in social and psychological research* (pp. 187-201). New York: Springer-Verlag.

Schwarz, N., Strack, F., and Mai, H.-P. (1991). Assimilation and contrast effects in part-whole question sequences: A conversational logic analysis. *Public Opinion Quarterly, 55,* 3-23.

Shadish, W.R., Cook, T.D., and Leviton, L.C. (1995). *Foundations of program evaluation: Theories of practice* (2nd ed.). Thousand Oaks, CA: Sage.

Teri, L., Truax, P., Logsdon, R., Uomoto, J., Zarit, S., and Vitaliano, P.P. (1992). Assessment of behavioral problems in dementia: The revised memory and behavior problems checklist. *Psychology and Aging, 7*(4), 622-631.

Tesch-Römer, C. (1997). Psychological effects of hearing aid use in older adults. *Journals of Gerontology Series B: Psychological Sciences and Social Sciences, 52B,* P127-P138.

Tombaugh, J., Lickorish, A., and Wright, P. (1987). Multi-window displays for readers of lengthy texts. *International Journal of Man-Machine Studies, 26*(5), 597-615.

Touron, D.R., and Hertzog, C. (in press). Strategy shift affordance and strategy choice in young and older adults. *Memory and Cognition.*

Vanderheiden, G.C. (1997). Design for people with functional limitations resulting from disability, aging, or circumstance. In G. Salvendy (Ed.), *Handbook of human factors and ergonomics* (2nd ed., pp. 2010-2052). New York: John Wiley and Sons.

Widaman, K.F. (1985). Hierarchically nested covariance structure models for multitrait-multimethod data. *Applied Psychological Measurement, 9,* 1-26.

Willett, J.B., Singer, J.D., and Martin, N.C. (1998). The design and analysis of longitudinal studies of development and psychopathology in context: Statistical models and methodological recommendations. *Development and Psychopathology, 10,* 395-426.

Wingfield, A., and Stine-Morrow, E.A.L. (2000). Language and speech. In F.I.M. Craik and T.A. Salthouse (Eds.), *The handbook of aging and cognition* (2nd ed., pp. 359-416). Mahwah, NJ: Lawrence Erlbaum.

Yin, R.K. (2002). *Case study research: Design and methods.* Thousand Oaks, CA: Sage.

Zigler, E., and Styfco, S.J. (2001). Extended childhood intervention prepares children for school and beyond. *Journal of the American Medical Association, 285,* 2378-2380.

Part III

Domain-Specific Papers

5

Addressing the Communication Needs of an Aging Society

Susan Kemper and *Jose C. Lacal*

COMMUNICATION NEEDS OF OLDER PEOPLE

The possibilities for using technology to meet the communication needs of an aging society are as broad as the communication needs of individual older adults. The ability to communicate is essential if older adults are to solicit assistance with daily living activities; fulfill lifelong learning goals; gain access to health and legal information from print, broadcast, or electronic media; or enjoy intergenerational contacts with family members. Older adults need to communicate with their families, friends, neighbors, and with their lawyers and physicians through face-to-face interaction and over the Internet.

Common barriers to communication include the declining sensory, cognitive, and physical abilities of older adults. Recent technological advances have led to the development of a dazzling variety of new technologies for assistive and augmentative communication for individuals with severe disabilities: Communication systems that recognize speech and translate it into American Sign Language displays in real time; "direct-select" speech synthesis systems with built-in 100,000 word vocabularies and concept- and grammar-based word prediction to speed message construction; communication systems that respond to a variety of inputs including "eye typing;" low-vision magnifiers with electronic page turners; portable optical character recognition programs that translate scanned or electronic text into speech or into Braille; talking picture books; telephones based on bone conduction; and laryngectomy speech amplifiers. These new technologies have dissolved communication barriers for children and adults with disabling conditions.

But search for communication devices that serve older adults who suffer only from normal aging with some hearing loss, some forgetfulness, some word retrieval problems, some slowing of cognitive function, and the list of communication aids suddenly shrinks. There are hearing aids, to be sure, and reading magnifiers to compensate for presbycusis and presbyopia; there are telephones with volume control and large buttons; but there is not much more currently available than these types of devices to amplify and magnify.

Charness (2001) suggested that "consumers of communication technologies are moving into something of a golden age" (p. 22). This golden age is to result from the rapid expansion of affordable, usable communication technologies such as videophones and web-based conferencing. However, this "golden age" of communication is likely to be tarnished unless these technologies are adapted to the needs of older adults who are likely, based on demographics alone, to constitute a significant proportion of their future users. One answer has been the proliferation of guidelines and standards for technology developers. Consider those of two recently issued white papers.

In 1999, the World Institute on Disability issued a bibliography on the use of telecommunications by people with cognitive disabilities. The report included a set of general design principles to overcome barriers to the use of telecommunication devices. Four "universal design" strategies were espoused:

1. Redundant, user-controlled modality, e.g., using diagrams as well as text descriptions, providing auditory as well as written information.

2. Streamlined, user-controlled amount and rate of information; user control of size and contrast of displays; user control of pitch, volume, rate, repetition of auditory information; reliance on recognition rather than recall for functionality.

3. Procedural support to reduce memory load, to counter distractibility, to support planning and sequencing.

4. Content organization: structure text for easy scanning, use hypertext anchors, support example and similarity-based search.

Many of these same recommendations were echoed by the 2002 National Institute on Aging (NIA) report *Older Adults and Information Technology* (Morrell, Dailey, Feldman, Mayhorn, and Echt, 2002) as a set of guidelines for web-site design:

1. Designing readable text, recommendations for typeface, type size, the use of color and backgrounds.

2. Increasing memory and comprehension of web-site content, using clear writing with illustrations, animation, and other text alternatives.

3. Increasing ease of navigation through consistent layouts, menus, site maps, and hyperlinks.

Both sets of guidelines are notable for their attempt to link specific recommendations to known barriers to communication with older adults, based on available research. It is not surprising that there is considerable overlap in the two sets of guidelines, as the World Institute on Disability considers aging to be a disabling "circumstance that *correlates* with cognitive impairments" (1999, p. 33). Nor is it surprising that these guidelines focus on overcoming issues of bad design with changes that would benefit all users, not just older or disabled users. What is surprising is that these guidelines focus primarily on design features, whether of web sites, voice mail systems, or cellular phones. All of these communication devices would indeed benefit from better design to enhance usability, and implementation of these design guidelines would undoubtedly benefit older users; however, they are insufficient. They will not address fundamental age-related barriers to communication.

Aging results in a number of sensory and cognitive changes that impose limits on communication; these limitations reach their most extreme when it comes to communicating with older adults with dementia. Note the overlap between these design guidelines for telecommunication devices and these recommendations for communicating with older adults with dementia (Bollinger and Hardiman, 1989) in Table 5-1.

Repetition, augmentation, amplification, and simplification are the recommended solutions to a variety of communication problems. The recommendations of Bollinger and Hardiman (1989) constitute a set of design guidelines for interpersonal communication. Yet these "guidelines" seem to be the very basis for the complaints of Anna Mae Halgrim Seaver in her posthumously published essay in *Newsweek* (Seaver, 1994, p. 11-12):

> Why do you think the staff insists on talking baby talk when speaking to me? I understand English. I have a degree in music and am a certified teacher. Now I hear a lot of words that end in "y." Is this how my kids felt? My hearing aid works fine. There is little need for anyone to position their face directly in front of me and raise their voice with those "y" words. Sometimes it takes longer for a meaning to sink in; sometimes my mind wanders when I am bored. But there's no need to shout.

Most guidelines for communicating with older adults stress amplifying and augmenting speech to compensate for hearing loss. Hearing loss is a major threat to the social integration and psychosocial well-being of older adults (Tesch-Römer, 1997; Wahl and Tesch-Römer, 2001). Yet hearing aids, even if used, do not remediate these problems, although hear-

TABLE 5-1 Processes Involved in Communication Requiring Message Modification for Optimal Communication with Demented Patients

Problem	Recommended Solution
Sensory loss	Amplify: to increase the strength of the stimuli by making louder, isolating, marking
	Augment: to add to by sending input through additional channels such as using spoken and printed words, gesture(s), and spoken words, touch and spoken word(s), and so on
Attention deficit	Amplify (see above)
	Structure: to make a task, activity, event, or physical surrounding organized, consistent, and predictable, decreasing need for cognitive analysis
	Augment (see above)
Perceptual changes	Exaggerate: to overemphasize by enlarging all segments of a message such as facial expression, intonation, loudness
	Label: to name or describe objects and events as they occur in the environment of a person with dementia
Reduced speed	Repeat: to present again in exactly the same manner and form
	Reduce rate: to slow the rate of presentation by increasing the interval between words and phrases; allowing more time for message from patient
Registration disorder	Repeat (see above)
	Reiterate: to present a previous message with the same content but with different form or structure
	Amplify (see above)
Memory reduction	Augment (see above)
	Repeat (see above)
	Decrease need: to assume an ability is not available thus providing a reminder, or performing the function for the person
Orientation disorder	Simplify: to reduce message to the basic form by shortening or deleting all nonessential words
	Repeat (see above)
	Reiterate (see above)
	Augment (see above)

Reasoning disorder	Simplify (see above)
	Eliminate need: if the task or message cannot be deleted from patient task, perform it for the patient
Language	Reiterate (see above)
	Simplify (see above)
	Amplify (see above)
	Augment (see above)
Speech deterioration	Reduce time pressure (see above)
	Augment (see above)
	Assist: to prompt the patient by proving cues or asking questions that will aid in achieving a response

SOURCE: Adapted from Bollinger and Hardiman (1989).

ing-aid use is associated with a reduction in self-perceived hearing handicap (Tesch-Römer, 1997). It is not surprising that audiologists (Cutler and Butterfield, 1991; Levow, 2002; Uchanski, Choi, Braida, Reed, and Durlach, 1996) and hearing-aid manufacturers (Oticon, 2003) have therefore attempted to promote the use of "clear speech" for individuals who are hearing impaired. "Clear speech" recommendations typically parallel those of Bollinger and Hardiman (1989): speak slowly, speak loudly, insert pauses between phrases and sentences, stress key words, pronounce each word precisely, reduce background noise.

Thus, even in the case of hearing loss, the technological remedy offered by hearing aids must be supplemented by recommendations to speak clearly. Age-related hearing loss involves more than just presbycusis. So too, the reading problems of older adults—on or off the communication highway—will not be remediated by technological guidelines that address only visibility, because older adults' reading problems result from more than just poor vision. Technological advances must move beyond considerations of visibility and amplification to address fundamental barriers to communication with older adults.

Three such barriers to communication with older adults are considered here: overaccommodations to aging, the prevalence of word retrieval problems, and the challenges raised by dual-task and multitasking environments. Each reflects a common source of complaints from older adults. Each has generated a considerable body of basic research. And each provides a potential access point for the application of technologies designed to enhance communication with older adults.

THREE BARRIERS TO COMMUNICATION

Overaccommodations to Aging

Ryan, Giles, Bartolucci, and Henwood (1986) identified two patterns that contribute to older adults' communication problems—underaccommodations and overaccommodations. Underaccommodations occur when the speaker or writer fails to consider how aging affects speaking and listening; overaccommodations occur when the speaker or writer is over-reliant on negative stereotypes of aging. Underaccommodations put older adults at risk for social isolation and neglect because they lead to comprehension failure and hence to the possibility of misunderstanding, deception, and exploitation. The guidelines and design standards reviewed above address underaccommodations to the sensory and cognitive limitations of older adults. But it is easy for these remedies to tilt too far in the other direction, giving rise to overaccommodations to aging. Overaccommodations also put older adults at risk because overaccommodations are often perceived by older adults as insulting and patronizing and so may disenfranchise older adults from full participation in a conversational interaction. Ryan et al. (1986) suggested that overaccommodations to aging may trigger negative self-assessments by older adults of their own communicative competence and thus contribute to a downward spiral of sociocognitive limitations.

Overaccommodations to aging are often marked by the use of a special speech register termed "secondary baby talk" or "elderspeak" in interactions between young adults and older adults (Kemper, Jackson, Cheung, and Anagnopoulos, 1994). Elderspeak is marked by a slow rate of speaking, simplified syntax, vocabulary restrictions, and exaggerated prosody. It resembles an extreme form of "clear speech" but also the sort of speech adults use with infants and small children. It occurs in hospitals and nursing homes but also in lawyers' offices, banks, senior centers, and grocery stores.

Research on elderspeak (Kemper and Harden, 1999) suggests that the short sentences and exaggerated prosody of elderspeak confer no positive benefit to older adults in terms of their performance on communication tasks. Using high pitch, a slow rate of speaking, and stressing important words may actually impair communication with older adults because this exaggerated prosody distorts vowels and other speech elements. Chopping up ideas into short phrases and simple ideas may eliminate causal and temporal connections essential for coherence and continuity. The exaggerated prosody and short choppy sentences of elderspeak also mimic baby talk. To be addressed in baby talk conveys the impression to older adults that they are cognitively impaired and childlike, reinforcing negative stereotypes.

This line of research has also shown that older adults benefit from redundancy and repetition, particularly of complex messages. Even when complex syntax is used, older adults are able to follow directions if they can interrupt to request repetition and clarification. Thus, some aspects of elderspeak may be beneficial to older adults if they can be divorced from those that are hurtful to older adults' self-esteem and those that simply are not helpful.

Implications for Technology

Although the core problem of the widespread use of elderspeak cannot be addressed by technology, technology can perhaps help with many of its manifestations. For example, the use of elderspeak over telephones and other electronic devices compounds many problems older listeners experience with these devices. Building in easy-to-use options for modulating pitch and amplitude might enable older adults to compensate for the high pitch that is characteristic of elderspeak. On-demand buffering of speech segments coupled with rate-adjustable playback might enable older adults to compensate for the slow rate of elderspeak (or too-fast rates of time-compressed speech typical of voice response systems and news broadcasts) so that an individual can adjust the rate of information transmission to their own processing rate. Buffering might also allow older adults to easily back up and replay critical segments, as repetition may be the necessary key to accurate comprehension. Speech-to-text capabilities might enable older adults to capture and record complex messages, instructions, or directions for later analysis.

Word Retrieval

Word retrieval problems are among the most common barriers to communication for older adults. Indeed, older adults cite problems remembering proper names as the most frequent effect of aging (Cohen and Faulkner, 1986; Sunderland, Watts, Baddeley, and Harris, 1986). They are the brunt of jokes about "senior moments" and the target of advertisements promising relief from the vexations of aging through herbal remedies and dietary supplements. Word retrieval failures disrupt conversations, impede orders and requests for services, and, for many older adults, raise the specter of dementia due to their alarming frequency and persistence. As one of the participants in Burke and Laver's (1990) study commented, "If you want to study something *really* useful, find out why I cannot remember the name of my friend of 20 years when I go to introduce her" (p. 281).

Diary studies and experimental investigations have documented that older adults experience word retrieval failures more often than young adults. Proper name failures predominate in older adults' diaries (Burke, MacKay, Worthley, and Wade, 1991), especially for names used infrequently and less recently. Burke and her colleagues have offered an explanation of word retrieval failures that also points to a role for technological intervention. The transmission deficit hypothesis holds that aging affects the strength of mental connections linking an idea to the pronunciation of a specific word—or in more formal terms, a network linking conceptual representations to phonological specifications. If one or more links between the idea and pronunciation is broken, a speaker will be able to retrieve the idea but be unable to translate that idea into an actual spoken word. The transmission deficit hypothesis model pinpoints the locus of the broken connection as between idea and word pronunciation, because speakers will often have partial phonological information about the target word as well as detailed information about the target idea. Older adults are more vulnerable to word retrieval failures because all network connections weaken with age; words are more vulnerable than ideas because words must be precisely articulated from a unique sequence of phonological features (pronouncing "cat" partially correctly might get you a "hat" instead) whereas ideas are redundantly specified by many converging associations and linkages (instead of thinking of a cat you might think of a lion or a tiger or Garfield). In a clever experiment, James and Burke (2000) (see also White and Abrams, 2002) asked young and older adults general-knowledge questions designed to promote word retrieval failures. The questions were embedded in a list of words. Sometimes these words shared phonological features with the target, sometimes they were unrelated to the target word. James and Burke report that fewer retrieval failures occurred when the target was preceded by phonologically related words than when it was not. For example, participants were more likely to correctly answer the question "What word means to formally renounce a throne?" [abdicate] when they had just read "abstract" than when they had read "reread." White and Abrams (2002) report that words sharing the first syllable with the target, e.g., "**ab**acus," "**ab**rogate," are most effective at reducing word retrieval failures, whereas other words sharing other phonological features with the target, such as "in**di**gent," "han**di**-cap," "edu**cate**," and "dupli**cate**" are ineffective.

Implications for Technology

One implication for technology developers is straightforward: Minimize opportunities for word retrieval failures by providing drop-down menus, lists of exemplars, and other options that are structured conceptually. Do not require someone to scroll through a list of names or retrieve a specific name, but provide conceptually organized options, e.g., relatives, friends, and business associates, and make creating that organization structure easy and transparent. A second implication is also clear: Accept partial phonological (or orthographic) information, especially word-initial fragments, in designing search engines, questionnaires, and other response formats. A third implication is less clear: Keep crucial phonological connections activated to avoid word retrieval problems. Based on the research of James and Burke (2000) and White and Abrams (2002), stimulating phonological connections maintaining linkages between ideas and words is the key to reducing word retrieval problems. Technology can potentially help with this—for example, by providing older adults with "talking memory books" that display visual, orthographic, *and* phonological information. Imagine preparing for a family reunion by scrolling through a family diary that displays photographs and biographic details while *pronouncing* the relative's name. Or creating a high school reunion directory by pairing digital photographs with a digital audio record of the classmate's name. Or ordering prescription medication by consulting a virtual pharmacist who displays the container and pill while *articulating* the brand name and generic name along with other medical information. Or "talking" name tags, perhaps linked to small optical scanners and miniaturized speakers embedded in eyeglasses. By activating phonological features, especially those used infrequently, such devices could spare older adults the communication disruptions triggered by word retrieval failures.

Dual and Multi-Tasking

Unlike computers, humans are poorly designed for dual and multi-tasking, and older adults are particularly prone to task disruptions when they are required to perform two or more tasks simultaneously (Sit and Fisk, 1999). This is nowhere more apparent than in common communication situations such as holding a conversation at a congregate meal site against a background of conversations at other tables or at home against a background of television or radio broadcasts. Sounds like "elevator music"; electronic hums and buzzes from computers and ventilation systems; and beeps and alarms from cell phones, pagers, and "smart" appliances all contribute to older adults' communication breakdowns. Older adults' difficulties understanding speech in noise are well documented (Schneider and Pichora-Fuller, 2000) and are often attributed to presbycusis as well as to age-related neuronal loss affecting noise dampening, frequency, and temporal resolution. There is also considerable evidence that age-related declines in attentional ability, specifically executive control over the ability to ignore distractions, also contribute to older adults' difficulties in understanding speech in noise (Tun, 1998; Tun and Wingfield, 1995, 1999). A similar breakdown in inhibitory processes has been implicated in other dual-task and multi-tasking situations. For example, visual distracters during reading may impact older adults more severely than young adults (Connelly, Hasher, and Zacks, 1991), talking on a cell phone while driving may be more hazardous for older adults than for young adults, and closed captioning of television broadcasts may be less helpful for older adults than for young adults (Tun, Wingfield, and Stine, 1991).

For example, Tun, O'Kane, and Wingfield (2002) asked young and older English-speaking adults to listen to lists of words while ignoring competing speech. They varied whether the competing speech was meaningful (read in English) or meaningless (read in Dutch by the same speaker). Although young adults were capable of ignoring the competing speech, the older adults' recall of the target words was severely impaired by the competing speech. This competing speech effect was greater for older adults when the competing speech was in English than when it was in Dutch (a language that closely resembles English phonology and prosody), suggesting that the effect is due to attentional factors. Indeed, controlling for hearing acuity did not eliminate this effect. Tun et al. conclude that young adults are able to filter out competing speech whereas older adults are less able to do so.

One exception to the general finding that older adults experience greater dual-task costs is a recent study of older adults' ability to perform simple tasks while talking (Kemper, Herman, and Lian, in press). They compared three motor tasks: simple finger tapping, complex finger tapping, and walking. Surprisingly, Kemper et al. report that young adults exhibited *greater* dual-task costs than the older adults. Analyses of young adults' language samples revealed reduced sentence length, grammatical complexity, and propositional content when talking while performing the motor tasks. In contrast, the older adults spoke more slowly during the dual-task conditions but their grammatical complexity and propositional content did not vary with dual-task demands. Based on these findings, Kemper et al. hypothesized that older adults, in response to age-related loss of processing speed and working memory capacity, have developed a restricted speech register that is buffered from many dual-task costs associated with simple motor and concurrent selective ignoring tasks.

However, when the walking task is only slightly more challenging (Kemper, Herman, and Nartowicz, 2002), older adults' speech quickly deteriorates. When asked to walk, talk, and carry a sack of groceries, older adults' rate of speaking slows further, and they use many more fillers such as "well" and "you know" to break their speech into short phrases and fragments. These fragments lack key elements of grammatical structure such as auxiliary verbs. Under similar conditions, young adults reduce their speech rate to accommodate for the increased task demands. Kemper et al. suggest that combining two tasks such as walking while talking falls within the range of older adults' reserve capacity, but task demands can quickly exceed their cognitive reserve capacity, whereas young adults can draw on sufficient reserve capacity to cope with the additional task demands. The idea of cognitive reserve capacity (Satz, 1993) is intended to capture the notion that trade-offs between two or more tasks may be revealed only when the tasks are performed under sufficiently challenging conditions. This concept of reserve capacity has proved useful for characterizing cognitive limits in older adults (Baltes and Baltes, 1980; Baltes, Dittmann, and Kliegl, 1986).

Implications for Technology

Although technology cannot increase older adults' reserve capacity, it can help minimize demands on it. FM broadcast systems, induction loops, and infrared systems, sometimes provided in public places such as concert halls, theaters, churches, and conference centers, may aid individuals who are hard of hearing by reducing or eliminating dual-task demands arising from poor acoustics, background noise, and competing voices and sounds. These systems typically require the listener to use a special receiver (some hearing aids can be tuned to pick up the signal generated by induction loops) to pick up a signal generated by a special microphone, amplifier, and transmitter.

Other forms of technology may also reduce dual-task demands and aid communication with older adults. Consider noise-dampening headphones. These devices are marketed for frequent travelers but they may also prove helpful for older adults. In one pilot study (Kemper, unpublished manuscript) it is suggested that older adults benefit from using noise-dampening headphones during reading. Older adults were tested in a small group in an ordinary classroom, acoustically "cluttered" by noise generated by the other participants, undergraduates passing by in the hallway, and a noisy ventilation system. When they wore noise-dampening headphones, their reading speed increased 20 percent and their comprehension improved approximately 15 percent. Young adults showed no improvement. Noise-dampening technology might benefit older adults in other situations, such as driving, writing, or preparing tax returns.

Voice-to-text technology might also benefit older adults by minimizing dual-task demands in situations where they are attending to speech while trying to remember or record details—such as names, phone numbers, and directions. Coupling the display and storage capacity of cell phones with automated speech-to-text capabilities could enable older adults to focus their attention on listening comprehension rather than on the need to find paper and pencil to record a name or a phone number, thus turning a dual-task situation into a single-task situation.

TECHNOLOGY TO EMPOWER OLDER ADULTS

Having covered some basic human needs, in this section we illustrate potential uses of communication technologies to address some of the needs identified above.

It is noteworthy that a large percentage of communication and computing technologies were originally designed for business uses. Those technologies then migrated to the consumer space once volume production allowed for the sale of the devices at significantly lower prices than those paid by the business "early adopters." Cellular phones were originally designed as a business tool, first tested in 1979. Personal digital assistants (PDAs) were first introduced into the business marketplace by Apple (the Newton) in 1993. Processing power has increased exponentially for both cell phones and PDAs since their launch in the business arena. Our thesis is that there is a significant opportunity to use these inexpensive, mass-produced, and very powerful devices to better serve the communication needs of an aging society by tailoring the devices' increasing processing capabilities to the specific strengths, needs, and capabilities of older users.

The growing power and sophistication of both cellular phones and PDAs present a unique opportunity to look at them as mobile communication and computing devices (MCCDs). Moore's law (Intel, 2002) is named after Gordon Moore, one of Intel's founders. He predicted the doubling of transistors in a CPU every couple of years. Moore's law is now applicable to MCCDs: CPU power and RAM capabilities double every 18 months. The devices can run an increasingly sophisticated range of software applications, using an expanding range of operating systems such as Windows CE, GNU/Linux, and Palm OS. Bandwidth is also increasing rapidly, allowing MCCDs to transfer most of the processing-intensive tasks, such as visual recognition and database storage and retrieval to remote servers to reduce demands on the local device. Battery life is the only area where the rate of improvement is slow.

A major challenge is that communication technology devices have traditionally been designed by young engineers (mostly male) targeting fellow young users. Older adults have traditionally been forced to adapt to these devices. However, some suggestions of how these devices can serve the needs of older adults are beginning to appear. For example,

Mann and Helal (2002) have demonstrated how emerging smart cellular phone technology can act as an effective booster of the utility of smart homes and other smart spaces. They present their vision of using smart phones as magic wands that can be used passively as remote control devices and proactively as intelligent companions offering advice, reminders, warnings, and calls for help. In the future, MCCDs, when properly designed, will increasingly have the power to

- Compensate for older adults' diminishing physical and mental capabilities. MCCDs can be designed to increase their "assistance level" as the individual's abilities change due to health conditions or situational factors, for example, by adjusting amplitude as well as pitch to the individual's hearing loss as well as the specific room acoustics.
- Emulate lost capabilities, such as a sense of direction. Some MCCDs are now able to use the global positioning system (GPS). A GPS-capable device can tell a user where he or she is (from a latitude and longitude perspective) with high accuracy. What is relevant here is the device's ability to correlate where the user is with what else is geographically close to the user to indicate a possible match or to make inferences that would compensate for a memory lapse: "You are near Mary's house. Do you need directions to get there?"
- Enhance current abilities, such as hearing or memory retrieval. An MCCD can assist the user by inconspicuously boosting the sound reception of the user. The device's camera might be used to match pictures of people at a meeting with their names and a list of past contacts with the user: "Hello Mary, how do you feel after your car accident 6 months ago?"
- Hide imperfections, such as slower comprehension speed. An MCCD can operate as a real-time recording unit that captures and stores other people's speech and then feeds it to the user at an appropriate rate and pitch for the user to better participate in the discussion.
- Reduce complexity, as by revising texts automatically. An MCCD can rewrite, paraphrase, elaborate, or annotate a text, providing background information to aid the reader or listener.
- Bridge distances, such as networking families. An MCCD can relieve loneliness by linking older adults with their families, social circle, and other caregivers.
- Replace other single-purpose assistive devices, such as hearing aids, note taking, audio recorders, cameras, etc. High-end MCCDs (such as the Compaq iPaq devices) are increasingly being used to perform multiple functions with a single device. This represents a boon for the user who has less hardware to lug around. On the flip side, this also means

that a user with a nonfunctioning MCCD could lose the functionality of multiple single-purpose devices.

• Represent older adults to the world as more competent individuals than their abilities allow them to appear unassisted. MCCDs bring older adults the opportunity to have a real-time "cheat sheet" technology available. Just as business executives learn to rely on their electronic "gizmos" to become more productive, older adults can use MCCDs to leapfrog some of their age-related challenges.

• Facilitate medical caregiving, by remote telemetry of an older adult by a caregiver. MCCDs are among the few electronic devices that are very close to or on a person's body during most of the day. These devices can be used to bridge on-the-body medical sensors with remote monitoring systems to give caregivers (and older adults themselves) peace of mind through active monitoring of the physiological signs of older adults.

Although all of the above-proposed features are technologically feasible, they range in potential availability from the short term to the distant future. This availability is predicated on both MCCDs and wireless communication technologies becoming increasingly ubiquitous. The most important barrier to overcome in the development and deployment of MCCDs for older adults is the business model hurdle. There is a definitive need for clear, concise, and defensible business proposals to secure the necessary funding to cover the development, manufacture, and deployment costs of MCCDs for older adults.

Predicting technological advances a few years out is a very risky proposition. A safer approach is to look at the features currently available in desktop personal computers and then to extrapolate when the hardware and software capabilities of today's MCCDs will be powerful enough to support those features. From this perspective, older adults will be able to acquire, at commodity prices, MCCDs that can

- convert text to speech and speech to text in real time;
- utilize nonvisual interfaces such as touch screens and speech recognition software;
- integrate on-board cameras with easy-to-use software and audiocapture to replace note taking;
- exploit GPS technology not only to inform people where they are but to remind them where they are going; and
- render visual information in increasing detail with built-in "zoom" and navigation capabilities.

One of the most exciting potentials of MCCDs is their ability to utilize alternative user interfaces. Highly complex devices such as cars have a standard basic interface. A person can drive nearly any car in the world with the driving skills he or she already has. That is not the case with most new technologies such as televisions, VCRs, microwave ovens, etc. Each such device places a demand on the user to learn the specific device's user interface features. MCCDs offer a third possibility: MCCDs could be envisioned as "personalized portable user interfaces" where the user controls target devices via the MCCD's interface, customized to fit the user's specific communication needs. Emerging research in nonvisual interfaces points toward a future in which older adults can interact with their MCCDs via different modes, depending on the user's choice: touch, enhanced voice commands (currently available in most new cell phones), and even by reading the lips of an emulated "talking head" on the device's display. (A talking head in this case is a visual caricature of a person that can simulate the facial expressions of a real person while speaking.)

Challenges to Be Overcome by MCCDs

A major technological challenge is that most MCCDs are becoming fashion statements: Users can choose from the titaniumlike PDAs or leather-clad cell phones. This trend poses some challenges for older adults as MCCDs are becoming ever smaller in overall size, with shrinking keypads and even color displays that are difficult to read under direct sunlight. To be useful to elder users, MCCDs must have clearly legible and audible displays and easy-to-use input devices.

A policy-related challenge is to ensure the privacy of older adults who use MCCDs. There are currently no clear regulations as to who owns the data generated by users of CCDs—for example, GPS coordinates obtained from tracking rental cars, data generated by remote monitoring, or digital telephone recordings. Issues of data privacy, levels of access, and data retention policies need to be addressed. The Health Insurance Portability and Accountability Act (HIPAA) of 1996 is a potential model to follow. For example, older adults must be made aware of the inherent risks of always being trackable, e.g., through cell phone use. HIPAA protects a person's right to keep his or her medical information private. Recent changes in banking regulations also force banks to seek their clients' permission before disclosing an individual's financial data to third parties. Unfortunately, in the area of telephone use, people's right to the privacy of their own data is not well established.

There are other specific areas that require further research and pending challenges that need to be addressed. In general, there is a need for more translational research to take the massive amounts of academic research and apply some of that knowledge to develop products and services that are useful to tomorrow's older adults. From a marketplace perspective, it is not clear that the significant social investment in both industrial and academic research and development has delivered a measurable benefit to America's older adults.

From a research perspective, there is a need for integrating life-span research on cognitive abilities and the design of adaptive technology so that the technology fits changing cognitive skills. Academics are advised to engage with electronic device manufacturers to build "cognitive flexibility" to ensure that devices will have several built-in operating modes, each of which places a different cognitive load on the user. That flexibility would be best expressed as a function of the percentage of the device's capabilities that are available to each member of a group of target users with different cognitive capabilities.

From a technological perspective, device manufacturers should pursue a closer alignment with the academic community to design products that address the needs of the growing older population. Such consultation should start at the initial design phase, not just as an add-on or packaging spin. The academic community (under the leadership of an appropriate organization such as NIA) should create a forum for the academic and business communities to come together and collaborate in the development of such user-friendly products and services for older adults. Specifically, the NIA should support the following activities:

• Fund translational research to transfer the most relevant academic research to private firms interested in developing products and services for older adults.
• Create an international clearinghouse for the compilation and dissemination of best practices relating to technological design for older adults.

CONCLUSION

We see a bright future for the use of new technologies to address significant communication barriers for older adults. MCCDs can be developed to address key issues, by moderating some of the deleterious effects of elderspeak, alleviating word retrieval problems, and reducing dual- or multi-task demands. MCCDs may also empower older adults by offsetting age-related sensory, physical, and cognitive limitations. However, we also see that these advances will come at some costs:

• Older adults' increasing use of technology-heavy devices will expose them to the vagaries of technology, such as frequent reboots, "hung" equipment, electronic tracking, "spam" mail, etc., that have plagued others who use similar devices.

• Device manufacturers must accelerate the development and commercialization of MCCDs that have truly usable multimodal interfaces, moving beyond the current trend for small graphic and keypad interfaces of today's devices.

• Older adults must become more vocal about their specific needs and constructively engage MCCD manufacturers to ensure that new generations of MCCD or similar devices truly meet their needs and expectations.

REFERENCES

Baltes, P.B., and Baltes, M.M. (1980). Plasticity and variability in psychological aging: Methodological and theoretical issues. In G. Gurski (Ed.), *Determining the effects of aging on the central nervous system.* Berlin: Schering.

Baltes, P.B., Dittmann, K.F., and Kliegl, R. (1986). Reserve capacity of the elderly in aging-sensitive tests of fluid intelligence: Replication and extension. *Psychology and Aging,* 1(2), 172-177.

Bollinger, R., and Hardiman, C.J. (1989). Dementia: The confused-disordered communicatively disturbed elderly. In R.H. Hull and K.M. Griffin (Eds.), *Communication disorders in adults* (pp. 61-78). Thousand Oaks, CA: Sage.

Burke, D.M., and Laver, G.D. (1990). Aging and word retrieval: Selective age deficits in language. In E.A. Lovelace (Ed.), *Aging and cognition: Mental processes, self-awareness, and interventions* (pp. 281-300). New York: Elsevier Science.

Burke, D.M., MacKay, D.G., Worthley, J.S., and Wade, E. (1991). On the tip of the tongue: What causes word finding failures in young and older adults. *Journal of Memory and Language, 30,* 542-579.

Charness, N. (2001). Aging and communication: Human factors issues. In N. Charness, D. Parks, and B.A. Sabel (Eds.), *Communication, technology, and aging.* New York: Springer-Verlag.

Cohen, G., and Faulkner, D. (1986). Memory for proper names: Age differences in retrieval. *British Journal of Developmental Psychology, 4,* 187-197.

Connelly, S., Hasher, L., and Zacks, R.T. (1991). Age and reading: The impact of distraction. *Psychology and Aging, 6,* 533-541.

Cutler, A., and Butterfield, S. (1991). Word boundary cues in clear speech: A supplementary report. *Speech Communication, 10*(4), 335-353.

Intel. (2002). *What Is Moore's Law?* Available: http://www.intel.com/labs/eml [December 3, 2003].

James, L.E., and Burke, D.M. (2000). Phonological priming effects on word retrieval and tip-of-the-tongue experiences in young and older adults. *Journal of Experimental Psychology: Learning, Memory, and Cognition, 26*(6), 1378-1391.

Kemper, S. (n.d.). Observations on the effects of noise-dampening headphones on mealtime conversations at Greenwood Village, unpublished document. University of Kansas.

Kemper, S., and Harden, T. (1999). Disentangling what is beneficial about elderspeak from what is not. *Psychology and Aging, 14,* 656-670.

Kemper, S., Herman, R.E., and Lian, C.H.T. (in press). The costs of doing two things at once for young and older adults: Talking while walking, finger tapping, and ignoring speech or noise. *Psychology and Aging*.

Kemper, S., Herman, R.E., and Nartowicz, J. (2002). Increasing the costs of doing two things at once. Unpublished manuscript. University of Kansas.

Kemper, S., Jackson, J.D., Cheung, H., and Anagnopoulos, C.A. (1994). Enhancing older adults' reading comprehension. *Discourse Processes, 16*, 405-428.

Levow, G.A. (2002). Adaptations in spoken corrections: Implications for models of conversational speech. *Speech Communication, 36*(1-2), 147-163.

Mann, W., and Helal, S. (2002). *Smart phones for the elders: Boosting the intelligence of smart phones*. (Report No. WS-02-02). Menlo Park, CA: American Association for Artificial Intelligence.

Morrell, R.W., Dailey, S.R., Feldman, C., Mayhorn, C.B., and Echt, K.V. (2002). *Older adults and information technology: A compendium of scientific research and web site accessibility guidelines*. Bethesda, MD: National Institute of Aging.

Oticon. (2003). *Clear speech*. Available: http://otikids.oticon.com/eprise/main/Oticon/com/SEC_AboutHearing/LearnAboutHearing/Products/SEC_OtiKids/Parents/Helping/_Index [December 3, 2003].

Ryan, E.B., Giles, H., Bartolucci, G., and Henwood, K. (1986). Psycholinguistic and social psychological components of communication by and with the elderly. *Language and Communication, 6*(1-2), 1-24.

Satz, P. (1993). Brain reserve capacity on symptom onset after brain injury: A formulation and review of evidence for threshold theory. *Neuropsychology, 7*(3), 273-295.

Schneider, B.A., and Pichora-Fuller, M.K. (2000). Implications of perceptual deterioration for cognitive aging research. In F.I.M. Craik and T.A. Salthouse (Eds.), *The handbook of aging and cognition* (2nd ed., pp. 155-219). Mahwah, NJ: Lawrence Erlbaum.

Seaver, A.M. (1994). My world now: Life in a nursing home, from the inside. *Newsweek, June 27*, 11-12.

Sit, R.A., and Fisk, A.D. (1999). Age-related performance in a multiple-task environment. *Human Factors, 41*(1), 26-34.

Sunderland, A., Watts, K., Baddeley, A.D., and Harris, J.E. (1986). Subjective memory assessment and test performance in elderly adults. *Journal of Gerontology, 41*(3), 376-384.

Tesch-Römer, C. (1997). Psychological effects of hearing aid use in older adults. *Journals of Gerontology Series B: Psychological Sciences and Social Sciences, 52B*, P127-P138.

Tun, P.A. (1998). Fast noisy speech: Age differences in processing rapid speech with background noise. *Psychology and Aging, 13*(3), 424-434.

Tun, P.A., and Wingfield, A. (1995). Does dividing attention become harder with age? Findings from the Divided Attention Questionnaire. *Aging and Cognition, 2*(1), 39-66.

Tun, P.A., and Wingfield, A. (1999). One voice too many: Adult age differences in language processing with different types of distracting sounds. *Journals of Gerontology Series B: Psychological Sciences and Social Sciences, 54b*(5), P317-P327.

Tun, P.A., O'Kane, G., and Wingfield, A. (2002). Distraction by competing speech in young and older adult listeners. *Psychology and Aging, 17*(3), 453-467.

Tun, P.A., Wingfield, A., and Stine, E.A. (1991). Speech-processing capacity in young and older adults: A dual-task study. *Psychology and Aging, 6*(1), 3-9.

Uchanski, R.M., Choi, S.S., Braida, L.D., Reed, C.M., and Durlach, N.I. (1996). Speaking clearly for the hard of hearing IV: Further studies of the role of speaking rate. *Journal of Speech and Hearing Research, 39*(3), 494-509.

Wahl, H.-W., and Tesch-Römer, C. (2001). Aging, sensory loss, and social functioning. In N. Charness, D. Parks, and B.A. Sabel (Eds.), *Communication, technology, and aging*. New York: Springer-Verlag.

White, K.K., and Abrams, L. (2002). Does priming specific syllables during tip-of-the-tongue states facilitate word retrieval in older adults? *Psychology and Aging, 17*(2), 226-235.

World Institute on Disability. (1999). *Telecommunications problems and design strategies for people with cognitive disabilities.* Oakland, CA: World Institute on Disability.

6

Technology and Employment

Sara J. Czaja and *Phyllis Moen*

DEMOGRAPHIC TRENDS RELATED TO AGING, WORK, AND RETIREMENT

How Many Older Adults Are There?

A number of demographic trends—including the aging of the population; changes in the labor-force participation of younger workers; the aging of the baby boom cohort; and changes in retirement policies, programs, and behavior—are fostering new interest in older workers. By 2010 the number of workers age 55+ will be about 26 million, a 46 percent increase since 2000, and by 2025 this number will increase to approximately 33 million. Although labor-force participation rates are projected to be slightly greater for older women than for older men, the labor-force participation rates for older males are also expected to increase. There will also be an increase in the number of workers over the age of 65 (Fullerton and Toossi, 2001; U.S. General Accounting Office, 2001) (see Figure 6-1).

Recently the trend experienced in the 1970s and early 1980s of workers permanently leaving the work force "early" has reversed (Costa, 1998; Purcell, 2002; Quinn, 2002). The traditional assumption that "retirement" from career jobs is isomorphic with workers' final exit from the labor force is increasingly obsolete, as people in their 50s, 60s, and 70s move in and out of paid (and unpaid) work. Retirement from one's full-time, primary career job can no longer be assumed to occur at the time of workers'

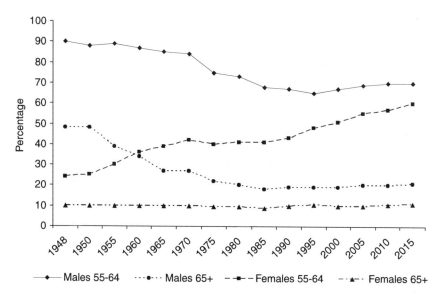

FIGURE 6-1 Labor-force participation rates for older workers, by sex, 1948-2015.
SOURCE: Adapted from U.S. General Accounting Office (2001, p. 9).

eligibility for Social Security benefits or to mean the total cessation of paid employment. Most older workers, according to a variety of studies (e.g., AARP, 2002), say they would prefer to continue to be engaged in some kind of work following their retirement, and a significant number of full-time retirees say they would like to be employed. Many workers view the years approaching retirement as a time for "midcourse corrections" (Moen and Freedman, 2003) rather than a final exit from employment. Instead of full-time leisure, workers and retirees in their 50s, 60s, and 70s (what Moen [2003] calls the "midcourse" years) are increasingly seeking more work options: reduced hours, more time off over the year, special project or contract work, part-time work, and even the opportunity to start second (or third) careers (including unpaid community service). In response, growing numbers of employers are providing a variety of options to bridge the passage from full-time career employment to full-time (complete) retirement (e.g., Watson Wyatt Worldwide, 1999). Programs like these may be especially beneficial for working caregivers who often need to decrease their work hours or have flexible work schedules to meet their caregiving responsibilities. The Cornell Retirement and Well-Being Study (Dentinger and Clarkberg, 2002) found that women caring for their husbands were five times more likely to retire than those without such care responsibilities. Currently, approximately 15 million American workers are involved in some type of caregiving for an older relative such as a parent or spouse (Family Caregiver Alliance, 2002).

Because of the projected increase in the aged dependency ratio (the ratio of the population age 65 and older to the working-age population age 20-64) (see Figure 6-2) and the average length of retirement, there have also been several changes in retirement policies to create incentives to work longer. For example, the Social Security Act was amended in 1983 to gradually increase the minimum age of full benefits for retirement from 65 to 67. The practice of reducing Social Security benefits when a person has earnings and has reached the normal retirement age has been eliminated, and the delayed retirement benefit for those who first claim benefits after normal retirement age is steadily being increased. In addition, the Age Discrimination in Employment Act was amended in 1986 to eliminate a mandatory retirement age for most occupational groups.

The Americans with Disabilities Act (ADA), which became law in 1990, also has important implications for the employability of older people. The passage of the ADA shifted the focus of disability policy in the United States from eligibility for public income transfers to ending discrimination and removing barriers (employers are to make "reasonable accommodations") that prevent people with disabilities from obtaining or remaining in paid work (Burkhauser and Daly, 2002). This oc-

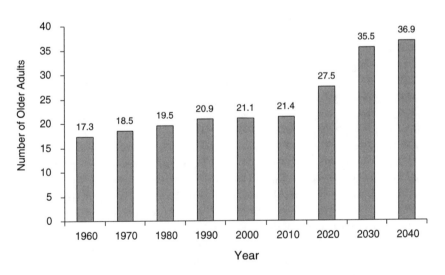

FIGURE 6-2 Past and projected older adults per 100 workers age 20-64.
SOURCE: Board of Trustees, Federal Supplementary Medical Insurance Trust Fund (1997, p. 148).

curred in tandem with technological advances and the growth of jobs in the service sector, both of which widened employment possibilities for those with disabilities.

As the work force ages, the number of people with a disabling health condition will increase. The onset of a disability often triggers an exit from the work force that leads to "total" retirement. Thus, understanding how assistive devices and adaptive technologies can be used to compensate for disabilities is critical to accommodating an aging work force. Disability, according to the ADA definition, includes those with a physical or mental impairment limiting one or more major life activities, with a history of or being seen as having an impairment. As we discuss in this chapter, "accommodations" can encompass a wide variety of changes in work environments.

Employers have also turned their attention toward older workers because of the slowed growth in the number of younger workers. Over the next few years the number of workers age 25-54 years is expected to decrease. This could create labor shortages, especially in skilled and managerial occupations. Some companies are turning to older workers to fill these positions and are providing flexible employment arrangements such as part-time work, telecommuting, and financial benefits to retain or recruit older workers.

Finally, many older people desire or need to continue working for financial or social reasons. In fact, findings from a recent survey (AARP, 2002) indicate that money and healthcare coverage were cited as the major reasons for the desire to continue to work. These findings are consistent with other data that suggest that workers with pension coverage are more likely to retire than workers without pension coverage and that those who would lose health insurance coverage are less likely to retire (Uccello, 1998).

Clearly there is a need to develop strategies to prepare for and accommodate an aging work force. This requires understanding (1) the characteristics of the older workers and the growing population of older adults who do not work; (2) the potential implications of aging for work and work environments; (3) the technological and social characteristics of existing jobs and work environments; and (4) the triggers, dynamics, and processes moving people into and out of employment. When addressing these issues we believe there is considerable value in distinguishing between "older" workers and retirees in their 50s, 60s, and early 70s and those in their late 70s, 80s, and 90s. Unfortunately, most extant studies of abilities and technology use tend to group people as 65+ or 55+. As the baby boomers move into and through their 50s, understanding the differences among the various subgroups within the older adult population will become increasingly important.

Characteristics of the Older Adult Population

In general, older Americans today are healthier, more diverse, and better educated than previous generations (Bass, 1995). Between 1970 and 2000 the percentage of adults aged 65+ who had completed high school increased by about 40 percent, and in 2000 at least 16 percent of people in this age group had at least a bachelor's degree. Increased levels of education should be beneficial for older workers, as higher levels of education are generally linked to higher income and increased employment opportunities. Occupations requiring a bachelor's degree are expected to increase by about 22 percent by 2010, and all but two (air traffic controllers and nuclear power reactor operators) of the 50 highest paying occupations will require a college degree (Bureau of Labor Statistics, 2002).

On some indices, today's older adults are healthier than previous generations. The number of people 65+ reporting very good health and experiencing good physical functioning, such as ability to walk a mile or climb stairs, has increased in recent years. Disability rates among older people are also declining (Federal Interagency Forum on Aging Statistics, 2001). However, the likelihood of developing a disability increases with age, and many older people have at least one chronic condition such as arthritis or hearing and vision impairments (*Clinical Geriatrics*, 1999) (see Figure 6-3). As discussed by Schaie (this volume), cognitive and memory impairments also increase with age.

Disability among older adults has important implications for workplace and job design. Employers may need to adapt workplaces or provide adaptive equipment or technology (such as low-vision aids) to workers who have functional limitations. Generally, labor-force participation rates are lower and retirement rates are higher for people with chronic conditions. People with disabilities, especially disabled elders and minorities with disabilities, are also less likely to use technology such as computers both at home and at work (Kaye, 2000; U.S. Department of Commerce, 2000) (see Figure 6-4).

Consistent with demographic changes in the U.S. population as a whole, the older population is becoming more ethnically diverse. The greatest growth will be seen among Hispanic persons, followed by non-Hispanic blacks. Work policies, programs, and services will require greater flexibility to accommodate this diverse population. For example, currently individuals from ethnic minority groups are less likely to own or use technologies such as computers. This implies that technology access and training programs need to be targeted for older minority populations. Computer and Internet use also tends to be lower in low-income households, although over the past several years both computers and Internet use have increased steadily across all income categories (U.S. Department of Commerce, 2002). This also points to the importance of

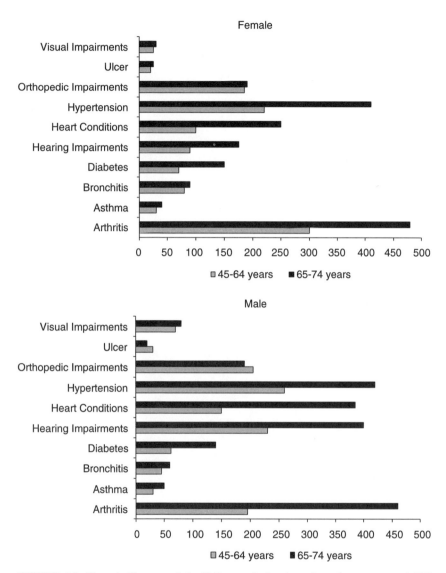

FIGURE 6-3 Chronic illness and the U.S. population (number of persons per 1,000). SOURCE: *Clinical Geriatrics* (1999, 8, p. 77).

ensuring that all people have equal access to technology and technology training.

Finally there are more older women than men, and the proportion of the population that is female increases with age (see Chapter 1 in this volume). The higher percentage of older females may have implications

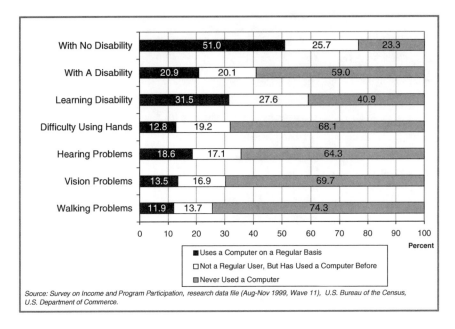

FIGURE 6-4 Personal computer use by disability status, 1999.
SOURCE: U.S. Department of Commerce (2000, p. 66).

for employment, as in recent years older women have been more likely to continue working or return to work than older men. Because of occupational differences, the use of computers at work is greater among females (~63 percent) than males (~51 percent). This difference is consistent across all ages (U.S. Department of Commerce, 2002). As we discuss below there are gender differences, in general, in computer use such that women aged 60+ are less likely than men to use computers (U.S. Department of Commerce, 2002) (see Figure 6-5). Thus, for the current cohort of older women returning to work, the need for computer training may be somewhat greater than for older males. In sum, health status, gender, race, educational background, cultural traditions, and economic circumstances may all influence employability and the adoption of new technologies that might prolong engagement in paid work.

Age-Related Changes in Abilities

Here we provide a brief summary of age-related changes in abilities that have relevance to work performance. A more detailed discussion of

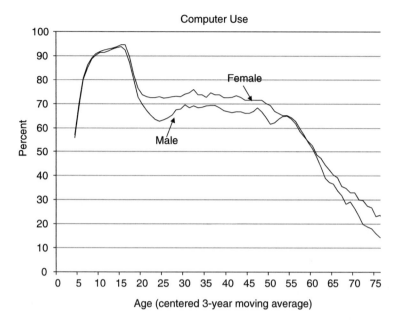

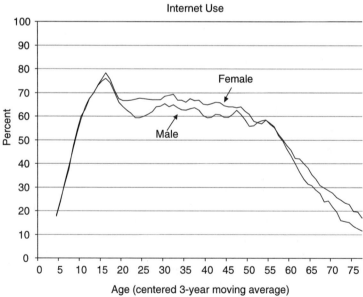

FIGURE 6-5 Computer and Internet use distribution by age and gender.
SOURCE: U.S. Department of Commerce (2002, p. 16).

these topics is provided in Chapters 2 and 3 of this volume. It is important to recognize that aging is associated with substantial variability, and older adults as a group are very heterogeneous. For many indices of performance there are greater differences within the older population than between older and younger age groups. Also, as noted, "older" workers and retirees in their "midcourse" years differ from what we think of as frail elders. Thus, although we can discuss age-related trends in abilities, predictions about an individual's ability to learn a new skill or perform a particular job should be based on that individual's functional capacity relative to the demands of that job or that skill rather than on chronological age.

As shown in Table 6-1, there are a number of changes in abilities associated with "normal" aging that have implications for work. Sensory impairments are common in older people (see Schaie, this volume). For example, currently about 17 million people in the United States over the age of 45 suffer from some type of visual impairment that is not corrected by glasses or contact lenses, and the incidence of visual impairment increases with age (Leonard, 2002). This has vast implications for today's computer-oriented workplace, given that interaction with computer systems is primarily based on visually presented information. Visual decrements may make it more difficult for older people to perceive small icons on toolbars, read e-mail, or locate information on complex screens or web sites. Age-related changes in vision also have implications for the design of written instructions and training manuals and for lighting requirements.

Many older adults also experience some decline in audition that has relevance to work settings. For example, older people may find it difficult to understand synthetic or compressed speech, as this type of speech is typically characterized by some degree of distortion. High-frequency alerting sounds such as beeps or auditory feedback on equipment may also be difficult for older adults to detect. Changes in audition may also make it more difficult for older people to communicate in noisy work environments. As we discuss below, a number of adaptive technologies are available to accommodate sensory impairments.

Aging is also associated with changes in motor skills, including slower response times, declines in ability to maintain continuous movements, disruptions in coordination, loss of flexibility, and greater variability in movement (see Ketcham and Stelmach, in this volume). The incidence of chronic conditions such as arthritis also increases with age (see Figure 6-3). These changes in motor abilities may make it difficult for older people to perform tasks such as assembly work that requires fine manipulation or to use common input devices such as a mouse or keyboard. Alternative input devices such as a light pen or speech recognition may be preferable

TABLE 6-1 Potential Implications of Aging for Work Activities

Impairment	Activity
Visual impairments	Read text, instructional manuals, computer screens
	Locate information on complex displays
	Perform tasks that involve fine visual discriminations (e.g., industrial inspection, microscope work)
	Lighting requirements
Auditory impairments	Comprehension of synthetic speech
	Detection of auditory signals or alerting sounds
	Speech communication (telephone or face to face)
Changes in motor skills	Performance of tasks that require small manipulations (e.g., fine assembly work)
	Use of computer input devices (e.g., mouse, keyboard)
Changes in cognitive abilities	Learning new skills or procedures
	Recall of complex operating procedures or instructions
	Time-sharing; performance of concurrent activities
	Locating information on complex displays
	Performance of paced tasks
Declines in strength and endurance	Reduced ability to perform physically demanding jobs (e.g., manual materials handling, construction)

for older people. Older adults also tend to have reduced strength and endurance and are generally less willing and able to perform physically demanding jobs.

Age-related changes in cognition also have relevance to work activities, especially in tasks that involve the use of technology. Adoption of new technology requires learning new skills and new ways of performing tasks. Declines in working memory may make it difficult for older people to learn new concepts or skills or to recall complex operational procedures. Declines in attentional capacity may make it difficult for older people to perform concurrent activities or to switch their attention between competing displays of information. They may also have problems attending to or selecting task targets on complex displays such as overly crowded web sites. Highly paced work or tasks that emphasize speed of performance, such as data entry tasks, may also be unsuitable for older workers.

Aging and Work Performance

The postulated relationships between age-related changes in sensory, motor, and cognitive abilities and work performance discussed above are primarily speculations. Although there is a great deal of information about aging as a process, there are limited empirical data on the practical implications of aging for work activities. The majority of studies regarding the impact of age-related changes in abilities on performance are based on laboratory tasks (e.g., Diehl, Willis, and Schaie, 1995; Salthouse, Hambrick, Lukas, and Dell, 1996; Czaja and Sharit, 2003). Typically, laboratory tasks fail to capture the contextual elements that are present in work environments and may not allow older people to evoke compensatory strategies that are used in real-world settings.

Common beliefs about older workers include that they are physically unable to do their jobs; have a high rate of absenteeism; have a high rate of accidents; are less productive, less motivated, and less receptive to innovations than younger people; and are unable to learn (Peterson and Coberly, 1988). Although these beliefs persist, data to support them are scarce; in fact, most research studies that are available indicate that these stereotypes are inaccurate.

With respect to age and productivity, the available data are limited, especially for technology-based jobs. Several extensive reviews of the literature on aging and work performance have been conducted (e.g., Rhodes, 1983; Waldman and Avolio, 1986; McEvoy and Cascio, 1989; Avolio, Waldman, and McDaniel, 1990), and the general conclusion of these reviews is that there is little evidence to suggest that work performance declines with age. It appears that the relationship between age and work performance is dependent on the type of performance measure, the nature of the job, and other factors such as experience. For example, studies that rely on supervisory ratings of performance may be biased if the rater has negative attitudes about older workers. In addition, many studies have methodological problems such as small samples or restricted age ranges, or they are cross-sectional—which may confound age effects with factors such as experience, education, or exposure to technology. Finally, the number of studies conducted in actual employment settings has been limited. Also much of the research pertaining to aging and work performance has not included a detailed analysis of contextual factors, such as opportunities for retraining, which have an impact on work ability (Avolio, 1992).

To date, there have only been a handful of studies that have examined the ability of older people to perform computer-based tasks that are common in work settings. Generally, these data suggest that, overall, older adults are willing and able to perform these types of tasks. However, there may be age differences in the performance of some tasks such as data entry where the emphasis is on speed and accuracy of performance (e.g., Czaja and Sharit, 1993, 1998, 1999). Importantly, the data also indicated that, similar to other age groups, there is considerable variability in performance of older people and that, with task experience, performance improves for people of all ages. In addition, the data clearly show that usability issues have an impact on performance and that design interventions such as redesigning the interface, providing on-screen aids, and reconfiguring the timing of the computer mouse can result in performance improvements. Finally, the data indicate that it is important to provide people (especially those with limited technology experience) with training on the use of the technology as well as the task.

With respect to other measures of job behavior, the findings, although limited, are more conclusive. Older workers tend to have lower accident rates than younger workers; however, older workers tend to remain off the job longer if they are injured (Panek, 1997). Absenteeism and turnover rates also appear to be lower for older adults (Martocchio, 1989).

Occupational Trends

Older workers, like younger ones, hold a wide variety of occupations; however, there is some variance according to age. For example, about the same percentage of workers in the age ranges of 40-54, 55-64, and 65+ are employed in white-collar occupations. However, a smaller proportion of workers age 65+ than of younger workers are in physically demanding blue-collar occupations. In the future the percentage of older workers will increase in all occupational categories, with the greatest increase occurring in white-collar occupations such as managers, healthcare professionals, administrative support, and sales (U. S. General Accounting Office, 2001) (see Figure 6-6).

General projections regarding the labor force can also be used to gain some understanding of employment opportunities for older people. In the next few years a gain of about 6.9 million jobs is projected for professional and related occupations such as computer and technical specialists and healthcare practitioners. The second largest growth rate will be seen in the service occupations, such as customer service representatives and healthcare support workers. Other occupations that will experience

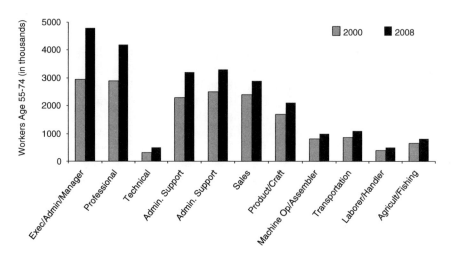

FIGURE 6-6 Projected change in the number of workers age 55+ by occupation, 2000 and 2008.
SOURCE: U.S. General Accounting Office (2001, p. 13).

growth include management and financial occupations, sales, office and administrative support operations, and technology maintenance and repair occupations, especially within the telecommunications industry (Bureau of Labor Statistics, 2002). If the labor-force distribution of older workers remains the same, older people will be in industries that are likely to experience growth. However, this does not necessarily mean that employment opportunities will expand for older workers. A number of factors such as the job and skill requirements of these occupations and receptivity to older workers by employers and organizations influence this equation. Almost two-thirds of the projected job openings in the next 10 years will require on-the-job training (Bureau of Labor Statistics, 2003).

The data also suggest that technology will have a major impact on the future structure of the labor force. Most workers including older workers will need to interact with some type of technology to perform their job. Computer occupations such as computer software engineers, computer support specialists, and network and computer systems administrators will account for 8 out of the 20 fastest growing jobs (Bureau of Labor Statistics, 2003); and the use of computers and other forms of technology is becoming more prevalent in other occupations. In 2001, more than half of the labor force used a computer at work (U.S. Department of Commerce, 2002). This number is expected to increase as developments in technology continue. Furthermore, the number of people who are telecommuting is rapidly increasing. In 1995 at least three million Americans were telecommuting for purposes of work, and this number is expected to increase by 20 percent per year (Nickerson and Landauer, 1997). Telecommuting may be particularly appropriate for older adults, as they are interested in alternative work schedules and are more likely than younger people to be "mobility impaired." Telecommuting allows for more flexible work schedules and more autonomy than the traditional workplace and is more amenable to part-time work. On the negative side, exclusive telecommuting from home may result in professional and social isolation. Employees may miss the opportunities for interacting with friends and colleagues and participating in and receiving the benefits of organizational membership. Managers often fear that it will be difficult to monitor people who work at home. To date, little research has been devoted to examining the social, behavioral, and organizational implications of telecommuting.

TECHNOLOGY AND AN AGING WORK FORCE

The Potential Impact of Workplace Technology on Older Workers

Given the widespread use of technology in most occupations, one important issue concerns how the influx of technology will affect employment opportunities for older workers. As discussed above, technology influences the types of jobs that are available, creating new jobs and opportunities for employment for some and eliminating jobs and creating conditions of unemployment for other workers. Technology also changes the way in which jobs are performed and alters job content and job demands. Often, existing job skills and knowledge become obsolete and new knowledge and skills are required. Workers not only have to learn to use technical systems, but they must also learn new ways of performing jobs. This will hold true for future generations of older adults, as technology by its nature is dynamic. For example, there have been dramatic changes in the design of cell phones, portable computers, input devices, and personal organizers over the past several years.

Issues of skill obsolescence and worker retraining are highly significant for older workers, as they are often bypassed for training or retraining opportunities (Griffiths, 1997). They may also be less willing to invest in retraining, as they may have a decreased expectancy of obtaining valued outcomes (such as promotion), or the value of these outcomes may diminish with age (Fossum, Arvey, Paradise, and Robbins, 1986). Today's older workers are also less likely than younger workers to have had exposure to technology such as computers (e.g., Czaja and Sharit, 1998). Older workers who lack certain skills or training may be seen as redundant and either encouraged or forced to leave the work force. Also, when technological changes in work reduce the number of workers needed, firms often respond by offering early retirement packages to "eligible" workers (those with a certain number of years' tenure or of a certain age) to avoid layoffs. For many older workers, the implicit message is to take the incentive package and retire, or else face layoff in the future. Women are less likely to receive such packages; many have moved in and out of the work force and do not satisfy the tenure requirements for eligibility (Han and Moen, 1999a, 1999b, 2001).

Problems with usability may also make it difficult for older workers to successfully interact with technology. Unfortunately, to date designers of most systems have not considered older adults as active users of technology and thus many interfaces are designed without accommodating the needs of this population (Czaja and Lee, 2002). Usability problems relate to screen design, input device design, complex commands and operating procedures, and inadequate training and instructional support. Although the usability of systems has improved substantially, current interfaces still exclude many people, such as those who are older or people with disabilities, from effective interaction with technology (National Research Council, 1997).

On the positive side, because in many cases technology reduces the physical demands of work, employment opportunities for older people may increase with the influx of workplace technologies. As discussed above, computer technology also makes work at home a more likely option and allows for more flexible work schedules. Finally, as we discuss below, advances in technology may also help older adults with disabilities or impairments

Technology to Support Computer Input

As shown in Table 6-2, there are a number of adaptive technologies that may make continued work more viable for older people, especially those with chronic conditions or disabilities. For example, there are a number of technologies available that can help people with blindness or low-vision problems function in the workplace. These technologies include portable Braille computers, speech synthesizers, optical character recognition systems, screen enlargement software, and video (closed circuit TV) magnifiers. Some computer users can be helped by using a screen with glare protection. Increasing the font size of text may also be necessary. This can be accomplished with font enlargement software or with the accessibility options available in operating systems. Conventional lens magnifiers can be used to help people with low vision access text and paper documents. Braille computers, small portable devices with a Braille keyboard, are also available to enable a person who is blind to

TABLE 6-2 Examples of Adaptive Technologies by Disability Type

Impairment	Adaptive Technologies
Visual	Screen enlargement software
	Braille input and output systems
	Speech synthesis
	Optical character recognition
	Video magnifiers
Hearing	Hearing-aid technologies
	Personal amplification devices
	Amplified telephone receivers
	Text telephones
Hand and mobility	Voice recognition software
	On-screen keyboard programs
	Touch screens
	Eye-gaze programs
Cognitive	On-line reminder systems
	Personal organizers and notebooks

take notes in a meeting. These computers frequently support speech synthesizers or Braille displays for output. Many Braille computers are also equipped with Braille printers or dynamic Braille displays. Braille translation programs are also available. Synthetic speech programs can be installed onto a computer to convert text to speech output, allowing people with visual impairments to review their input as they type. Optical character recognition systems can be directly connected to a computer so that print can be immediately reviewed and edited or converted to speech. Screen-reading software is available that reads aloud information displayed on computer monitors including text, menu selections, and graphical icons (AbilityHub, 2003). Similarly, speech recognition systems allow people to interface with technology such as computers using their voice rather than a mouse or keyboard.

Similar technologies are available for people with other types of impairments. For example, recent advances in hearing-aid technology such as digital hearing aids have improved the effectiveness of hearing aids for persons with sensorineural hearing loss. Personal amplifying devices and amplified telephone receivers can be also used to aid persons with hearing loss. Amplification devices can also be attached to the computer. However, it is important when using any type of amplification device to provide personal headsets to avoid disturbing others in the workplace. Text telephones, such as the telecommunication device for the deaf (TDD), and software that allows a computer with a modem to emulate a TDD are also available that allow persons with hearing impairments to communicate over phone lines. Computers can also be used as educational tools for individuals who are hearing impaired and aid with learning written language (e.g., grammar, proper use of terms). They can also be used in speech therapy and to aid in the translation of sign language to written or spoken English (AbilityHub, 2003).

Technology to Support Computer Output

There are a number of adaptive devices available to aid persons with movement or mobility impairments. Voice recognition software, on-screen keyboard programs, or touch screens may be beneficial for persons who have limited ability to use traditional input devices such as a mouse or keyboard because of hand or finger limitations. "Sticky keys" allow a user to execute commands with one hand that involve simultaneous key pressing. Eye-gaze systems allow people with severe motor impairments, such as those who have suffered a stroke, to use their eyes to operate their computer. There also are personal organizers and reminder systems to aid people with memory impairments. For example, software is available to aid people in the planning and performance of complex activities. The Planning and Execution Assistant and Training System (PEAT) (AbilityHub, 2003) is a program that provides cueing and planning assistance for people with memory problems. PEAT helps users plan daily tasks and maintain a schedule. The software includes graphic and auditory reminders of when to start and stop tasks and "scripts" that describe hierarchical, multistep activities. As discussed in Dishman, Matthews, and Dunbar-Jacob (in this volume), there are new developments in biomedical engineering on the horizon that may also help older people or people with disabilities function independently in the workplace. For example, biosensors that detect and communicate information about irregularities in bodily functions may help someone monitor and control a chronic condition such as diabetes. Gluco Watch, a device similar to a wrist watch that provides general glucose readings and necessary doses of insulin, is an example of the new generation of biosensors (Herrera, 2003). In the near future systems like these will become available for people suffering from other types of diseases that require close monitoring. Other systems that actually deliver the needed medication may also become available.

Clearly there are a number of technologies that can improve the ability of older adults to function in work environments. However, the availability of these technologies does not guarantee their success. The degree to which these technologies improve the work life of older persons depends on the usability of these technologies, the availability of these technologies within organizations, the manner in which these technologies are implemented (e.g., training), and the willingness of older people to use these devices.

Acceptance and Use of Technology by Older Adults

A commonly held belief is that older people are resistant to change and have negative attitudes toward the use of technology. However, the available data dispute this stereotype and indicate that, in general, older people are receptive to using technology if they perceive the technology as useful, if the technology is easy to use, and if they are provided with adequate training and support (Czaja, 1997). Although they may experience more anxiety and less "technology efficacy," older people's attitudes toward technology and comfort using technology are largely influenced by experience and the nature of their interactions with these systems. Experience with computers generally increases user comfort and confidence.

Although there are a number of settings such as the workplace, the home, healthcare, and service settings where older people are likely to encounter technology, such as computers, use of technology among people over the age of 55 is still low compared with other age groups (see Figure 6-5). Generally, the percentage of people who use a computer at work also steadily declines with age. Use of the Internet among older people is also lower than that of younger age groups (see Figure 6-5). Only 30 percent of people age 50+ were Internet users in 2000; and although the number of Internet users in this age group is increasing at the same rate as the overall population, Internet users age 50+ are still less than half of users aged 16-40 (U.S. Department of Commerce, 2002). The picture may be different for future generations of older adults with respect to computers and the Internet, however. It will be interesting to observe if the relationship between age and technology use will be maintained for new and emerging forms of technology.

Factors that limit the use of computers and other forms of technology by older people include lack of access to the technology, lack of knowledge, and cost (Morrell, Mayhorn, and Bennett, 2000). For example, recent data (U.S. Department of Commerce, 2002) indicate that, although the use of computers and the Internet is growing across all segments of the population, use of computers is lower among low-income households, persons with lower educational attainment, persons who are unemployed, and minority populations. Generally, the current cohort of older adults has less income, less education, and higher rates of unemployment than younger people. Also, as noted, older adults are often bypassed for retraining opportunities or are less motivated to invest the time and resources needed to acquire new skills. A challenge for work organizations and policy makers is to develop strategies to ensure that older adults are provided with equal access to technology and to the training needed to acquire the skills to interact with these technologies. In the following subsection we discuss the issue of training older adults to interact with new technologies.

Can Older Adults Learn to Use New Technologies?

Given that the majority of older workers will need to interact with some form of technology such as computers, a critical issue is whether they will be able to acquire the skills necessary to successfully interact with these systems. Generally, the literature on aging and skill acquisition indicates that older people have more difficulty acquiring new skills than younger people and that they often achieve lower levels of performance (Park, 1992). This is especially true for tasks that represent unfamiliar domains.

A number of studies (e.g., Elias, Elias, Robbins, and Gage, 1987; Gist, Rosen, and Schwoerer, 1988; Zandri and Charness, 1989; Czaja, Hammond, Blascovich, and Swede, 1989b; Czaja, Hammond, and Joyce, 1989a; Charness, Schumann, and Boritz, 1992; Morrell, Park, Mayhorn, and Echt, 1995; Mead, Spaulding, Sit, Meyer, and Walker, 1997) have examined the ability of older adults to learn to use technology such as computers. These studies span a variety of computer applications and also vary with respect to training strategies such as conceptual versus procedural training (Morrell et al., 1995). The influence of other variables, such as attitude toward computers and computer anxiety, on learning has also been examined. Overall, the results of these studies indicate that older adults are, in fact, able to use technology such as computers for a variety of tasks. However, they are typically slower to acquire new skills than younger adults and generally require more help and "hands-on" practice. Also, when compared with younger adults on performance measures, older adults often achieve lower levels of performance. However, the literature also indicates that training interventions can be successful in terms of improving performance and it points to the importance of matching training strategies with the characteristics of the learner. Clearly, greater attention needs to be given to the design of training and instructional materials for older learners. The potential use of technology as a training aid also needs to be examined. For example, older people may benefit from multimedia systems or interactive on-line training programs that allow for self-paced learning. However, careful attention needs to be given to the design of such packages. The current cohort of older adults might also need training on basic concepts such as mouse and windows management, in addition to training on the application area of interest. Finally, employers need to ensure that older adults are provided with access to retraining programs and incentives to invest in learning new skills and abilities. Consideration also needs to be given to the scheduling and location of training programs and potential for industry-community partnerships. As noted, issues related to usability and workplace design are also critical to the successful adoption of technology by older people.

The Role of Technology in the Work-Retirement Transition: Rethinking the Role and Contribution of Older Adults

Americans of all ages are coming to realize that they will navigate their way through a series of jobs during their lives. Fewer workers can count on stable, upwardly mobile jobs with a single employer throughout their working life. American men and women at all ages and of all ethnic backgrounds—professionals and managers as well as clerical, service, and production workers—are less likely to hold "secure" jobs, regardless of how many years they have been with their employers. Nevertheless, the lockstep pattern of contemporary life—first education, then paid work, and then retirement—remains the norm throughout Europe and Asia as well as the United States. This is not simply a matter of cultural expectations; the lockstep template both shapes and is shaped by social policies still geared to full-time continuous paid work as the key to economic and occupational success, and is crucial for achieving eligibility for disability benefits, unemployment insurance, and pensions. Age-related role expectations on the part of American employers and workers themselves mean that they are less likely than younger workers to participate in education and training (Hamil-Luker and Uhlenberg, 2002). This vulnerability is not found in some countries. For example, although Canada, Germany, and other countries in the European community have experienced high unemployment rates, they also maintain "safety nets" of unemployment benefits and training options not found in the United States.

Individuals are thus shaping their retirement in unique ways—by changing occupations, starting their own businesses, becoming active as volunteers, going back to school, learning a new craft. All of these strategies can be enhanced by technological applications, such as, for example, distance learning. But most retirement (e.g., the Social Security Act) policies are out of step with the growing heterogeneity of a baby boom workforce population that is moving beyond the conventional career building years, but will not go quietly into old age.

Negotiating the Transition(s) from Work to Retirement: Technology Can Play a Role

Technological advances can have an impact on retirement trends and serve to foster both retention and replacement of older workers. As discussed above, technological applications can also provide accommodations needed to permit older workers or workers with health problems or limitations to continue in their jobs. A key role of information technologies can also be to promote organizational change in the temporal structure of work, making more flexible work schedule options both technically and practically feasible. Thus the new information technologies can play a key role in fostering the view of retirement as not a state but a process, involving a series of work-hour or job changes over a period of years. Technological systems can also be used to provide education and applications related to workers' choice and decision making—from early planning, to midcourse transitions in and out of the work-force (due to health limitations or for other reasons), to second or third careers, to life in (final) retirement. For example, software programs could be developed to facilitate the retirement planning process by making retirement planning information, tools, and models easily available so that workers can make informed choices about issues such as finances, second careers, (re-)employment, (re-)training, or community service. New employment-type agencies or career planners might specialize in the career development of older workers. Technology transfer in the form of research, education, and applications can help these planners open up the possibilities of life "midcourse corrections." Also, a large proportion of the 31 percent of doctoral scientists and engineers in the United States in 1997 who were over 55 were employed (94 percent of those 55-59, 80.3 percent of those 60-64, 53.2 percent of those 65-69, and 28.2 percent of those 70-75). This group of older workers is key to the nation's knowledge development and training; they represent fully one-fourth of the doctoral scientist and engineer work force in the United States. Not only can these workers continue to work productively, but they might also be used to train the upcoming younger workers or become mentors for those who are still in school. These programs can be easily implemented with the technology that is used for video-conferencing or distance learning applications.

The necessary infrastructures that would make these options available have yet to be developed, but it is clear that technological applications—for data acquisition and management as well as for organizational solutions—will be necessary to make these possibilities real in the twenty-first century.

Computer-based tools and programs can also provide workers with privacy and anonymity when they are gathering information and planning for retirement. Workers seldom discuss retirement plans with co-workers. Only about half of prospective retirees in the Cornell Retirement and Well-Being Study (Moen, Erickson, Agarwal, Fields, and Todd, 2000) say they attended employer-sponsored sessions. This might mean that workers are reluctant to discuss retirement out of fear of being "encouraged" to leave their jobs. Software programs can help workers (1) create choices around the work-retirement transition, (2) obtain knowledge of these options, and (3) facilitate their ability to make informed decisions about the choices that are available.

Information technologies also make it feasible for both employers and governments to keep track of the variations in work-hour and career path arrangements as well as the consequences of nontraditional paths for retaining older workers and attracting retirees back into the work force. Tools can be developed to assess the costs and benefits of alternative options for workplace productivity and efficiency and employee equity and life quality. In the Cornell Couples and Careers Study (Moen, 2003) there was limited knowledge among human resource personnel about the number of employees who were working part time or on some form of flextime or about the firm's policies regarding issues such as phased retirement.

What can we conclude about the changing nature of retirement planning and its implications for retirement behavior? The growing heterogeneity of the work force, in terms of age, gender, and ethnic background, along with the changing social contract linking job security with seniority, underscore the fact that the traditional lockstep career-retirement template is increasingly obsolete. It will be interesting to observe the ways in which these forces play out in the actual work-force exits of contemporary workers. Clearly, using technology to increase the availability of information and planning tools can facilitate the retirement process and encourage older workers to consider a range of possibilities, rather than simply trading full-time work for full-time leisure.

Will private-sector employers accommodate the needs and goals of older workers and retirees by using technological advances to create new ways of doing business? They are more likely to do so if, in fact, the projected labor-force shortage occurs and if they are provided with tax incentives. Moreover, the idea of phased exits may seem compelling to policy makers who themselves are in or can anticipate their midcourse years and old age. What is required, we believe, is not simply a "retirement track" of jobs of limited and uncertain duration and narrow skill requirements, but also a way of using information and tracking technologies to (1) redesign existing "full-time" jobs in ways that make them more flexible and attractive with a range of work-hour options and (2) redesign existing career paths to include multiple options for exiting and reentering.

In many ways, the aging work force raises challenges that can be seen as variants on the larger theme of "person-job fit," but at a time when both people and jobs are in transition. Technologies can be used to facilitate the accommodation of the job to the abilities and needs of individuals, to promote older workers' health and safety, to communicate to workers the range of alternative work arrangements available to them, to prepare (screen and train) people who move into or out of various health impairments to adjust their work to these new circumstances, to prevent the onset of impairments in the first place, and to lessen the work load and work hours of those unwilling or unable to put in the time or effort currently expected of "regular" employment. The issue is therefore how to use technological applications both to accommodate the worker to existing job arrangements and to accommodate existing job arrangements to workers' shifting needs and preferences.

AREAS OF NEEDED RESEARCH

The topic of aging and work is increasingly important given current demographic trends, but the empirical data regarding the impact of aging on work performance are limited, especially for present-day jobs and those likely to exist in the public sector in the future. There is a critical need for further research in this area.

Overall, we need more information on the relationship between age-related changes in functioning and job performance. Although there are age-related declines in some functions, the changes are gradual and most jobs do not demand constant performance at the level of maximum capacity. The majority of the population of older adults remains healthy and functionally able until very late in life. One important area of needed research is developing a knowledge base that links age-related changes in skills and abilities to specific skill requirements of jobs. For example, currently the relationships among aging, cognition, and work productivity are unclear. A more complete understanding of these relationships would help direct the development of intervention strategies for older workers. This underscores the need to investigate differences in health, abilities, workplace performance, and technology use by cohort and by finer age categories, as well as to follow particular subgroups over time.

Using a human factors engineering framework, the issue becomes one of determining the degree of fit between job demands and the capabilities of older persons. This type of framework would identify specific components of jobs that are limiting for older adults and target areas where workplace interventions could be used to enhance the ability of older people to meet their job requirements. These interventions might include job redesign, workplace and equipment redesign, or the development of innovative training strategies. Where age-related declines exist, many performance decrements can be reduced by changes in design. Studies are needed to identify the locus of the age differences in work performance and how workplace and job design and training and technological interventions can help mitigate them.

We also need sound research-based information about the impact of technology on an aging work force and how technology might be used to promote employment opportunities for older people. In addition we need knowledge about how technology can be used to facilitate career and employment transitions. It is also important to understand how to design technology so that it is useful and usable for older adult populations, especially those with impairments. All too often designers restrict their "vision" of user groups to young, able-bodied populations. Research also needs to be directed toward examining the cost-effectiveness of technological interventions.

Organizations and policy makers also need to turn their attention to issues related to successful retirement and recruitment of older workers. Issues of worker retraining and skill obsolescence are also critical. The work preferences of older people as well as the benefits of alternative work arrangements and financial incentives need to be understood. In addition, the potential benefits and pitfalls of telecommuting for older workers need to be investigated, and we need information on how other factors such as family caregiving impact on work performance.

In general, research attention directed toward those aspects of work that could become more difficult, less productive, or less satisfying with age could make a worthwhile contribution to improving the work life of older adults. Such research would also help to assure the availability of appropriate employment opportunities for older people and broaden the pool of potential employees for public agencies competing for increasingly scarce labor.

Socioeconomic and organizational trends and existing research evidence point to the importance of documenting the processes and predictors of workers' decision making and planning. The aging of the baby boom generation, along with increases in longevity and ongoing debates over Social Security, savings, and early retirement, make it important to distinguish between retiring from a job and exiting the work force completely. This is a central policy issue. Identifying factors associated with thoughtful planning, including various technology applications, can help identify what facilitates, motivates, or constrains effective retirement exits that are gradual rather than total. A key research agenda is understanding how plans for retirement reflect the intersections of choice processes (agency), opportunity structures (e.g., social and organizational policies and practices), the changing demography of the work force, and local situational conditions (e.g., such as buyout offers and corporate mergers).

We also need information on the role of coworkers and workplace cultures in worker decision making. Clearly, cultures of particular occupations, professional associations, unions, and firms have implicit as well as explicit rules and routines regarding retirement planning and timing. Research is needed to understand the impact of organizational demographics, customs, and norms about retirement timing on the retirement timing expectations and experiences of individual workers. Currently little is known about the personal or organizational impacts of (1) past experiences of downsizing and early retirement incentives, (2) customary or emerging norms within the organization as to retirement planning and timing, (3) workers accepting phased retirement or buyout options, or (4) the role of information dissemination technologies in shaping these impacts.

CONCLUSIONS

Inequality in the distribution of paid work by age is a recent phenomenon. Contemporary social and corporate policy and research on organizations and occupations have not kept pace with the fact that the nation is experiencing a graying of the work force. We believe that a confluence of forces—demographic, technological, medical, cultural—are producing a new life stage in the middle of adulthood between the early years of career building and old age (Moen, 2003). In fact, an unprecedented proportion of the work force is moving to, and through, the *midcourse* years and either contemplating or experiencing retirement. Many workers are also considering ways to scale back their "first" careers or to start second or third careers. Technological change may well make its greatest contribution by aiding and encouraging adjustments in human resource and accounting practices to move work-force policies beyond the narrow choice between long hours of work and total retirement.

What is required is a distinction between first and final retirement and an emphasis on the supports, options, and safety nets that will assist older workers to pursue new and more flexible possibilities for social interactions and to build portfolios for retirement that include paid work. We believe the ways to foster this continued attachment to the work force require new social as well as technical inventions that permit temporal as well as physical accommodations. Such options might move us closer to an age-integrated society (Riley and Riley, 2000), one in which education, employment, and leisure are possibilities throughout the life course.

REFERENCES

AARP. (2002). *Staying ahead of the curve: The AARP work and career study.* Washington, DC: AARP.

AbilityHub. (2003). Assistive technology solutions. Available: http://www.abilityhub.com [December 3, 2003].

Avolio, B.J. (1992). A levels of analysis perspective of aging and work research. In K.W. Schaie and M.P. Lawton (Eds.), *Annual review of gerontology and geriatric* (pp. 239-260). New York: Springer-Verlag.

Avolio, B.J., Waldman, D.A., and McDaniel, M.A. (1990). Age and work performance in nonmanagerial jobs: The effects of experience and occupational type. *Academy of Management Journal, 33,* 407-422.

Bass, S.A. (1995). *Older and active: How Americans over 55 are contributing to society.* New Haven, CT: Yale University Press.

Board of Trustees, Federal Supplementary Medical Insurance Trust Fund. (1997). *The 1997 annual report of the Board of Trustees of the Federal Supplementary Medical Insurance Trust Fund.* Washington, DC: U.S. Government Printing Office.

Bureau of Labor Statistics. (2002). *Occupational outlook handbook, 2002-2003.* (Bulletin #2540). Washington, DC: U.S. Government Printing Office.

Bureau of Labor Statistics. (2003). *Occupational outlook handbook.* Washington, DC: U.S. Department of Labor.

Burkhauser, R.V., and Daly, M.C. (2002). U.S. disability policy in a changing environment. *Journal of Economic Perspectives, 16*(1), 213-224.

Charness, N., Schumann, C., and Boritz, G.M. (1992). Training older adults in word processing: Effects of age, training technique, and computer anxiety. *International Journal of Technology and Aging, 5*(1), 79-106.

Clinical Geriatrics. (1999). Trend Watch: Chronic illness and the aging U. S. population. *Clinical Geriatrics, 7,* 78.

Costa, D.L. (1998). *The evolution of retirement.* Chicago: University of Chicago Press.

Czaja, S.J. (1997). Computer technology and the older adult. In M. Helander, T. Landauer, and P.V. Prabhu (Eds.), *Handbook of human-computer interaction* (pp. 797-812). Mahwah, NJ: Lawrence Erlbaum.

Czaja, S.J., and Lee, C.C. (2002). Designing computer system for older adults. In J. Jacko, and A. Sears (Eds.), *Handbook of human-computer interaction.* Mahwah, NJ: Lawrence Erlbaum.

Czaja, S.J., and Sharit, J. (1993). Age differences in the performance of computer-based work. *Psychology and Aging, 8*(1), 59-67.

Czaja, S.J., and Sharit, J. (1998). Ability-performance relationships as a function of age and task experience for a data entry task. *Journal of Experimental Psychology: Applied, 4*(4), 332-351.

Czaja, S.J., and Sharit, J. (1999). Age differences in a complex information search and retrieval task. Paper presented at the Annual Meeting of American Psychological Association, Boston.

Czaja, S.J., and Sharit, J. (2003). Practically relevant research: Capturing real world tasks, environments, and outcomes. *Gerontologist, 43*(1), 9-18.

Czaja, S.J., Hammond, K., and Joyce, J.B. (1989a). *Word processing training for older adults.* (Report No. Grant 54 AG04647). Bethseda, MD: National Institute on Aging.

Czaja, S.J., Hammond, K., Blascovich, J.J., and Swede, H. (1989b). Age related differences in learning to use a text-editing system. *Behaviour and Information Technology, 8*(4), 309-319.

Dentinger, E., and Clarkberg, M. (2002). Informal caregiving and retirement timing among men and women: Gender and caregiving relationships in late midlife. *Journal of Family Issues, Special Issue: Care and Kinship, 23*(7), 857-879.

Diehl, M., Willis, S.L., and Schaie, K.W. (1995). Everyday problem solving in older adults: Observational assessment and cognitive correlates. *Psychology and Aging, 10*(3), 478-491.

Dishman, E., Matthews, J., and Dunbar Jacob, J. (2004). Everyday health: Technology for adaptive aging. In National Research Council, *Technology for adaptive aging* (pp. 178-206). Steering Committee for the Workshop on Technology for Adaptive Aging. R.W. Pew and S.B. Van Hemel (Eds.). Board on Behavioral, Cognitive, and Sensory Sciences. Division of Behavioral and Social Sciences and Education. Washington, DC: The National Academies Press.

Elias, P.K., Elias, M.G., Robbins, M.A., and Gage, P. (1987). Acquisiton of word-processing skills by younger, middle-aged, and older adults. *Psychology and Aging,* (2), 340-348.

Family Caregiver Alliance. (2002). *Fact sheet: Selected caregiver statistics* Available: http://www.caregiver.org/factsheets/selected_caregiver_statistics.html [June 27, 2003].

Federal Interagency Forum on Aging Statistics. (2001). *Older Americans 2000: Key indicators of well-being.* Bethesda, MD: NIA/NIH.

Fossum, J.A., Arvey, R.D., Paradise, C.A., and Robbins, N.E. (1986). Modeling the skills obsolescence process: A psychological/economic integration. *Academy of Management Review, 11,* 362-374.

Fullerton, H.N., and Toossi, M. (2001). Labor force projections to 2010: Steady growth and changing composition. *Monthly Labor Review,* (November), 21-38.

Gist, M., Rosen, B., and Schwoerer, C. (1988). The influence of training method and trainee age on the acquisition of computer skills. *Personnel Psychology, 41*(2), 255-265.

Griffiths, A. (1997). Aging, health, and productivity: A challenge for the new millennium. *Work and Stress, 11,* 197-214.

Hamil-Luker, J., and Uhlenberg, P. (2002). Later life education in the 1990s: Increasing involvement and continuing disparity. *Journals of Gerontology Series B: Psychological Sciences and Social Sciences, 57B*(6), S324-S331.

Han, S.K., and Moen, P. (1999a). Clocking out: Temporal patterning of retirement. *American Journal of Sociology, 105*(1), 191-236.

Han, S.K., and Moen, P. (1999b). Work and family over time: A life course approach. *Annals of the American Academy of Political and Social Science, 562,* 98-110.

Han, S.K., and Moen, P. (2001). Coupled careers: Pathways through work and marriage in the United States. In H-P Blossfeld and S. Drobnic (Eds.), *Careers of couples in contemporary societies: From male breadwinner to dual earner families* (pp. 201-231). New York: Oxford University Press.

Herrera, S. (2003). *I've got you under my skin.* Available: http://www.redherring.com. [December 3, 2003].

Kaye, H.S. (2000). *Computer and internet use among people with disabilities.* Washington, DC: National Institute on Disability and Rehabilitation Research, U.S. Department of Education.

Ketcham, C.J., and Stelmach, G.E. (2004). Movement control in the older adult. In National Research Council, *Technology for adaptive aging* (pp. 64-92). Steering Committee for the Workshop on Technology for Adaptive Aging. R.W. Pew and S.B. Van Hemel (Eds.). Board on Behavioral, Cognitive, and Sensory Sciences. Division of Behavioral and Social Sciences and Education. Washington, DC: The National Academies Press.

Leonard, R. (2002). *Statistics on vision impairment: A resource manual.* New York: Lighthouse International Foundation.

Martocchio, J.J. (1989). Age-related differences in employee absenteeism: A meta-analysis. *Psychology and Aging,* 4(4), 409-419.

McEvoy, G.M., and Cascio, W.F. (1989). Cumulative evidence of the relationship between employee age and job performance. *Journal of Applied Psychology,* 74(1), 11-17.

Mead, S.E., Spaulding, V.A., Sit, R.A., Meyer, B., and Walker, N. (1997). Effects of age and training on World Wide Web navigation strategies. Paper presented at the Human Factors Society 41st Annual Meeting, September 22-26, Albuquerque, NM.

Moen, P., Erickson, W.A., Agarwal, M., Fields, V., and Todd, L. (2000). *The Cornell Retirement and Well-Being Study: Final Report.* Ithaca, NY: Bronfenbrenner Life Course Center, Cornell University.

Moen, P. (2003). Midcourse: Navigating retirement and a new life stage In J. Mortimer and M.J. Shanahan (Eds.), *Handbook of the life course.* New York: Plenum.

Moen, P., and Freedman, M. (2003). Midcourse corrections. Unpublished document. Cornell University.

Morrell, R., Mayhorn, C.B., and Bennett, J. (2000). A survey of World Wide Web use in middle-aged and older adults. *Human Factors,* 42, 175-182.

Morrell, R.W., Park, D.C., Mayhorn, C.B., and Echt, K.V. (1995). Older adults and electronic communciation networks: Learning to use ELDERCOMM. Paper presented at the 103 Annual Convention of the American Psychological Association, New York.

National Research Council. (1997). *More than screen deep: Toward every-citizen interfaces to the nation's information infrastructure.* Washington, DC: National Academy Press.

Nickerson, R.S., and Landauer, T.K. (1997). Human-computer interaction: Background and issues. In M.G. Helander, T.K. Landauer, and P.V. Prabhu (Eds.), *Handbook of human-computer interaction* (2 ed., pp. 3-32). North Holland, Amsterdam: Elsevier Science.

Panek, P. (1997). The older worker. In A.D. Fisk and W.A. Rogers (Eds.), *Handbook of human factors and the older adult* (pp. 363-394). New York: Academic Press.

Park, D.C. (1992). Applied cognitive aging research. In F.I.M. Craik and T.A. Salthouse (Eds.), *The handbook of aging and cognition* (pp. 449-493). Mahwah, NJ: Lawrence Erlbaum.

Peterson, D.A., and Coberly, S. (1988). The older worker: Myths and realities. In R. Morris, and S. A. Bass (Eds.), *Retirement reconsidered: Economic and social roles for older people* (pp. 116-128). New York: Springer-Verlag.

Purcell, P.J. (2002). *Older workers: Employment and retirement trends.* Washington, DC: Congressional Research Service.

Quinn, J.F. (2002). Retirement trends and patterns among older American workers.. In S.H. Altman and D. Shactman (Eds.), *Policies for an aging society* (pp. 293-315). Baltimore: Johns Hopkins University Press.

Rhodes, S.R. (1983). Age-related differences in work attitudes and behavior: A review and conceptual analysis. *Psychological Bulletin,* 93(2), 328-367.

Riley, M.W., and Riley, J.W. (2000). Age integration: Conceptual and historical background. *Gerontologist,* 40(3), 266-70.

Salthouse, T.A., Hambrick, D.Z., Lukas, K.E., and Dell, T.C. (1996). Determinants of adult age differences on synthetic work performance. *Journal of Experimental Psychology,* 2(4), 305-329.

Schaie, K.W. (2004). Cognitive aging. In National Research Council, *Technology for adaptive aging* (pp. 43-63). Steering Committee for the Workshop on Technology for Adaptive Aging. R.W. Pew and S.B. Van Hemel (Eds.). Board on Behavioral, Cognitive, and Sensory Sciences. Division of Behavioral and Social Sciences and Education. Washington, DC: The National Academies Press.

Uccello, C.E. (1998). *Factors influencing retirement: Their implications for raising retirement age.* Washington, DC: AARP, Washington Public Policy Institute.

U.S. Department of Commerce. (2000). *Falling through the net: Toward digital inclusion.* Washington, DC: Economic and Statistics Administration, National Telecommunications and Information Administration.

U.S. Department of Commerce. (2002). *A nation online: How Americans are expanding their use of the Internet.* Washington, DC: U.S. Government Printing Office.

U.S. General Accounting Office. (2001). *Older workers: Demographic trends pose challenges for employers and workers.* Washington, DC: U.S. General Accounting Office.

Waldman, D.A., and Avolio, B.J. (1986). Meta-analysis of age differences in job performance. *Journal of Applied Psychology, 71,* 33-38.

Watson Wyatt Worldwide. (1999). *Phased retirement: Reshaping the end of work.* Bethesda, MD: Watson Wyatt Worldwide.

Zandri, E., and Charness, N. (1989). Training older and younger adults to use software. *Educational Gerontology,* 15(6), 615-631.

7

Everyday Health:
Technology for Adaptive Aging

Eric Dishman, Judith Matthews, and *Jacqueline Dunbar-Jacob*

This new structure is indicated . . . by the minute but decisive change, whereby the question: "What is the matter with you?" with which the eighteenth-century dialogue between doctor and patient began . . . was replaced by that other question: "Where does it hurt?" in which we recognize the operation of the clinic and the principle of its entire discourse. *Michel Foucault, The Birth of the Clinic*: An archaeology of Medical Perception, 1973, p. xviii.

The archetypical question "Where does it hurt?" still governs most patient-provider encounters today and still serves as the basis for how we conceive of and operationalize healthcare within our society. As we enter the twenty-first century, it is fast becoming clear that we need a new way to think about the body, about healthcare, and especially about aging as we face the challenge of caring for the largest worldwide population of elders in human history. We need, perhaps, to ask a different question, "How can we help you live your life well?"

Strategies for addressing the everyday health concerns of our aging population increasingly rely on advances in technology to prevent, detect, and treat the complex health problems prevalent among older adults living in the community. Novel approaches range from implanted and wearable technology to distributed networks embedded in the living environment to in-home delivery of health services from remote locations. These technologies target several pressing health needs of older adults, including promoting physical function and social interaction, facilitating early diagnosis, enabling self-monitoring of health status, and assuring adequate treatment. At the personal level, they contribute to preserving older adults' health and well-being and support their oft-stated preference for remaining independent as long as possible. At the population level, their value lies in helping to compress morbidity, in keeping with the goal of *Healthy People 2010* (U.S. Department of Health and Human Services, 2000) to increase the quality and years of healthy life.

Just as advances in science and technology converged to spawn invention of the health clinic in the 1700s,[1] contemporary developments in these same arenas may herald the birth of a new era in which healthcare is increasingly based in the home and community, enabled by a range of pervasive, embedded computing and communications technologies. This evolutionary—if not revolutionary—shift from clinic-centric to community-centric healthcare will move us away from infrequent exam room encounters to everyday activities of health and wellness that put the burden of responsibility on an informed, proactive citizenry. This shift will likely coincide with revised notions of healthy aging. Traditionally associated with regular visits to the doctor to keep body parts and functions in working order, healthy aging may evolve into a more holistic process through which optimal function and life quality are achieved using an array of health-related technologies that augment human interaction and support.

But how will we get there? What kinds of problems need to be solved? How should we be conducting research to bring forth a new way of thinking about healthy aging? This chapter is about provoking questions more than providing answers—questions about how next-generation technologies should be designed and developed to support the needs of the next generation of elders. Here we express a perhaps extreme position in arguing for a shift to primary healthcare in the home—for a deep focus on aging-in-place technology research—as an antidote to the historical naturalization that put the clinic and the health professional at the center of our health and wellness universe. We ask, how can we develop evidence-based technologies for the home to enable better prevention, detection, adherence, and caregiving for the "age wave"? How can these tech-

---

[1]According to cultural theorist Michael Foucault (1973), the invention of the clinic in the eighteenth century changed the way we conceived of the body and its care. At that historical moment, biological science, the architecture of the clinic, and the treatment of health problems became mutually reinforcing cultural forces that mapped the human body into a divide-and-conquer grid of classified tissues, organs, and systems. This nosological carving up of the body—this "way of seeing" in John Berger's (1991) terminology—was evident in the division of academic departments (cardiovascular, neurological, etc.), was reified by the architecture of medical clinics (cardiology wing, brain unit, etc.), and became the normal way of doing the business of caring for one's health.

nologies shift the burden of healthcare from tertiary to primary prevention? What kinds of solutions will expand the functional domain from a
main emphasis on health status to more holistic notions of everyday
health? And how do we expand the repertoire of available technologies to
include devices that are more personal and embedded in our home environment as opposed to having to travel elsewhere for care? Informed by
knowledge of normal aging and its attendant health conditions and
guided by a conceptual model of health-related technology, the ensuing
discussion points to some high-level opportunity areas for further thinking and action by a diverse set of researchers with sights set on these
important sociotechnological challenges.

AGING AND ASSOCIATED HEALTH CONDITIONS

Deterioration occurs in almost all physiologic systems as people age,
often accompanied by structural or anatomical changes. Some of these
changes are due to lifestyle over time and some to environmental expo-
sures, whereas others are a function of the aging organism. There is wide
variation in the rate of decline among individuals and across systems.
Changes in cognitive function and mobility are described in detail elsewhere in this volume, yet exhaustive discussion of aging anatomy and
physiology is beyond the scope of this chapter. Nevertheless, several sys-
temic changes that occur gradually over time, and their functional implications, are briefly presented here.[2]

With age, skin becomes thinner, less elastic, and more likely to tear,
thus more prone to infection. Wounds heal more slowly, and the scars
that form are weaker. Epidermal changes increase susceptibility to blis-
tering and abrasion from minor trauma, decrease vitamin D synthesis,
and heighten sensitivity to sun exposure. Cellular and vascular changes
in the dermis reduce the skin's capacity to respond to extremes in tem-
perature and mute its inflammatory response to allergens, ultraviolet ir-
radiation, chemical irritants, and microbial invasion. Loss of subcutane-
ous fat further decreases the skin's capacity to insulate and protect the
body (Gilchrest, 1999).

Blood vessels become thicker and more rigid with age, with blood
pressure fluctuating more widely in response to catecholamines, exercise,
and postural changes. Healthy older adults maintain their cardiac stroke
volume and output while at rest through a cascade of adaptations that

---

[2]See Blass, Ettinger, Halter, and Ouslander (1998) for a comprehensive discussion of aging changes and age-related disorders.

include enlargement of the left ventricle of the heart, augmentation of systolic arterial pressure, and prolonged myocardial contraction. However, aerobic capacity to support increased activity decreases. Similarly, stiffening of the chest wall, loss of lung elastic recoil, and distortion of lung excursion due to vertebral decalcification have little effect on normal breathing in healthy older adults. Yet decreased cardiac and pulmonary *reserve capacity* limits stamina when older adults perform daily activities and lessens their resilience in response to physical demands posed by exercise and stress (Johnson, 2000; Lakatta, 1999).

The ratio of fat-to-lean body mass increases due to loss of muscle, bone, and organ tissue, further compromising reserve capacity, altering metabolism of essential nutrients and medications, and predisposing individuals to pain, deformity, falls, and fractures. This change in body composition also lowers energy requirements and increases the risk of micronutrient deficiency, glucose intolerance, and immune dysfunction. Although increased fat mass may protect older adults from hip fracture and hypothermia, it is an independent risk factor for many chronic disorders (e.g., heart disease, stroke, cancer, diabetes, and osteoarthritis) and functional limitations (e.g., exercise intolerance and functional dependency) prevalent among older adults (Singh and Rosenberg, 1999).

Sensory changes diminish acuity of hearing, vision, taste, and smell. Perception of pressure, vibration, and touch also decreases, raising the pain threshold (see Schaie, this volume, for a full discussion of sensory changes). These changes, along with diminished proprioception, increase the likelihood of injury (Gilchrest, 1999). In addition, joints become destabilized, stiff, and painful due to wear and tear and inflammation of component structures, limiting older adults' mobility and further increasing their risk of falls.

Loss of bone mass beginning around age 40 is associated with impaired osteoblast (bone-forming) activity that continues over the remaining years of life, predisposing older adults—particularly older women—to fractures. Yet fractured bones typically take no longer to heal in older adults than in their younger counterparts (Khosla, Melton, and Riggs, 2000). Slower reflexes and muscular atrophy affect endurance, speed, gait, and balance, in turn affecting safe performance of motor activities such as lifting, walking, and driving (see Ketcham and Stelmach, this volume, for full discussion of changes in motor function.)

Decreased efficiency of the immune system translates to greater susceptibility to communicable diseases, reduced responsiveness to antibiotic treatment and immunizations, and longer recuperation when infections take hold. Most prominent among many factors contributing to age-related immune dysfunction are changes in the T-cell and B-cell populations. These changes include decreases in delayed-type hypersensitivity reactions, impaired proliferation of peripheral blood mononuclear cells in response to T-cell activation, and altered cytokine production. Typically, the immune response to vaccination or infection is less robust, even when antibody production levels rival those observed in younger adults (Murasko and Bernstein, 1999).

Gradual weight gain that peaks in the forties (for men) and fifties (for women) commonly reverts to weight loss after age 70 (Lipschitz, 2000). Inadequate intake, absorption, and metabolism of fluids and nutrients may predispose older adults to constipation, dehydration, electrolyte imbalance, and malnutrition. Thirst drive and appetite may be reduced at a time in life when opportunities to share meals with others become less frequent. Renal function becomes less efficient and may result in slower excretion of unwanted substances (including medications) through the kidneys, poorer urinary concentration, and acidosis (Feest, 2000).

Superimposed on these changes associated with aging are a multitude of chronic disorders that may further threaten function and wellbeing. The most common include arthritis, coronary artery and peripheral vascular diseases, cancer, and diabetes, as well as obstructive and restrictive pulmonary disorders and osteoporosis. The prevalence of neurologic disorders such as stroke, Parkinson's disease, and Alzheimer's disease, which variously cause deterioration in sensorimotor function, communication, emotional stability, and cognition, also increases with age. In addition, several geriatric syndromes, including frailty, falls, infection, incontinence, and depression, result from the complex interplay among physiologic, pharmacologic, and psychosocial factors.

Change is the operative word in geriatric healthcare in that any deviation from an older adult's *usual* cognitive status, behavior, or ability to function is a red flag suggesting the need for prompt investigation and action. Older adults may not exhibit the classic signs and symptoms of a disorder that are the hallmarks of the same condition in younger adults. For example, a young adult with a urinary tract infection would likely spike a fever and experience painful urination, but an older adult might merely present with confusion or lethargy. Such nonspecific symptomatology makes diagnosis of occult conditions more difficult and treatment delays likely.

Compared with younger individuals, older adults are more likely to have multiple comorbid conditions and complicated prevention and treatment regimens. Medications may be prescribed by several different clinicians and contribute to polypharmacy, or consumption of a large number of medicines with possible additive or interactive effects. Older adults use more health resources despite access barriers that include transportation difficulties, lack of proximity to health providers and facilities, and high out-of-pocket costs for uninsured expenses. Social support may be distant and dwindling, as older adults outlive their peers and their widely dispersed families become less available for in-home help and supervision. Due to complexity, cost, isolation, and lack of access or understanding, they may *not* adhere to health practices capable of improving their health and well-being. In the process, they may neglect—even endanger—themselves and, in so doing, increase their need for medical intervention and assistance with self-management.

There is wide variability in health status and function among older adults. Although most exhibit remarkable vitality, when deterioration occurs the consumption of health resources and the need for support increase considerably. Changes in lifestyle may also result, as when fear of falling undermines confidence in walking and leads to deconditioning or when embarrassment about memory loss or urinary incontinence causes withdrawal from social contact.

The debilitating effects of age-related disorders have an impact not only on affected elders, but also on family members who become their informal caregivers. Whether close at hand or far away, family members often provide extraordinary amounts of supervision and assistance to compensate for older adults' diminishing capacities to manage independently. Caring family members may be in the position to provide tangible help with hygiene, household chores, and monitoring of health status, as well as medical appointments and medication management. Or they may be limited by time and distance to infrequent visits home to assess how the older adult is managing, patch together local resources, and then follow up with periodic, if less than ideal, phone contact. In either case, the strain on families can be substantial, with evidence that the most strained caregivers are themselves at risk for premature illness and death (Schulz and Beach, 1999).

MODEL OF HEALTH-RELATED TECHNOLOGY

Health-related technology is moving toward increasingly sophisticated ways of meeting the challenges that aging, disease, and disability pose for community-residing older adults and their families. New applications are being made of old technologies not originally developed for health purposes (e.g., using the telephone for health monitoring, information, and reminders). On the horizon are aging-in-place technologies that involve new interfaces or interaction paradigms (e.g., receiving reminders and information from unconventional—even multiple— sources, such as through the television, computer, and other household appliances). In addition, new core technologies and scientific capabilities are being developed (e.g., domestic robots, "lab on a chip" (LOC) technology, and personal electronic health records).

Technological innovation threatens to evolve inefficiently, even haphazardly, if it is not informed by a guiding framework. Thus, a model is proposed that conceptualizes health-related technology for older adults in three dimensions: level of prevention, adaptation domain, and site of operation (see Figure 7-1). Consistent with the taxonomy developed by Leavell and Clark (1965), some devices may help preserve health (primary prevention), whereas others may reduce disease risk or enable its detection and treatment as early as possible (secondary prevention). Still others may control or slow the advance of a disease (tertiary prevention). At each level of prevention, health-related technologies help older adults adapt to changes in the domains of health status, physical function, cognitive function, and social interaction. In terms of location, devices may be implanted in, worn by, or within reach of an older adult. They may be part of an embedded network of devices within the living environment, or even provide in-home access to resources based some distance from

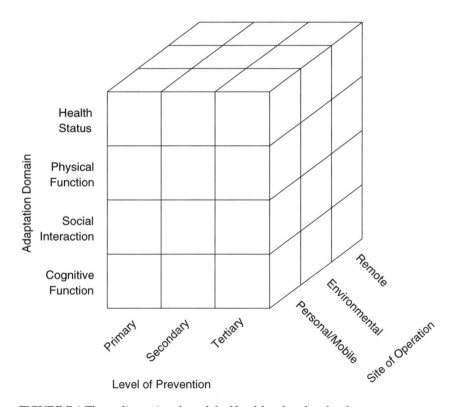

FIGURE 7-1 Three-dimensional model of health-related technology.

the home. In this model, increased emphasis is placed on primary and secondary prevention, multiple functional domains are supported, and technologies are designed more for the home and personal mobile uses.

FROM TELEMEDICINE TO EMBEDDED
HEALTH TECHNOLOGIES

The most developed area of home-oriented technologies is "telemedicine" or "telehealth," where remote connectivity and remote diagnostics have been the two primary foci. Advances in telemedicine are both exciting and promising, especially because the kinds of home portal devices marketed by companies like American TeleCare and Cybercare will begin to build consumer expectation of devices and services that work for them from the comfort of their own homes. But it is important to recognize that the understood paradigm of care here assumes that a medical professional and facility *have* to be in the mix. Certainly many of the potential applications for aging-in-place technologies have a medical component to them, but these technologies have the potential for greater impact when conceived as—and developed for—more broadly supporting daily health and wellness behaviors of elders in their homes. For example, the same infrastructure needed to support videoconferencing between home and clinic—a broadband Internet connection, personal computer, and video camera—can be used to connect elders with each other and their family members in elaborate, informal care networks.

Several technologies are today in their infancy but help to point the way to interesting research areas for successful aging technologies. Even after the demise of many health-related Internet start-ups, we see large informational web sites like WebMD, health-related chat and support groups, the emergence of e-mail and even instant messaging between doctors and patients, and on-line disease management planners. Instead of the push for videoconferencing as the holy grail of connecting with elders in their homes, we need research that examines all of the communication channels afforded by today's technology to see which ones work best to support, motivate, and track healthy behaviors at home. Sometimes a low-bandwidth connection that lets a person know someone on the other end of the line is "there" may be more powerful than an immersive, high-bandwidth video link. Similarly, the adoption of multimedia technologies such as DVD, personal videorecorders, and mobile "entertainment" devices means that elders will increasingly have multiple channels through which health information, coaching, and social support can reach them. How can these devices, ostensibly adopted for entertainment purposes, provide a platform for everyday health and wellness as well?

The explosion of mobile devices today, especially with the expanding and diversifying repertoire of diagnostics that can be plugged into them, is an important trend toward personal, home-based care for older adults. The market for diabetics seems to be the most developed at this point, with a vast number of glucometers and nutrition analysis programs that work in personal digital assistants (PDAs) and personal computers (PCs). Tools like pulse oximeters are moving from large, stand-alone devices in hospitals to PC cards for laptops or even small, compact flash plug-ins for PDAs. Most of these devices are being targeted for use by medical professionals, but as they become cheaper and more available, and as even simple household devices like bathroom scales, thermometers, and blood pressure cuffs are being connected to the Internet, consumers will begin to purchase and use this kind of equipment, whether or not their physicians are prepared to deal with that fact. More and more, devices are becoming embedded into "everyday technologies" like cell phones that can monitor heart rate, PDAs that know how many steps we have taken, or clothing such as the VivoMetrics Lifeshirt™ system that tracks "Every Breath, Every Heartbeat."[3]

As much as we need to move beyond clinic-centric thinking, it is clear from the kinds of technologies mentioned above that we also need to escape our past conceptions of computing and communications technologies. Not that many years ago the prospect of a PC per household was unimaginable, so we have to ask ourselves: Where are computing and communications technologies going? What technology paradigms are just over the horizon of our current imaginations? And what are we shifting *to*?

There are many visions of the future of computing and communications technologies, but the recurring themes include embedded, pervasive technologies that surround us: intelligent, assistive, and even proactive technologies that work on our behalf and personalized, adaptive, customized technologies that fit our individual needs and preferences. Marc Weiser, considered the father of "ubiquitous computing," defined the paradigm this way:

> Ubiquitous computing names the third wave in computing, just now beginning. First there were mainframes, each shared by lots of people. Now we are in the personal computing era, person and machine staring uneasily at each other across the desktop. Next comes ubiquitous computing, or the age of *calm technology*, when technology recedes into the background of our lives.[4]

---

[3]See http://www.vivometrics.com/site/system.html.

[4]This is a widely used quote from Weiser, found in articles and on the Internet, including http://www.ubiq.com/hypertext/weiser/UbiHome.html.

Perhaps the best way to capture this post-PC paradigm shift is in the word "embedded," which carries an important double meaning in this chapter. First, it suggests technologies that are embedded more naturally and easily into our everyday lives and environments. Second, it suggests our movement toward a community-centric agenda of embedding health and wellness activities into everyday routines. The National Research Council (2001, p. 6) describes this new technology paradigm as "embedded networks," or "EmNets" for short, indicating that

> Computing and communications technologies will be embedded into everyday objects of all kinds to allow objects to sense and react to their changing environments. Networks comprising thousands of millions of sensors could monitor the environment, the battlefield, or the factory floor; smart spaces containing hundreds of smart surfaces and intelligent appliances could provide access to computational resources.

Research Topics and Technology Capabilities for Aging in Place

Few of the embedded network technologies needed for the age of aging in place have to be created explicitly for the purposes of everyday health and wellness. It is doubtful that economic or business models would support such a path of innovation anyway. These technologies will already be embedded into people's everyday lives, just as cell phones and Internet access have become reliable "norms" for people of a certain socioeconomic class in many parts of the world. We need research that explores what new capabilities for home health are afforded by these increasingly commonplace technologies. The "connected home"—meaning not just the literal house but also the car, the workplace, and the public places people regularly frequent with their personal mobile technologies—is an infrastructure being built and motivated in most cases by digital entertainment and high-definition TV, by cellular networks for anytime communication with others, and by the need for more robust home security systems.

Given the wide range of tools that will be available to impact health status, physical and cognitive function, and social interaction, what should we be doing with them? What outcomes are really needed to drive independent living and a good quality of life for tomorrow's elders? And given those outcomes, which of these technologies can be brought to bear to achieve these outcomes? A quick review of much of today's health intervention and outcomes research seems to suggest that things are backwards. So many studies begin with a "new" technology like a web site or a PDA and ask, "What is this technology good for? Can it do this, or that, and how well?" But first we need to know the behaviors and activities to

---

BOX 7-1
Sarah: Living Alone with Chronic Heart Disease

It has been more than 10 years since Sarah's husband died of lung cancer. For the first 5 years she stayed in the four-bedroom rural home on the outskirts of St. Louis that they had lived in for almost three decades. But the house became too much to manage as her heart disease progressed, so 5 years ago she moved into the ground-floor apartment of a complex that is closer to town. Except for holidays or the rare event when she pays for a cab to take her to the theatre, Sarah, age 84, lives a rather lonely existence with her two cats. Her daughter Judy lives about 6 hours away, works full time, takes care of two young children, but still tries to check in with Sarah several times a week. Sarah wishes it were several times a day. She is prone to weeks-long bouts of depression, especially in the winter, when she cannot go outside to enjoy her small patio garden. During those down times, she tends to hibernate in bed or at the television, eating very little and getting little more exercise than going to the bathroom or answering the door for her meals-on-wheels delivery.

---

support, and then we can design—or more often repackage—technologies that are most likely to achieve the desired goal.

Perhaps the greatest challenge for aging-in-place research is matching up the diversity of human needs with the palette of technological capabilities that are emerging in our time. Looking through the lens of two case studies (or vignettes) about elder households helps to address both the human and the technological components. One is about 84-year-old "Sarah" who has chronic heart disease and lives alone in an apartment (see Box 7-1). The other is about "Jim" and "Jennie" who still live together in their home in spite of Jim's multiple health problems: high blood pressure, diabetes, and increasing cognitive decline due to Alzheimer's (see Box 7-2).

These examples, based on two households observed by social scientists in Intel's recent "Proactive Health" study,[5] provide the context for describing numerous capabilities—and related research issues—that are ripe for elaboration by real prototype development and outcomes studies. These should not be taken as "prescriptions" for real products in any way, but as foils for discussing key technology research areas that are critical to an aging-in-place agenda.

The Sarah scenario is a sad but too-frequent story of the severe social isolation, depression, and decline in health status that accompanies retirement for many millions of elders, especially once they leave their own

---

[5]See http://www.intel.com/research/prohealth for a general description of the kinds of research Intel is conducting to understand aging-in-place needs and technology opportunities.

BOX 7-2
Jim and Jennie: Aging in Place with Alzheimer's Assistance

Jim, age 78, and Jennie, age 81, live in their suburban home of 50 years in Charlotte, North Carolina. Their one adult child lives in California, so they rarely see him, but he calls every Sunday evening. They have been quite active in their retirement years with travel to the nearby coast and mountains with friends. That is, until Jim began forgetting names and repeating things almost 2 years ago. A few weeks ago, Jennie finally drove him to the doctor—she only drives during daylight hours—only to discover that he has Alzheimer's. It makes sense to her, given how much Jim has declined over the past 2 months—so much so that she has to leave him sticky notes everywhere and to remind him of just about everything, especially to take his medications for high blood pressure and diabetes. The only upside is that he does not seem to get bored with the healthy meals she fixes him because he forgets they had the same thing the day before. Jennie still feels pretty healthy and energetic—she walks daily because it helps with her mild arthritis. But she grows tired more easily, especially having to monitor Jim's every move. Fortunately, Martha, a neighbor, stops to check in on them daily, and Peter, a home health nurse, comes to the house to give Jennie a few hours twice a week to go shopping.

---

homes for an apartment, assisted living facility, or nursing home. It allows us to explore the possibilities of technologies not only to help Sarah manage her heart disease, but also to increase her opportunities for social engagement and intellectual stimulus. The Jim and Jennie scenario, perhaps not as bleak as Sarah's situation, provides fodder for examining the complex changes that take place as couples grow old together, especially when someone like Jim, with multiple ailments, begins to decline much more rapidly than Jennie. In their story, a nearby neighbor and a home-care nurse serve as foils to illustrate the issues of multiple-household connectivity and care. In the discussion that follows, we weave the stories of Sarah and Jim and Jennie into the fabric of a conversation about core technologies and capabilities that are emerging in an embedded networks paradigm. The list of nine research areas below (see Table 7-1) is hardly exhaustive, and many of the categories overlap.

Wireless Broadband

Aside from her two cats, Sarah's biggest companion is the television—it is, in fact, the center of gravity in her small apartment, especially since "downsizing" forced her to give up her computer-craft room from her previous home. What would it mean for Sarah to have computing anywhere in the home? Or for her television, connected to the Internet, to become her resource for learning how to manage her heart disease? How

TABLE 7-1 Selected Core Technologies and Their Capabilities

Technology	Values to Aging in Place
Wireless broadband	Anywhere in the home, any device connectivity Rich and multiple streams of health information delivery
Biosensors and bodily diagnostics	Real-time, routine chemical analysis Targeted drug delivery and effects analysis
Activity sensors and behavioral diagnostics	Location, object, and person tracking around the home Regular activity and activities of daily living measurement and assessment
Information fusion and inference engines	Personal baselines and alerts to meaningful deviations Reliable data even from temperamental technologies
Personal health informatics	Central repository for personal and professional health information Tools for easy visualization of long-term trends
Ambient displays and actuator networks	Lightweight ways to notice "okayness" of loved ones Smart home controls of all devices and appliances
Agents, assistants, coaches, companions	Reminding and coaching of activities of daily living that are declining Companionship for intellectual stimulus and support
Adaptive, distributed interfaces	Any device interactivity—do not have to use a personal computer to compute Interface experience personalized for familiarity and function
Remote community and collaboration	Multiple modes and media for communicating across distance Ways of representing and feeling "presence" at lonely times

might Sarah, like so many elders, better manage her long list of medications if reminders could track her down on whatever device she is closest to and most familiar with? What are the opportunities for her to watch her favorite childhood shows again, perhaps at the same time and with a shared audio connection with a long lost friend who lives two time zones away? How would such a network get installed, who would care for it, and what would happen in the event of its failure if it were to become Sarah's lifeline to the rest of the world?

Wireless broadband for the home is one of the foundational technologies for EmNets, as it provides a building block for many of the capabilities described above. With the emergence of WiFi (wireless fidelity) networks in the United States and the explosion of cell phone technology throughout much of the world, we are moving soon to a technoscape filled with high-speed wireless "anywhere" connectivity that will change the ways health systems can diagnose, track, convince, engage, and assist us. High-speed data transfer will allow for richer content (Sarah's favorite shows from the past "downloaded" to her network) as well as multiple data streams to multiple devices simultaneously (a pill reminder propagating from the alarm clock to the TV to the PDA). The always-on aspect of the network will afford constant real-time monitoring of activities of daily living, and the anywhere-in-the-home connectivity will mean every device and location can become a locus for gathering or delivering health-related information without running wires everywhere.

With the Health Insurance Portability and Accountability Act (HIPAA) and future legislative mandates protecting private data, security technologies must be built into these wireless networks to protect everything from low-bandwidth raw data (a sensor tracking how often someone uses the restroom or how restless he or she is at night) to high-bandwidth information (a multimedia coach providing instruction about physical therapy exercises through a PDA or personal medical record information being delivered on a television). Again, this kind of functionality will not necessarily be installed because of aging care needs. But once installed, what does it have to offer to new ways of caring for ourselves and our loved ones? We need research programs that move beyond testing outcomes of web-site- and CD-ROM-based interventions to ones that prototype and experiment with an entire "connected home" infrastructure.

Biosensors and Bodily Diagnostics

Given her heart problems, would Sarah's eating habits change if she had access to an ongoing analysis of her cholesterol? If there were an easy, noninvasive way for Jim to track hormones and other chemicals in his body, would he allow his wife and doctor to track the progression of his Alzheimer's? What would be the trade-offs to knowing "What's next?" in his likely decline versus just letting things unfold? We already see the advent of new home diagnostic equipment to support telemedical applications. Over the next decade, we will see an explosion of smaller and cheaper biosensor technologies that can detect and track various aspects of bodily function. These will help give older adults, their family caregivers, and health professionals an awareness of health status and disease progression that was never before possible. From "on-the-body" diagnostic equipment—wearables like watches, patches, clothing, and shoes—to "in-the-body" technologies—consumables, injectables, implantables—there will be a wide selection of biosensors available for in-home diagnosis.

Two important areas of research in this domain are in microelectromechanical systems and LOC technologies. Microelectromechanical systems will include microscopic motors that can flow through the bloodstream to a particular location and monitor some key organ or chemical activity. LOC technologies are chips that can externally (through blood, urine, sweat, saliva, and other fluid samples) and internally do chemical analyses to help understand what is going on. Numerous social questions emerge in such a world of biosensors. In what cases will people like Sarah or Jim view the diagnostic data themselves? Under what circumstances should the data be sent out to a family caregiver or health professional, and who decides? What types of people will change their behaviors as a result of having access to such detailed, ongoing biological data? What can researchers learn about the aging process itself by having access to a widespread database of longitudinal biological data?

Activity Sensors and Behavioral Diagnostics

Although biosensors have become a headline- and venture capital-grabbing topic, a smaller but equally important technology research area is *activity* sensors that enable a kind of everyday behavioral diagnostics that may redefine how we engage in prevention and early detection and monitor adherence to treatment. Jennie knows that Jim is becoming more dependent on her as his memory fails, so much so that she finally takes him to the doctor for an official diagnosis of Alzheimer's, but can a system help determine more reliably which functions are failing? Jennie feels she has to be there at every moment to help Jim with even the simplest of activities of daily living—putting on clothes in the morning, helping him microwave soup for lunch, or reminding him to do a few laps around the basement to stay fit, given his diabetes and obesity. What are the possibilities of a system tracking and assisting Jim's activities over a long period of time—perhaps even developing behavioral baselines and "signatures" that reveal potential decline long before Jennie or Jim recognize or admit to it? What would be the value or detriment of such forecasting for Jim, his family, and his physician?

Many homes today already have alarm systems that include simple activity sensor networks. They may consist of equipment as simple as today's motion (light) or badge sensors (usually infrared or radio frequency) that, when networked together and focused more on the internal activities of the household (as opposed to just keeping criminals out), have the potential for us to create monitoring systems that give us a new lens on our own behaviors. Would Judy come by to see her mother more often if a location system alerted her that Sarah has not left the house for days and, in fact, has not even gotten up from the sofa except for occasional bathroom and kitchen trips? More complex sensor systems, such as high-resolution cameras used for three-dimensional tracking, may provide a diagnostic capability that could eventually change how we treat physically disabling diseases in the home. For example, Jennie may well be willing to put up with a system monitoring her gait and movements around the house if it might offer her an early warning that her arthritis has gotten worse or that she needs to see a doctor because her stride length has radically decreased over the past month. Clearly the privacy and control issues of such systems are a key component for researchers to tackle—and we need to realize that different generations, cultures, and individuals may have extraordinarily different reactions to a sensor network that is recording, analyzing, and perhaps even "publishing" their every move.

Information Fusion and Inference Engines

Although Sarah, Jim, and Jennie are unlikely to know or care about the underlying "artificial intelligence" technologies used in their sensor networks, it is important to mention the need for computer science research to transform raw sensor data, both biological and behavioral, into useful, meaningful information. Neither Sarah's daughter nor her primary care physician is likely to want every bit of raw data in the weight and motion sensors that could be placed in her bed to monitor how well she is sleeping. But both of them may well want to know that over the past month Sarah has become more agitated while sleeping (multiple weight sensors in the bed), has tripled the number of times she gets up to go to the bathroom at night (location tracking), has lost about six pounds (weight sensors), and has initiated a lot fewer phone calls or e-mails than normal (everyday device tracking). The important capability here is for systems to establish baselines using multiple data sources and then to alert the appropriate people of deviations from those baselines. And they should do so even in light of the network and sensor failures that are bound to happen in Sarah's home: the infamous ice storms of St. Louis wiping out electricity for a few hours, her cats jostling various sensors and sleeping on her bed at times, or Sarah herself, feeling irritated that "Big Brother" is watching, unplugging the weight sensors from the network.

The computing technologies to create reliable trending, often from unreliable and "noisy" sensor data, will have to be quite advanced to deal with the complex rhythms of home life, which are often much less controlled and routine than in nursing homes or hospitals. Multiple approaches to classic artificial intelligence problems are likely to be needed for different purposes in the system: dynamic Bayesian networks and other statistical approaches, hierarchical approaches, and learning-based systems that may be comparing a current activity or behavior to a decade's worth of prior data. Experts in information fusion and sensor networks will have to work hand in hand with medical experts of all kinds—gerontologists, biochemists, psychologists, etc.—to identify classes of activities that need to be tracked and the sensor approaches that can even begin to provide the raw data to such an inference system.

Personal Health Informatics

In an age when Sarah is still trying to get her complete medical record from her old doctor, now that she has found a new physician closer to her new apartment, and Jennie finds it difficult to know all of the medicines that Jim is supposed to be taking for his diabetes, high blood pressure, and Alzheimer's, it is almost impossible to imagine the kind of lifelong database needed—and created—by embedded networks in the home. Given that most hospitals and clinics have failed to adopt data standards to enable ubiquitous electronic medical records, what are the strategies and issues for doing this for electronic personal medical records that Sarah or Jim might accumulate over a lifetime? How can Jennie keep an accurate record of all of Jim's activities as his doctor has requested, but more importantly, how can she be empowered to decide whether or not she wants to share all of that personal information about her husband with her health plan? As XML and other metadata standards are developed, and as HIPAA-compliant data transfer systems are honed, we are finally likely to see the beginnings of powerful systems to support personal health informatics. This will likely explode as genetic testing and genomics advance and consumers pay much more attention—and want access—to their extended families' medical histories.

Even if we had all of the data in one place today, there are a host of research questions about people's abilities to *use* those data. What are the most effective, useful, understandable, meaningful ways to display personal health and wellness data to different consumers? Certainly the commonplace problem of visual decline suggests the need for larger and higher-contrast screens for many elders, but how might information display be designed with their needs in mind? What are the most appropriate ways to display large data sets—such as activity sensor logs for the entire household, long-term trend analyses of someone's sleep habits, or changes in an individual's exercise regimen over decades—to people who often are not experts at reading traditional charts and graphs? Most people already feel overloaded by information. So research into personal health informatics has many challenges, including simplifying, personalizing, and contextualizing data into information that consumers can themselves act on.

Ambient Displays and Actuator Networks

Much of the above discussion of biobehavioral sensor networks has been about how data are input into the system automatically and routinely, how the data are translated into information and inferences about behavior or health status, and how the data might be stored and used in some sort of personal health informatics database. But what is the *output* of such systems? If a wireless broadband sensor network allows for distributed input, it also affords distributed, highly customizable output. Research is needed to show us the possibilities for "ambient displays"— that is, for more passive displays of information embedded into everyday objects and devices.

Medication reminders on the television or instructions for Jim to dress himself presented through his radio alarm clock are certainly plausible interactions in the near future, but what about more abstract, even sometimes playful, displays? Given Sarah's heart condition and sedentary, solitary lifestyle of late, and as Jim grapples with obesity from his diabetes, both of them may benefit from an at-a-glance means of noticing "how are my eating habits this week?" This nutritional prompting and trend analysis could certainly be displayed directly on a computer monitor or TV, but it is not far-fetched to consider the whimsical, more haptic example of the refrigerator door becoming harder to open to privately signal to Jim or Sarah that they have been there too often lately. Different people are likely to respond to different kinds of prompts or reminders, and many may well prefer something more abstract, private, even playful. The refrigerator is an excellent example of how the home network can not only afford sensor input, but also serve as an actuator network—as a means of controlling and animating the environment far beyond today's home control networks used for lighting, heating, and music.

The research of Mynatt and colleagues (2001) on ambient photograph frames provides a provocative example of using a simple digital photograph frame of a grandparent with iconic butterflies surrounding the image to represent the general well-being of a distant relative.[6] How might a distant caregiver respond to such an abstracted, at-a-glance display? Does it provide enough information and reassurance? Or would more detailed data be needed? We can apply the concept to Sarah and her daughter Judy who lives about 6 hours away. What new social interac-

---

[6]See http://www.cc.gatech.edu/fce/ecl/projects/dfp/index.html.

tions would emerge if Judy had a photograph frame—or equivalent display on one of her television channels for that matter—that displayed Sarah's general "okayness": that she has eaten properly today, taken her meds, gotten a little bit of exercise, but had very little social contact?

Sometimes even simpler displays bring people closer together or allow them to check in on a faraway loved one. For example, Ambient Devices sells Ambient Orb™— a small plastic orb-shaped light that can be made to represent whatever data set the user wants.[7] Increasingly pressed to care for Jim's every need as his Alzheimer's progresses, Jennie may well get a sense of moral support just by having her lamp glow whenever her neighbor Martha is at home. This can be instrumented today with a simple motion sensor in Martha's house to cue the orb in Jennie's living room, or even with regular lamps through smart home networking technologies like X-10 that can be found at almost any Radio Shack.

Agents, Assistants, Coaches, and Companions

Most of today's personal computing experiences might be thought of as reactive or interactive computing in that the user has to go to the computer and enter all of the data to be able to get something useful back from the system. Proactive computing, a term coined by Tennenhouse (2000), calls for a paradigm in which embedded networks of multiple kinds of computing devices allow systems to act more proactively on our behalf when we want them to. This transition is more necessity than nicety because there will be hundreds if not thousands of computing elements in our homes, and no human will be able to pay attention to each and every component.

But how will tomorrow's elders and their caregivers interact with the kind of "intelligence" needed to support proactive systems? A continuum of increasingly intelligent systems will prove crucial to the future of aging-in-place technologies: from existing "agents" or software "bots" that do our bidding on information searches on the web to more capable online "assistants" that we rely on for certain kinds of expertise, to more media-rich and responsive "coaches" that may help watch and guide our actions, to eventual "companions" that may provide meaningful social interaction at times. An extended example using Jennie's predicament as an elder caregiver for her husband with Alzheimer's helps to elucidate this continuum. Her husband Jim has a commonly complex healthcare

---

[7]See http://www.ambientdevices.com.

situation with his high blood pressure, obesity, diabetes, and now Alzheimer's. In supporting his everyday health needs, Jennie may well activate an on-line agent to search for highly customized information that takes into account all of Jim's conditions and potential drug interactions. Eventually, the information may become so difficult for her to track and translate from medical jargon that she may consult a virtual personal medical assistant, much like the one being developed at the University of Rochester Center for Future Health,[8] regarding which medication she should administer to Jim for his headache.

Many Alzheimer's family caregivers experience severe burnout, depression, and exhaustion because of the around-the-clock care demanded by their charges. Jennie has to be concerned about her own increasing arthritis pain, especially now that she has to help Jim get in and out of bed every day, but she hates taking the pain pills prescribed to her because they make her drowsy. An exercise coach on her computer, using a network of cameras and wearable sensors, may guide Jennie in doing proper physical therapy exercises to help her alleviate her pain without drug therapies. Although this sounds like science fiction, researchers at a number of universities are already working on sensor networks and software to allow for this very kind of interaction.[9] Finally, if Jennie's own physical disability increases as she ages, it is conceivable that a robotic companion, equipped with a sophisticated surveillance and reminder system, may be of help by carrying items from one place to another, keeping track of Jim's whereabouts when he is elsewhere in the house, and serving as a walker capable of autonomous navigation if she (or Jim) needs it. The collaborative Nursebot Project[10] at the University of Pittsburgh, Carnegie Mellon University, and the University of Michigan is a perfect example of research going on today to make this kind of robotic companionship a reality.

In addition to the host of technical research needed to build out this agents-to-companions continuum, numerous usability, social, and psychological research topics warrant investigation. We know very little about how people in general will prefer to interact with "intelligent" systems, if at all. How will the baby boomer cohort take to the idea of

---

[8]See http://www.futurehealth.rochester.edu/.

[9]Researchers at the Massachusetts Institute of Technology Media Laboratory and the Center for Future Health have been working on video-monitored systems to help people conduct proper Tai Chi exercises. See press articles at http://www.rochester.edu/pr Review/V62N2/featur2a.html and at http://www.rochester.edu/pr/releases/med/future. htm.

[10]See http://www-2.cs.cmu.edu/~nursebot/ for details about the Nursebot research project.

having more explicitly proactive software tools working on their behalf? What are effective strategies for representing that intelligence in the home? Will some elders prefer a centralized source for intelligence—some sort of computing companion that cuts across all of their applications from entertainment to healthcare? And will others want each device or each application domain to have its own intelligence and representation? How important are anthropomorphism and conversational interaction with these systems? Much of this is uncharted territory because very few research platforms exist to answer these kinds of questions. But even with today's "artificial intelligence" in video game characters and with early consumer robots like the playful AIBO® from Sony or the vacuuming Roomba™ from iRobot,[11] we can begin to craft research programs that will help us understand the potential of agents, assistants, coaches, and companions to the future of health-related technologies for aging in place.

Adaptive, Distributed Interfaces

The issues surrounding how people will interact with robots and online coaches suggest a larger question: What are the trade-offs to having adaptive, distributed interfaces in an embedded, networked world? Embedded networks will afford mass customization so that each device can adjust its interaction paradigm according to the needs and preferences of the user. At the simplest level, Sarah's "connected home" can know which room she is in, which device she is closest to, and which device or interface she prefers based on a trend analysis of her past usages. If her computing time is concentrated all in one place—such as the living room where her television is located—rather than distributed across multiple everyday devices, will she spend even more "screen time" parked on her sofa instead of getting exercise to help with her heart condition? The benefits and detriments of distributed interfaces have yet to be determined to any significant degree, but many of the component technologies are here today and could be integrated into test-bed environments to begin to research these important issues.

Someone like Jim needs more than a distributed system. Adaptability is imperative. As his Alzheimer's progresses, he is likely to first lose his abilities to use newer devices (like a PC or PDA), but is it possible for him to use familiar, overlearned devices like his telephone and TV for new capabilities? For example, if his activities of daily living monitoring system were also to remind him to take his numerous medications on time,

---

[11]See http://www.aibo.com/ for Sony's AIBO® robot and http://www.roombavac.com/ for iRobot's Roomba™.

would he respond to prompts inserted between commercials on his TV or delivered to him as a verbal reminder over the phone? The answer is probably "yes" for some persons with Alzheimer's and "no" for others, with the factors leading to lucidity one day and confusion the next not well understood.

That very variability suggests that a system to help Jim has to adapt not only its locus (the device on which the prompt appears) but also its modality (the type of prompt—text, verbal, video, or all of the above) and its level of support (simple reminding versus step-by-step instructions for locating and taking his pills). Even more important, how can such a system wait to deliver its prompt until the last possible moment in hopes of Jim remembering on his own accord so that he does not become prematurely dependent on his cognitive computing aid? Of course, while Jennie is alive and well, she is likely to be Jim's pill reminding "system," but many people with cognitive decline are not lucky enough to have a full-time caregiver with them at every moment. For those who do not, how might they interact with support systems—through what devices and modalities—and what kinds of interface paradigms will lead to the best possible outcomes? How can those systems adapt and "grow old" with a person to meet increasing needs for medical, physical, cognitive, and social support?

Remote Community and Collaboration

This last but certainly not least important research area for aging in place concerns the social interaction domain. Social support and intellectual engagement, so often overlooked in the clinic-centric view, are two of the most pressing needs for many people in their retirement years. The depression described in the Sarah scenario is all too common. The move to her apartment took her away from longtime neighbors and nearby friends. Her daughter Judy loves her very much, but she lives 6 hours away and is dealing with a full-time job and a family of her own. So as not to be a burden, Sarah often tells Judy, "Everything is fine, dear" on the phone, hiding the sedentary, solitary nature of her existence. How might EmNets and proactive computing technologies give Judy a clearer view of her mother's plight? How might they afford new virtual and co-present social interactions for Sarah so that her sofa is not a cave for hibernation but Grand Central Station for connecting her with people all over the world?

In a world where "connected television" is commonplace, Sarah should be able to find people her own age or with her own interests in theatre and crafts who can "watch" TV together over an open audio link, or just chat while doing a craft or eating a meal. Text-based instant messaging today begins to show us the ways in which these open, always-on channels with other people start to provide new comfort and new ways to "be together." But how will people interact with or through other modalities like audio, video, audio plus occasional stills, even abstracted animations? How can Sarah safely show her availability and interests to a select group of potential companions? Perhaps a "connected telephone" is all that is needed in the short term for Sarah and Judy's situation. If Judy gets an e-mail from the system telling her that her mother has had no phone or e-mail contact with anyone this week, would she be more likely to call or perhaps even ask a friend who lives nearby to visit? There are clearly technological, social, privacy, and interface issues in such scenarios, but tools already exist to begin testing outcomes of such capabilities, which go well beyond the web-site and e-mail studies commonly done today.

For someone like Jennie, these same technologies may simply offer comfort in knowing that someone else is there for her, even if she never actually asks them for assistance. Might she find solace and strength, for example, in seeing her small "social network" ticker tape at the bottom of her TV screen, showing that Peter, the home-care nurse, and her neighbor Martha are available at that exact moment if she should need them? How might Peter be able to optimize his "quality time" during home visits to Jim by looking in advance at the behavioral and medical data accumulated since his last home visit? Is Jennie willing to let Martha have access to some kind of real-time warning system that shows the overall well-being or stress of Jim and Jennie's household so that Martha may stop by when Jennie is having a bad day?

Jim, at least on his most coherent days, may well avail himself of these kinds of communication technologies to help maintain his sense of purpose in life. Even though it is unsafe for him to continue using his basement saws to do woodworking, he can use the same infrastructure installed for today's "telemedicine" to conduct his own "telementoring" sessions with high school students who may be taking shop. Or he can collaboratively browse old photos or genealogy web sites with his son who lives in California. The competing TV commercials in the Internet battle between software titans AOL and MSN show that many of these social networking technologies are already here. The seeds of these more advanced collaborative capabilities are planted in today's data-sharing, peer-to-peer software programs such as Napster, Groove, and the numerous collaboration tools for businesses and professionals. Granted, today's elders may not have access or abilities to use solutions like these, but we need to begin research today to build evidence for or against the utility of embedded network capabilities applied to aging-in-place challenges. These technologies can be reworked to start to test some of these new social support and caregiving paradigms—and to build a body of knowledge around radically new computing experiences that can begin to address the epidemic of social isolation expected to spread widely over the coming decades.

CHALLENGES FOR HEALTH-RELATED
TECHNOLOGIES RESEARCH

Technology development in isolation is unlikely to get us very far in constructing evidence-based systems that can transform the way we care for our aging population. We suggest six strategies, each of which should occur concurrently and collaboratively, for approaching research that involves engineering, computer science, and the health and behavioral sciences.

Imagination: Moving Beyond Today's
Clinical and Computing Models

The largest challenge facing anyone trying to transform the future of everyday health in aging is not technology but *imagination*. Hence, celebrating the "birth of a new era" is meant to challenge us to begin to go beyond our clinic-centric notion of *disease* care to a community-centric notion of healthy aging, in step with the birth of new technological approaches incorporating embedded networks and proactive computing. The three-dimensional model of health-related technology presented in this chapter further suggests that some research resources be taken "out of the box" of tertiary prevention in clinics and hospitals and dedicated to finding creative solutions for promoting health and preventing disease in community-residing older adults.

Identification: Finding and Prioritizing Problems to Pursue

Recognizing that research resources are limited, we must ask: What are the most important, high-impact problems that embedded network technologies and proactive computing should try to address? Within each of the support domains, what kinds of behavioral changes and interventions are most needed to improve health status, physical and cognitive function, and social interaction? How can social engagement, intellectual stimulus, and personal motivation be supported through embedded technologies? How will the needs, daily activities, and everyday technologies for today's elders compare with those of the baby boomers moving into retirement? How will cultural, political, socioeconomic, and gender differences affect development and diffusion of such technologies?

These kinds of questions call for a range of qualitative and quantitative techniques (focus groups, surveys, anthropological fieldwork, demographic analysis, segmentation analysis, cross-cultural comparison) to be used to understand the daily lives and often unarticulated needs of older adults. One of the biggest challenges is to examine the entire household—situated within a particular community—as the unit of analysis.

Iteration: Concept Testing and Refinement

Iterative design is crucial to development of home-based systems that will help with aging in place. Long before major investments are made to develop and deploy embedded health technologies, we need research conducted on conceptual and experiential prototypes[12] that are quicker and cheaper to build. Small-scale outcomes studies of experiential prototypes are needed prior to engaging in larger studies that incorporate more thoroughly developed systems.

These can be done by human factors experts, interaction designers, and social scientists working with engineering teams and health professionals to create an array of artifacts for "testing" with elders, their informal care networks, and their professional caregivers. A rigorous, iterative process from simple sketches or storyboards to "vision videos" to on-screen animations to "informances"[13] to concept prototypes (often called "wizard-of-oz" prototypes) to usable prototypes should yield useful results all along the way and help to ensure that the final products are technological interventions that deliver positive outcomes. Many technology components are available today to begin testing models and interfaces, even if the economies of scale have not made them cheap enough for mass distribution or the applications have not made them compelling enough for mass consumption.

Infrastructure: Deep Dives on Enabling Technologies

Much of the engineering research needed to develop these technologies will—and should—occur independent of aging-in-place applications.

---

[12]Prototypes built from current off-the-shelf technologies to enable consumers to experience enough of some future technology that reliable consumer feedback is attainable.

[13]Informances, or informative performances, involve live actors enacting future technology scenarios to elicit consumer reaction. This innovative research methodology is usually used because the concepts of interest are so futuristic that today's consumers do not have an understanding of—or frame of reference for—the technologies (see Dishman, 2003).

But a portion of this enterprise should examine the unique needs of this domain, such as potential legislative mandates for home-based data security (next-generation HIPAA?) that must be built into the core architecture. What capabilities have we missed or mischaracterized that will likely impact the home health "platform" over the coming decade? Also, what core technologies and capabilities will be developed for other applications like digital entertainment and home security that can be exploited for home health and aging-in-place purposes? Finally, it is crucial to understand how aging-in-place technologies will be developed and diffused differently in different parts of the world, where key underlying technologies (e.g., cable networks versus cellular networks) may differ radically as a result of historical, social, and economic conditions.

Interfaces: Exploration of Human-Machine Interaction

Well before usability research is conducted on a fully implemented application or device, we need *plausibility* and *livability* research that examines the likely uptake of these new technologies by their intended audiences, as well as the "fit" of the technologies into their daily lives. An overarching principle of importance here is "mass customization," not only of the graphical user interface, but of the whole interaction paradigm. The devices or form factors (size and type of display such as on a laptop versus a desktop computer), input and output paradigms, adaptive interfaces, multiple modalities, and interface personalization and dispersion will create a level of interface customization—and potential confusion—that we have never seen before. Interfaces for the aging population will need to move beyond today's limited "access" approach to interface strategies that support people with different and changing cognitive and physical function.

Integration: Testing Whole Systems in Situ

True systems integration research will be essential to the development of successful aging-in-place technologies. Treating the entire home as a "system" means doing technology research into interoperability and adaptive architecture like we have never seen before. Because EmNets involve input (from intentional user input to automatic sensor input) and output throughout and across multiple devices, form factors, and interfaces, testing of single devices in isolation will be insufficient, if not impossible. It will be necessary to test the synergy of many connected, intelligent devices as part of a larger system. This will present enormous installation challenges, both for researchers and for end users, especially in the many years required to retrofit older homes and earlier networks.

Furthermore, outcome studies that require large numbers of households for randomized clinical trials will likely be infeasible. Instead, researchers will need to rely on quantitative strategies, single case studies, and small-sample intervention designs to evaluate consumer satisfaction and utility.

Collaboration in conducting true systems integration research will require teamwork not only across multiple disciplines, including healthcare, gerontology and other social sciences, and technology, but also across multiple organizations—industry, government, and academe. Funding for such ambitious endeavors will require more jointly sponsored initiatives by the National Institutes of Health, the National Science Foundation, and the National Institute of Standards and Technology. Greater utilization of cooperative agreements and contracts will be needed to bring together the various players who can develop and evaluate these complex technologies. Several questions arise: How can "open-source" research platforms for the home be constructed across competing universities and businesses to help accelerate home health research and development efforts? Given the diversity and scale of players who must cooperate to do good, successful aging technology research, it is also clear that we will need to negotiate new models of intellectual property and new incentive structures to help organizations maintain a competitive spirit while also collaborating with their competitors.

Diffusion of these technologies will alter the structure and function of our healthcare system and have implications for educational preparation of older adults, their families, and our work force. The shift toward remote sites handling older adults' primary care needs and simple conditions, with clinics and hospitals focusing almost exclusively on diagnosis and treatment of complex acute and chronic conditions, will necessitate training a new cadre of individuals with expertise in home installation and systems maintenance. Training will also be needed to ensure that healthcare professionals and paraprofessionals know how to employ these tools appropriately in the home and from remote sites, particularly in light of their poor adoption of existing technologies (e.g., Internet and e-mail, CD-ROMs, PDAs) for use with older adults and their families. Although the upcoming baby boomer cohort may be more tech-savvy than their elders, they will not necessarily be more sophisticated in understanding complex technologies. It will be incumbent on technology developers to work toward maximally intuitive interfaces. Likewise, we will need to do a better job educating older adults and their families about the capabilities and limitations of health-related technologies and about how to use them—as utilization is now largely limited to the most aggressive consumers—thus promoting realistic expectations of performance and not *over*selling the prospect of promising results.

Ethical issues related to the use of these technologies will need to be considered, but they should not be any more complex than those encountered in our current system of healthcare. Just as individuals are now responsible for their own lifestyles, treatment regimens, and follow-up at specified intervals, so too will they retain control over whether to heed recommendations for changing their behavior and adhering to prescribed regimens. As is true for health-related technology in the home today, understanding who is capable of using what technology will be important, and ongoing reassessment of its appropriateness and adequacy in relation to a person's functional and motivational status will continue to be imperative.

Ensuring privacy will pose a difficult, although arguably surmountable, challenge. Safeguarding personal data, including designating who can have legitimate access to those data, will likely entail broadening the current HIPAA mandate. Protection will be needed for the raw data gathered from a variety of nontraditional sources (e.g., opening of the refrigerator door, periods of ambulation, pressure applied to a chair or bed) from which inferences are made about an individual's health status, physical function, cognitive function, and social interaction. The economic benefit of these health-related technologies remains an open question. In a best-case scenario, preventing or slowing physical and cognitive decline and reducing complications from chronic disorders could result in significant cost savings. Lower costs would conceivably result from fewer office visits, lower hospitalization rates, and lower rates of institutionalization, more than offsetting the cost of the technologies themselves. Medication noncompliance is now estimated to account for 6 percent of all emergency room visits (Toh, Low, and Goh, 1998) and 11 percent of hospital admissions (Col, Fanale, and Kronholm, 1990). The economic impact of reducing this problem alone could be enormous. Although such improvements would provide welcome budgetary relief, the downside is that healthcare workers may consider their jobs threatened and healthcare organizations may fear for their continued viability. These concerns would likely be resolved through job reorganization and modification of facilities to accommodate the new roles and services necessitated by the shift from clinic-centric to community-centric healthcare.

Although our focus in this chapter has been largely on the United States, it is important to recognize that the challenge of dealing with the "age wave" is not unique to the United States. Given that other countries are already facing—and dealing with—the aging crisis, we need to consider that technologies and expertise may come into our culture from abroad and that cultural differences in the treatment of elders may mean that many technologies and contexts of care do not necessarily translate well across geopolitical boundaries. In the transition from the archetypical medical question "Where does it hurt?" to "How can we help you live your life well?" perhaps we will discover that the promise of everyday health through embedded technologies is not only about improving the health and well-being of our older population, but is about enabling all of us to live the well-lived life.

REFERENCES

Berger, J. (1991). *Ways of seeing* (3rd ed.). New York: Penguin Books.

Col, N., Fanale, J.E., and Kronholm, P. (1990). The role of medication noncompliance and adverse drug reactions in hospitalizations of the elderly. *Archives of Internal Medicine,* *150*(4), 841-845.

Dishman, E. (2003). Designing for the new old: Asking, observing, and performing future elders. In B. Laurel (Ed.), *Design research: Methods and perspectives* (pp. 41-48). Cambridge, MA: MIT Press.

Feest, T. (2000). Renal disease. In J.G. Evans, T.F. Willliams, B.L. Beattie, J.P. Michel, and G.K. Wilcock (Eds.), *Oxford textbook of geriatric medicine* (pp. 654-663). Oxford, England: Oxford University Press.

Foucault, M. (1973). *The birth of the clinic: An archeology of medical perception.* New York: Random House.

Gilchrest, B.A. (1999). Aging of the skin. In W.R. Hazzard, J.P. Blass, W.H. Ettinger, J.B. Halter, and J.G. Ouslander (Eds.), *Principles of geriatric medicine and gerontology* (pp. 573-590). New York: McGraw-Hill.

Hazzard, W.R., Blass, J.P., Ettinger, W.H., Halter, J.B., and Ouslander, J.G. (1998). *Principles of geriatric medicine and gerontology.* New York: McGraw-Hill.

Johnson, B.D. (2000). Age-associated changes in pulmonary reserve. In J.G. Evans, T.F. Williams, B.L. Beattie, J.P. Michel, and G.K. Wilcock (Eds.), *Oxford textbook of geriatric medicine* (pp. 483-497). Oxford, England: Oxford University Press.

Ketcham, C.J., and Stelmach, G.E. (2004). Movement control in the older adult. In National Research Council, *Technology for adaptive aging* (pp. 64-92). Steering Committee for the Workshop on Technology for Adaptive Aging. R.W. Pew and S.B. Van Hemel (Eds.). Board on Behavioral, Cognitive, and Sensory Sciences. Division of Behavioral and Social Sciences and Education. Washington, DC: The National Academies Press.

Khosla, S., Melton, L.J., and Riggs, B.L. (2000). Involutional osteoporosis. In J.G. Evans, T.F. Williams, B.L. Beattie, J.P. Michel, and G.K. Wilcock (Eds.), *Oxford textbook of geriatric medicine* (pp. 617-625). Oxford, England: Oxford University Press.

Lakatta, E.G. (1999). Circulatory function in younger and older humans in health. In W.R. Hazzard, J.P. Blass, W.H. Ettinger, J.B. Halter, and J.G. Ouslander (Eds.), *Principles of geriatric medicine and gerontology* (pp. 645-660). New York: McGraw-Hill.

Leavell, H.R., and Clark, E.G. (1965). *Preventive medicine for the doctor in his community* (3rd ed.). New York: McGraw-Hill.

Lipschitz, D.A. (2000). Nutrition and ageing. In J.G. Evans, T.F. Williams, B.L. Beattie, J.P. Michel, and G.K. Wilcock (Eds.), *Oxford textbook of geriatric medicine* (pp. 139-150). Oxford, England: Oxford University Press.

Murasko, D.M., and Bernstein, E.D. (1999). Immunology of aging. In W.R. Hazzard, J.P. Blass, W.H. Ettinger, J.B. Halter, and J.G. Ouslander (Eds.), *Principles of geriatric medicine and gerontology* (pp. 573-590). New York: McGraw-Hill.

Mynatt, E.D., Rowan, J., Craighill, S., and Jacobs, A. (2001). Digital family portraits: Providing peace of mind for extended family members. In *Proceedings of the 2001 ACM conference on human factors in computing systems* (CHI 2001). Seattle, WA: ACM.

National Research Council. (2001). *Embedded, everywhere: A research agenda for networked systems of embedded computers.* Washington, DC: National Academy Press.

Schaie, K.W. (2004). Cognitive aging. In National Research Council, *Technology for adaptive aging* (pp. 43-63). Steering Committee for the Workshop on Technology for Adaptive Aging. R.W. Pew and S.B. Van Hemel (Eds.). Board on Behavioral, Cognitive, and Sensory Sciences. Division of Behavioral and Social Sciences and Education. Washington, DC: The National Academies Press.

Schulz, R., and Beach, S.R. (1999). Caregiving as a risk factor for mortality: The Caregiver Health Effects Study. *Journal of the American Medical Association, 282*(23), 2215-2219.

Singh, M.A., and Rosenberg, I.H. (1999). Nutrition and aging. In W.R. Hazzard, J.P. Blass, W.H. Ettinger, J.B. Halter, and J.G. Ouslander (Eds.), *Principles of geriatric medicine and gerontology* (pp. 81-96). New York: McGraw-Hill.

Tennenhouse, D. (2000). Proactive computing. *Communications of the ACM, 43*(5), 43-50.

Toh, S.L., Low, C.L., and Goh, S.H. (1998). Drug related visits of geriatrics to the emergency room. Abstract of presentation at American Society of Health-System Pharmacists Annual Meeting 55 INTL-3.

U.S. Department of Health and Human Services. (2000). *Healthy People 2010.* (Conference Edition in Two Volumes). Washington, DC: U.S. Department of Health and Human Services.

8

Technology and Learning in Current and Future Older Cohorts

Sherry L. Willis

SunTrust Equitable Securities recently issued a report evaluating companies involved with technology-enabled learning on the Internet. The report provided some interesting information on the financial world's perspective. It stated "although the Internet's impact on commerce . . . will be notable, ultimately we believe the improvements on how we learn will be the single greatest change that the Internet has on our society" (Close, Humphreys, and Ruttenbur, 2000, p. 5).

In this chapter I consider the current and future role that technology can play in the learning activities undertaken by older people in our society. Learning is typically defined as the acquisition of new information through practice or experience (Howard and Howard, 1997). Of particular interest in this chapter is learning that occurs in everyday life and that often occurs in response to a need or problem. For example, the older adult acquires new information on various treatment options as a first step toward medical decision making. When technology is involved in acquiring this information, the older adult must not only learn the new substantive information, but may also need to acquire knowledge and skills required to use the technology.

In this chapter, two major domains of technology-based learning are considered: the use of technology to acquire knowledge and skills related to substantive topics (e.g., healthcare, leisure activities, job skills) and the knowledge and skills required to use technology (e.g., Internet searches, e-mail). In the commercial and public sectors, technology-based learning is often referred to as "e-learning." E-learning has been defined as learning experiences delivered or enabled by electronic technology (Commission on Technology and Adult Learning, 2001). Because this chapter is concerned with the use of technology to support and enhance the learning activities of older adults, the terms learning or e-learning will refer to learning in a technology-based context.

The potential impact of e-learning is large, given the importance of education and the current resources allocated to education in our society. The United States currently spends more than $700 billion annually in the education and knowledge arena—the education industry is the second largest, behind healthcare (Close et al., 2000). The education market for kindergarten through grade 12 is considered the largest (59.6 percent), followed by the postsecondary sector (36.3 percent). Although the corporate training market (16.1 percent) is currently third in importance, it is projected that technology-based learning will penetrate the business world at a faster rate than any other educational sector. The corporate spending figure does not include the $40 billion plus spent by the government on training. The smallest and newest arrival in the education industry is the lifelong learner. The lifelong learning market (3.9 percent) is projected to develop into a prominent segment within the technology-based learning marketplace as the Internet occupies a larger presence in citizens' daily lives (Close et al., 2000). Of particular concern in this chapter is this lifelong learning segment.

A major purpose of this chapter is to consider current knowledge and research in the area of cognitive aging as it applies to learning in a technology-based context. I begin, therefore, by discussing cognitive processes and skills that have been studied in cognitive aging research. I briefly review traditional views of learning, problem solving, and decision making and distinguish between well-structured versus ill-structured learning tasks. I discuss research on expertise and examine differences between experts and novices in how they learn and solve problems. The similarities between the novice's approach to learning and the approach of many older adult learners and of the typical Internet user searching for information are considered. The various segments of the e-learning industry are briefly described, and their potential role in addressing the learning needs of older adults is discussed. I then consider conceptions of learning evolving within the e-learning context and the potential benefits and challenges of the technology-based environment for the older adult. The role and challenge of the electronic technology context for learning and information seeking are briefly considered.

COGNITIVE PROCESSES INVOLVED IN LEARNING: INFORMATION SEEKING AND PROBLEM SOLVING

At the heart of complex, long-term learning activities is the ability to acquire and retain relevant information and to solve problems. Acquisition of information involves learning, whereas retention and recall of acquired information involve memory. Problem solving involves assessing the present state, defining the desired state, and finding ways to transform the former to the latter. Decision making refers to the evaluation of possible solutions and the selection of one for implementation (Reese and Rodeheaver, 1985; Reitman, 1964).

Problem solving as studied in the laboratory has tended to focus on well-defined problems that are relatively short term and have clear-cut solutions. Examples of well-defined structured problems include older adults' learning of computer-based tasks, such as using an ATM (Rogers, Cabrera, Walker, Gilbert, and Fisk, 1996), an electronic bulletin board (Morrell, Park, Mayhorn, and Echt, 1995), or text editing (Czaja, Hammond, Blascovich, and Swede, 1989). However, the types of problems associated with learning that the older adult often encounters in the real world may vary along a continuum from very well-defined problems with "right answers" to problems that are highly ambiguous, ill-structured, and either have multiple possible solutions or have solutions based on personal choice or consensus among problem solvers (Willis, 1996). Real-world problem solutions often take longer and involve an iterative process (Leventhal and Cameron, 1987; Willis and Schaie, 1993). An example of an ill-defined, poorly structured task is the seeking of health information on the Internet and use of this information in decision making regarding a medical problem. Table 8-1 presents characteristics of well-defined versus ill-defined problems as defined by researchers (Sinnott, 1989; Willis, 1996). Problems vary along this continuum, but the distinction is an important one in discussing the use of technology for learning.

TABLE 8-1 Characteristics of Well-Defined Versus Ill-Defined Problems

Well-Defined Problem	Ill-Defined Problem
Problem is well framed, easily understood	Problem is ambiguous, ill-defined
All or most information needed to solve the problem is available or knowable	Not all information is available, knowable, or agreed upon
Often there is a well-defined procedural knowledge or plan relevant to the problem	No well-defined or agreed procedural knowledge or plan for "solving" theproblem
Often there is one "correct" or agreed-upon solution to the problem	Multiple possible solutions; solutions based on choice or consensus, not on "fact"

SOURCES: Chi (1985); Reitman (1964); Sinnott (1989); Willis (1996).

In this section I describe some of the findings from survey research on the approach of the typical Internet user who is seeking information on line. Because health information is one of the more common topics for an Internet search, I describe survey findings on health information searches, based on the Pew Internet and American Life Project (Fox and Rainie, 2000, 2002). Over 25,000 adults were surveyed including over 4,000 adults over the age of 65; both older Internet users and nonusers were surveyed. The Internet search behaviors described below have been reported for older Internet users, as well as users in general.

I then relate the search behaviors of the typical Internet user to experimental studies on expertise and problem solving (Chi, 1985; Hershey, Walsh, Read, and Chulef, 1990; Meyer, Russo, and Talbot, 1995). Expertise involves not only substantive knowledge of a domain, but also an understanding of how to organize and use the knowledge in solving a problem within the domain. Experts and novices differ in their possession and use of both. Although many people use the Internet quite often, the search behaviors of the typical Internet user are similar to the approach taken by novices, rather than experts. Importantly, the search behaviors of older adults have some resemblance to those of experts, but also some similarities to those of novices.

Searching for Health Information on the Internet

Most health information seekers go on line without a definite search plan (Fox and Rainie, 2000, 2002). They typically start with a global search engine, not a medical site, and visit two to five sites on average, spending 30 minutes on a search. About one-fourth of those who seek health information are vigilant about verifying a site's information; another fourth are concerned about the quality of the information they find but follow a more casual protocol; and half rely on their own common sense and rarely check the source of the information, the date when the information was posted, or a site's privacy policy. The average information seeker reports feeling assured by advice that matches what they already know about a health condition and by statements that are repeated at more than one site. Age is a factor in the perceived success of a health information search. Although 37 percent of young adults report always finding the information they were looking for, only 19 percent of those over 50 years report such a high rate of successful searches (Fox and Rainie, 2000, 2002).

Declarative Knowledge

I now discuss prior experimental research on differences between experts and novices in information seeking and problem solving and relate these research findings to search behaviors of the typical Internet user. A major difference between experts and novices is in their possession and use of two forms of knowledge: declarative and procedural knowledge. Declarative knowledge involves knowing what facts and information are relevant in solving a particular problem (Anderson, 1985; Chi, 1985). It is one's knowledge of the subject matter. Three aspects of declarative knowledge are considered: size of the knowledge base, organization, and relevance and quality of knowledge.

Size of Knowledge Base

Subject-matter experts are believed to have a large body of domain-specific knowledge (Hershey et al., 1990). In contrast, novices have been shown to have a very limited knowledge base. Although it is certainly the case that older adults have large knowledge bases in many domains, sometimes the data do not bear out conventional wisdom on this point. For example, older women who are diagnosed with breast cancer might be expected to have a larger amount of knowledge than younger women because of prior reading or discussions with friends and relatives. In a study of decision making, however, older women with breast cancer had no greater domain-specific knowledge than young or middle-aged women (Meyer et al., 1995). Moreover, they remembered less of the information regarding breast cancer that was presented during the study and so their knowledge base did not grow to the same degree as in younger adults.

Organization of Knowledge

The knowledge domains of experts are organized hierarchically with information indexed via meaningful interrelations, allowing experts to scan their memory of a topic quickly and efficiently (Chi, 1985; Hershey et al., 1990). In contrast, novices in a subject area have only a limited body of relevant declarative knowledge. Because novices are just acquiring the relevant information, they have less understanding of how to efficiently organize information on a topic, and the organization of their knowledge base is therefore less hierarchical and integrated. Older adults with experience in a subject domain would be expected to have declarative knowledge bases that are hierarchically organized and well integrated (Hershey et al., 1990). However, research on learning and memory indicates that older adults often do not organize or chunk information efficiently for recall, even when they are dealing with familiar subject matter (Smith, 1996). They fail to use mnemonics such as superordinate categories spontaneously, suggesting that information is not always organized hierarchically.

Search behaviors of Internet users seeking health information suggest that they do not begin the search with a well-organized body of knowledge, nor do they search in a manner useful to building a systematic hierarchical, integrated knowledge base (Fox and Rainie, 2000, 2002). Most Internet users reported starting with a general search engine. Almost half of information seekers started with the first search results on the retrieved list and worked their way down, reflecting neither hierarchical organization of knowledge nor an understanding of the most relevant information regarding a problem. Many information seekers did not know that search engines may be paid to list sites in a prominent position. Only one-third reported ever book-marking a health-related web site (Fox and Rainie, 2000, 2002).

Quality and Relevance of Information

Experts have the ability to select quickly the most relevant information for a particular problem, obviating the need for a more exhaustive and time-consuming search through their declarative knowledge. In contrast, novices are less adept at differentiating higher-order versus lower-order information, and thus they have difficulty determining the most relevant information for a particular problem (Hershey et al., 1990; Staudinger, Smith, and Baltes, 1992).

Some research suggests that older adults also have difficulty determining what information is particularly relevant to the current problem (Labouvie-Vief and Hakim-Larson, 1989). Older adults often base the decision of whether information is relevant in solving a current problem on whether the information was useful in solving previous problems. They fail to consider similarities between the current problem and prior problem-solving experiences. The expertise literature suggests that the organization of the knowledge base is critical in quickly identifying the most relevant information for a given problem. The inability of older adults to identify the most relevant information may suggest limitations in the organization of their knowledge base or limitations in their ability to reorganize their knowledge base to address a new problem. Investigators have also found that older adults, as compared with young adults, focus more on pragmatic, concrete, subjective information based on or compatible with their own past experiences (Sinnot, 1989). Their approach is characterized as being sensitive to the interpersonal context and focused on inner and personal experience as the way of thinking and knowing.

In a similar vein, Leventhal and Cameron (1987) argue that a distinction should be made between two types of declarative knowledge. They distinguished between semantic memories, which represent the individual's conceptual knowledge about the problem, and episodic memories, or autobiographical information, based on the subject's prior experiences with respect to a particular problem domain. The former (i.e., semantic memories) is similar to the typical use of the term declarative knowledge. However, the more personalized knowledge (i.e., episodic memories) may be particularly relevant for older adults, given that they would be expected to have a more extensive bank of experiences and thus would be more disposed to employ this personalized knowledge in problem-solving situations. Leventhal and Cameron suggest that there may be a conflict between the two types of knowledge in solving a problem. For example, with regard to medical decision making, the more objective, semantic knowledge may inform a person that certain diseases (e.g., heart disease) are asymptomatic and hence one cannot rely on how one feels in making decisions regarding the efficacy of medications or when to see a doctor. In contrast, the personalized knowledge based on episodic memories may argue that, in the past, sickness is related to not feeling well (e.g., symptoms); hence, if there are no symptoms, then one is not sick. Different decisions and problem solutions will be reached depending on which knowledge system is utilized. Leventhal and Cameron (1987) found that personalized knowledge (episodic memories), not the more objective declarative knowledge, is the more critical and predictive of seeking medical attention and complying with prescribed medical treatment. The individual's own personal belief system or representation of the problem appears to become increasingly salient in the solution of problems when the goal of the problem is less clearly defined and there are less well-determined heuristics or algorithms (i.e., procedural knowledge) to employ in solving the problem (Leventhal and Cameron, 1987).

Information seekers using the Internet have been found in survey research to be remarkably confident regarding the validity and quality of information on the web, particularly regarding healthcare (Fox and Rainie, 2000, 2002). Almost three-fourths of those engaging in self-directed searches of health information think that one can believe all or most of the health information that is found on line. What are the major mechanisms information seekers employ to determine the quality of information? First, if the information fits with facts they already know, they are more likely to believe what they read. Thus, Internet information seekers are somewhat like older adults in that they rely inordinately on their own prior knowledge or psychologically meaningful data in determining the validity of information. Whereas the expert quickly identifies the specific unit of prior knowledge that is relevant to a given situation, older adults and the Internet user seeking health information often draw on prior knowledge indiscriminately, whether or not it is relevant to the current problem. Second, if they read the same "facts" on several different sites, their trust in the site information increases. Many information seekers are not aware that information is often syndicated and appears on multiple sites (Fox and Rainie, 2000, 2002).

Procedural Knowledge

Procedural knowledge represents the individual's understanding of how to go about solving a particular problem—how declarative knowledge relevant in a particular situation can be combined to produce a solution (Anderson, 1985; Chi, Feltovich, and Glaser, 1981). Often the procedural knowledge involves performing a set of operations or following an algorithm. Deficits in procedural knowledge are generally seen as more serious than lack of declarative knowledge in problem solving. Two aspects of procedural knowledge are discussed: extensiveness of the search and the plan.

Extensiveness of Search

One of the most interesting distinctions between experts and novices is that experts attend to fewer pieces of information than novices. However, the information attended to by experts is usually higher-order information within the hierarchical knowledge base (Hershey et al., 1990). Because experts have both well-organized knowledge hierarchies and well-honed strategies for solving problems, they are more efficient in selecting only the most relevant information and plugging it into the problem strategy. Experts arrive at problem solutions faster than novices. This finding appears to be due not only to the more extensive declarative and procedural knowledge of experts, but also to greater efficiency in using this knowledge (Hershey et al., 1990; Meyer et al., 1995).

Novices, particularly young adult novices, in contrast to experts, engage in more time-consuming information searches and amass large amounts of data in the early stages of problem solving. Novices' intensive and lengthy searches often are due to their limited understanding of what particular information is most relevant to solving a given problem. Having accumulated a mass of information, novices are more likely to reexamine the same information more than once, because the information is poorly organized and the novice may have insufficient command of the topic to hierarchically organize the information. Moreover, the information sought by novices is often at a lower level in the hierarchical structure of domain-specific knowledge constructed by experts (Chi, 1985).

There is a superficial similarity between experts and older adults in that both groups conduct more limited searches and reach decisions or problem solutions more quickly than younger novices (Leventhal, Leventhal, Schaefer, and Easterling, 1993; Meyer et al., 1995). This finding of a similarity between elders and experts in the brevity of their searches is interesting because often older adults are making decisions relatively quickly even though they have relatively limited information regarding the problem. In contrast, experts are making decisions quickly based on extensive declarative knowledge.

Some researchers have suggested that the similarity between experts and older adults in the speed of making decisions reflects very different processes. Leventhal et al. (1993) found that the speed of seeking medical attention is associated with older adults' increased need to conserve physical and emotional resources. The strategies that adults use in dealing with health threats are believed to change and to become more efficient with age. These strategies include being strongly motivated to detect and avoid threat as soon as possible and to do so with minimal resource expenditure. Thus, the brief searches and quick decisions by experts are a reflection of their knowledge of the domain. In contrast, the decisions of older adults reflect urgency, even in the absence of knowledge.

Plan, Script, or Algorithm

One of the hallmarks of the expert is quick development of an appropriate plan to go about seeking relevant information and solving a particular problem. The expert "plugs in" the relevant information to the plan or script. In contrast, novices spend much time developing or discovering a plan as they go about solving a problem.

The Pew Internet survey findings indicate that Internet users have relatively little in terms of a plan (procedural knowledge) at the beginning of a search. This lack of a plan is reflected in their starting a search with a general search engine and going consecutively down the list of sites rather than scanning for the most relevant or high-quality sites (Fox and Rainie, 2000, 2002). Reports that Internet users do not routinely bookmark sites or return to these sites for further information also reflect lack of a plan. They depend on the algorithms of global search engines rather a preconceived plan of their own. Table 8-2 provides a summary of the similarities and differences between expert, novice, elder, and the typical Internet user with regard to declarative and procedural knowledge.

Declarative and Procedural Knowledge in Training on Computer Skills

The literature on training older adults to use computer technology illustrates the salient features of declarative and procedural knowledge discussed above. Research on the most effective training methods supports the salience of hierarchically organizing the information to be

TABLE 8-2 Similarities and Differences Between Expert, Novice, Elder, and Typical Internet User

Characteristic	Expert	Novice	Older Adult	Typical Internet User
Declarative knowledge				
Size of knowledge base	Large and relevant	Limited	Large?	Limited
Organization of knowledge base	Dense, well-integrated, hierarchical	Bottom up; sparse; not well-integrated	Top down; not always hierarchical; focus on gist, not detail	Bottom up; incremental
Quality and relevance of information	Highly selective of information Larger chunks of information	Cannot differentiate lower- from higher-order information; many small bits of information	Emphasis given to personal experience, meaning; values experience over scientific findings	Limited quality check of information; evaluates quality based on own prior knowledge
Procedural knowledge				
Extensiveness of search	Limited search; attends to selected, highly relevant information	Extensive search; attends to many bits of information; seeks second opinions	Limited search; attends to few bits of information; is information most relevant?	Brief search—30 minutes; searches two to five sites
Plan, script, or algorithm	Well-developed plan; plugs problem information into predetermined plan	Time spent developing plan	Overuse of heuristics and strategies that have worked in past	No apparent plan; begins with general search engine and works down list of sites consecutively

SOURCES: Fox (2001); Fox and Rainie (2000); Hershey, Walsh, Read, and Chulef (1990); Meyer, Russo, and Talbot (1995); Sinnott (1989); and Willis (1996).

learned, proceeding in training from simple to more complex or higher-order concepts and skills, and highlighting for the older learner the most salient information and skills to be acquired. In addition, the particular importance of procedural knowledge is supported in the training studies.

Zandri and Charness (1989) found that use of advanced organizers was particularly effective for older adults learning to use a calendar and notepad system without a training partner. Czaja et al. (1989) reported that older adults learning text editing profited from a goal-oriented approach in which elements of text editing were introduced in an incremental fashion, moving from simple to more complex tasks. Rogers et al. (1996), in teaching older adults to use automatic tellers, found that an on-line tutorial that provided specific practice on task components was superior to written instructions.

The particular importance of procedural knowledge in learning a task was supported in several studies. Morrell et al. (1995) reported a procedural instructional method to be more effective in learning to use an electronic bulletin board system. "Hands-on" training methods, which imply an emphasis on procedural knowledge, have been shown to be more effective than verbal descriptions of navigational tools for older adults who were learning to navigate the web (Mead, Spaulding, Sit, Meyer, and Walker, 1997). Likewise, behavioral modeling of use of a software package followed by actual practice with the package has been employed successfully with older learners (Gist, Rosen, and Schwoerer, 1988).

Rogers (2000) has provided a summary of training recommendations for older adults. Although they were not developed from the same declarative and procedural knowledge framework within which this chapter is organized, it is relatively easy to see that, in following them, both types of knowledge would be gained and applied with greater efficiency. They include the following:

(1) Allow extra time for training; self-paced learning is optimal.
(2) Ensure that help is available and easy to access.
(3) Ensure that the training environment is free from distractions.
(4) Training material should be well organized and important information should be highlighted.
(5) Provide sufficient practice with task components.
(6) Provide an active learning situation.

CHALLENGES IN E-LEARNING AND E-INSTRUCTION

Emphasis on Content by the E-Learning Industry

The e-learning industry considers content to be the most critical component of learning through the Internet, and the greatest financial resources and effort in the e-learning industry are often being targeted at content (Close et al., 2000). High-quality content is seen as the feature that is most likely to attract individuals to learning on the Internet. Why is content viewed as so important by the e-learning industry? It is believed that extensive, in-depth content will (a) encourage customers to spend more time on the Internet, (b) attract more site visitors, (c) increase interaction among learners, and (d) foster customer loyalty to a site. At some sites, users play a role in the development of content via chat rooms and threaded e-mail; the content of a site may increase as a result of user input.

Content as conceived in the e-learning industry appears to place primary emphasis on declarative knowledge. The findings discussed above indicate that a focus solely on the volume and depth of declarative knowledge is insufficient for successful learning. Of critical importance is the industry's ability to organize content in ways that facilitate information searches and to highlight the relevance of particular content for a specific task. Moreover, the average problem solver or information seeker has serious deficits in procedural knowledge, a deficit that is shared by most current e-learning resources.

Synchronous, Asynchronous, and Blended Learning Settings

E-learning content can be delivered by several methods, including synchronous, asynchronous, and blended settings. These settings differ in the amount of interactivity between the learner and instructor and among the learners (Close et al., 2000).

Asynchronous learning, where learners and facilitators are not on line at the same time, can involve self-paced courses or can involve asynchronously scheduled classes with interaction between students and teachers that falls short of the virtual classroom. Interaction between participants includes threaded discussions and e-mails. In contrast, synchronous e-learning enables all users to participate simultaneously. Thus, while one person is presenting material, others can often ask questions of both the presenter and the other participants. Frequently, synchronous e-learning environments allow shared applications and workspaces (e.g., whiteboards) for brainstorming, revision, etc.; full audio and video capabilities; shared web use; and archiving for recordkeeping, quality assurance, and later reference.

What are some of the strengths and limitations of each approach? Asynchronous settings require more up-front preparation and time on the part of the developer or instructor. Synchronous e-learning requires less physical course design for trainers and instructional designers. In asynchronous e-learning, reproducing all of the information that is in the head of the trainer or subject-matter expert in a manner that is engaging for a self-study learner can be hard work. Synchronous e-learning eliminates part of the work by putting the trainer or subject-matter expert back into the picture.

At the same time it should not be assumed that teaching in a synchronous setting is identical to teaching in a traditional classroom (Duckworth, 2001). Both the instructor and the students must learn somewhat different communication skills in a virtual classroom. Learners will need instruction on how to take turns (e.g., when asking for help), the use of features that foster interactivity, and instruction on course content. Thus, learners will be multitasking in ways that are unfamiliar to them. This may be particularly challenging for older learners. At the same time older adults may find having an instructor on line particularly helpful to organize and pace the presentation of material. Unlike the traditional classroom, however, instructors teaching on line may be less able to read participants' confused expressions when a new concept is perplexing. There would appear to be more burden on students to monitor their own learning and to initiate questions for clarification. Although there is always the need for an instructor to continually ask questions to increase interactivity and to monitor students' progress, continually diagnosing each learner's particular strengths and limitations would seem more challenging in a virtual than a traditional classroom (Duckworth, 2001).

The freedom to learn asynchronously may require extra motivation and time management skills on the part of the learner (Tang, 2000). The student must take the initiative to determine the time and place to cover course material. Ironically, asynchronous learning settings may offer greater opportunity for highly individualized instruction. Personal electronic "tutors" can offer different pathways (sound, virtual depictions, alternative explanations) to help learners grasp what was not clear the first time around. Visualization technologies may enable instructors to model and present many different types of material in dynamic ways to help people learn by doing rather than observing. However, this personalized approach to instruction appears to depend on interactive high-speed technology that is often not available in the older learner's home. Without this interactive, personalized technology, asynchronous learning would seem to place a greater burden (than synchronous settings) on students to monitor their progress, to determine how much time and emphasis to give to various course materials, and to determine when errors have been made. These executive planning and monitoring skills that appear to be needed for self-paced instruction have been shown to exhibit some age-related decrements (Czaja, 2001).

The Costs of E-Learning

Although terms such as cost-effectiveness, learner control, interactivity, and accessibility are frequently used to describe the benefits of e-learning, the bottom line is that quality e-learning is labor and time intensive.

E-learning instructor guides recommend that a technical assistant, in addition to the instructor, be available for synchronous learning settings (Duckworth, 2001). Multiple assistants may be required if multiple sites are involved. A live e-learning session can be derailed when one participant calls because he cannot load the plug-in, another sends a message to say she is having trouble with the audio, etc.

More time is needed at the beginning of an e-learning course. Time is needed for students to master interactive technology. Time is needed to establish "netiquette" (Tang, 2000). Time is needed to establish rapport and group identity. Time is needed to solve problems such as incompatibility of student and program technology and interruptions in transmission. Moreover, discussion and teamwork often take more time in e-learning than in the traditional classroom. Work is often asynchronous and it takes extra time for group members to respond to messages and reach agreements.

USING TECHNOLOGY FOR SYNCHRONOUS, DISTRIBUTED LEARNING

In the previous sections I have discussed some of the cognitive processes required for the efficient use of technological innovations such as the Internet that support long-term learning. Throughout this treatment, the importance of declarative and procedural knowledge has been emphasized both as a means of understanding individual differences between expert and nonexpert learners and as a critical framework for training people in the use of technology to foster their own learning. A concrete example is in order. What follows is a brief case study, an illustration of one type of learning affordance available to older people through current technologies. After describing the system, some of its strengths and weaknesses relative to the needs and capacities of the older user are discussed.

Figure 8-1 depicts the CentraOne™ system, a desktop-based environment for allowing multiple users to interact with each other. Although it can be used for purposes other than learning (e.g., social interaction or support groups), it has been developed primarily as a learning environment. It combines recent developments in web-based telecommunications and applications sharing with established forms of content delivery. Course outlines, lecture notes, discussion questions, and the like are often

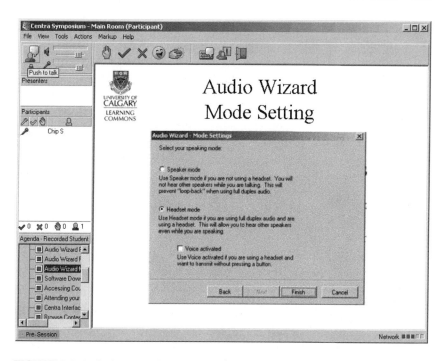

FIGURE 8-1 A desktop, multipoint, synchronous e-learning environment.

presented visually but, in addition, multiway audio and video communication is possible. A shared virtual whiteboard is available for brainstorming and team work, and other applications resident on participants' workstations or the web can be shared among users. There are mechanisms for the control of communications, provision of synchronous feedback to the coordinators, entry of new participants, etc. All of these resources are also available in breakout groups. Archiving of "meetings" allows recordkeeping, and archives can be accessed by those unable to attend. This system and other similar products available today get high marks on several grounds. They can provide the vocational, avocational, social, and affective benefits of group learning for all older adults, even those who are homebound, mobility impaired, or simply not attracted to the traditional classroom. They rely on many familiar conventions in the use of icons and allow integration with very common applications for word processing, presentations, and web browsing. They are not overly technical, and many of the tools are labeled well or have easily recognized meanings. Still, as can be seen from Figure 8-1, there is a good deal of learning that must go on before one can even begin to use the environment, and this learning will be more of a challenge for the older user.

First, there is the matter of learning what operations and interactions are allowed by the system. A user cannot be expected to engage in text chat, propose an ad campaign in a shared whiteboard, or signal that they are temporarily leaving the group if they do not know that this functionality is available. Some tools are not visible in the default configuration, and confusion results when facilitators assume users can make use of these tools when, in fact, the users do not know they exist or where to find them. Even if they know that the system is capable of these functions, accessing them is not always intuitive or transparent. For example, many people might assume that the upraised hand icon is intended to signal a desire to stop some action. In fact, it signals the facilitator that there is someone who wishes to speak and puts that person in a queue to be given speaking privileges. And what the heck is that person with the exclamation mark on his or her shoulder intended to convey? It should come as no surprise that a 2-hour tutorial is needed to bring relatively technology-savvy people to a reasonable comfort level in using the system at an introductory level. Learning to deliver content and dynamically control delivery and user interactions takes considerably longer.

Returning to the declarative versus procedural knowledge framework that has guided much of this chapter, there are myriad facts that must be learned to use this system well. These include "what" and "where" information about logging in, participation in conversations, feedback, and developing content. Whereas some of this information may have been learned previously and so falls under the heading of semantic declarative knowledge (Leventhal and Cameron, 1987), other facts are linked uniquely to this particular product and so, at least during the acquisition phase, are rightly considered episodic declarative knowledge. It is unlikely that older adults will have the same semantic declarative knowledge as their younger counterparts, and well-known deficits in episodic learning (see Kausler, 1991) will slow their learning of new material.

The same might be said for procedural knowledge. Many of us learned long ago that there are generic algorithms or scripts for taking turns in a guided group discussion. The algorithm involves signaling to the facilitator, frequently by raising one's hand, that one wishes to speak and then waiting for the facilitator to provide a visual or auditory signal that one's turn has come. This algorithm works in the learning environment illustrated, and one might expect people to adopt it rather easily. Before this occurs, however, users must integrate superficial differences in the environment with the general constraints of the algorithm. For example, the users need to know that it is by accessing the raised hand icon that they signal a desire to speak. They must also learn that their microphone will not be enabled unless they execute a specific key press while talking. Facilitators must learn additional actions that they must perform to allow users to speak sequentially. Each of these components to the specific instantiation of the algorithm must be learned and remembered to use the system well. That is, there is an episodic component even for those cases in which semantic procedural knowledge is available.

When procedural knowledge is not stored in semantic memory, cognitive demands can be overwhelming, particularly for older adults who have limitations in dividing attention (McDowd and Shaw, 2000), memory (Salthouse, 1991), and learning (Kausler, 1991). Consider, for example, setting audio controls so that one can hear and speak clearly in the environment. Some of the instructions for setting these controls, labeled an Audio Wizard Mode Setting in Figure 8-1, are puzzling, to say the least. Would the typical older adult know the meaning of terms such as "voice activated" or "full duplex audio"? Would they know that, on a system with an internal microphone, using an external microphone produces considerable feedback? Would users even know that they have an internal microphone? Not likely. Furthermore, many people do not have general experience in setting controls that would transfer readily to this setting.

Complicating matters further, both declarative and procedural knowledge can be important in learning both the content being delivered and the tool being used to deliver that content. Recent research by Laberge and Scialfa (under review) showed that content and technology knowledge made independent contributions to individual, age-related differences in search rates. Greater knowledge of local geography helped older adults search a web site, but they were hindered by less experience with the World Wide Web. Thus, expertise with both the material being learned and the means of delivery will impact the older user.

Although it has not been a focus of this chapter, there is good reason to mention age deficits in attentional deployment in the context of using technology to foster long-term learning. The environment that serves as the basis for this case study has the capability to use several active areas simultaneously. That is, feedback on a critical question can be collected, tallied, and displayed in one area while groups of users are working on an outline in a second area and when a presenter is progressing through content in a third. Facilitators often make the assumption that users are attending to these multiple regions optimally so that they register critical state changes shortly after they occur. This is a naive assumption at best, particularly for the older user, who will have difficulty dividing attention, sustaining attention when information changes at a rapid rate or is embedded in noise, and switching attention once it is focused on a particular subtask or region (see McDowd and Shaw, 2000).

Because it is covered in other chapters (see Schaie, this volume), the role of sensory and perceptual aging is not treated in detail here. However, it is critical to bear in mind that when developers focus on content, they frequently do it at the expense of signal-to-noise ratios. Print is reduced and sound quality is compromised. White space is eliminated to allow for more links, action buttons, and the like. Such changes are likely to hamper older adults in learning to use these tools and in using them efficiently once they are mastered. Although there have been numerous recommendations for universal design that would make technology user friendly for people of all ages, adherence to these recommendations is not common practice today. As a consequence, for older adults, learning through technology will continue to fall short of its potential.

THE CONTEXT FOR E-LEARNING

An issue relevant to both current and future older e-learners concerns the contexts in which most adults have access to technology, learn to use it, and more importantly update their technological skills. Technological competence, access, and use are significantly associated with being in the work force or being in a household with someone in the work force. In addition, interaction with younger generations is important to learning and updating computer skills (U.S. Department of Commerce, 2002). Older adults are at a disadvantage because they are less likely to have regular contact with the workplace, educational settings, or to intergenerational exchanges with the young.

Approximately three-fourths of the work force (73 percent) today report using a computer and 65 percent use the Internet at work (U.S. Department of Commerce, 2002). However, prevalence of computer-related activities in the work place does vary with age; only 25 percent of workers aged 65 years or over use the Internet or e-mail. There appears to be "spillover" from work to family in computer use (U.S. Department of Commerce, 2002). The presence of someone in the household who uses a computer or the Internet at work is associated with substantially higher computer ownership and use at home of the computer or the Internet. This spillover also occurs for those over age 55 years with greater Internet use in the home if someone in the household uses the Internet at work (U.S. Department of Commerce, 2002).

In addition, family households with children under age 18 are more likely to use the Internet than family households with no children. Nonfamily households, composed primarily of persons living alone, have the lowest use of the Internet. With increasing age, adults are less likely to live in households with the younger generation and are more likely to live alone. Forty percent of older women age 65+ live in a nonfamily household (Administration on Aging, 2002). It is these older women living alone who may most benefit from proficiency in various forms of technology in order to maintain an independent lifestyle (U.S. Department of Commerce, 2002).

Broad and equitable access to e-learning is possible only when an appropriate infrastructure is in place, involving high-speed telecommunications and connectivity for individuals and communities (Commission on Technology and Adult Learning, 2001). Broadband Internet services that give e-learning its revolutionary potential are still relatively limited, particularly among low-income, poorly educated people. Community services such as those offered through libraries may provide access to technology in low-income communities.

For e-learning to become widely accessible, consensus will have to be reached on shared technical standards for key features of the e-learning environment. Common standards for such things as metadata, learning objects, and learning architecture will ease communications among different platforms, operators, providers, sites, and learners. Common standards can reduce the time and cost of producing high-quality content and applications. Standards exist; the challenge is for government and business to adopt consensus standards.

Finally, use of e-learning systems is driven largely by the technology available to the participant. The use of state-of-the-art video and audio streaming can lead to delays when used with a slower Internet connection. The "fit" between the user's technology and the technology required for a given program or course is critical for a positive learning experience.

REFERENCES

Administration on Aging. (2002). *A profile of older Americans: 2002.* Washington, DC: U.S. Department of Health and Human Services.

Anderson, J.R. (1985). *Cognitive psychology and its implications* (2nd ed.). New York: W.H. Freeman.

Chi, M.T.H. (1985). Interactive roles of knowledge and strategies in the development of organized sorting and recall. In S. Chipman, R. Segal, and R. Glaser (Eds.), *Thinking and learning skills: Current research and open questions* (Vol. 2). Mahwah, NJ: Lawrence Erlbaum.

Chi, M.T.H., Feltovich, P.J., and Glaser, R. (1981). Categorization and representation of physics problems by experts and novices. *Cognitive Science, 5,* 121-152.

Close, R.C., Humphreys, R., and Ruttenbur, B. (2000). *E-Learning and knowledge technology: Technology and the Internet are changing the way we learn.* New York: Sun Trust Equitable Securities.

Commission on Technology and Adult Learning. (2001). *A vision of E-learning for America's workforce.* Washington, DC: American Society for Training and Development.

Czaja, S.J. (2001). Technology change and the older worker. In J. Birren and K.W. Schaie (Eds.), *Handbook of psychology and aging* (5th ed., pp. 547-568). San Diego, CA: Academic Press.

Czaja, S.J., Hammond, K., Blascovich, J.J., and Swede, H. (1989). Age related differences in learning to use a text-editing system. *Behaviour and Information Technology, 8*(4), 309-319.

Duckworth, C.L. (2001). An instructor's guide to live e-learning. *Learning Circuits: American Society for Training and Development Online Magazine. All about E-learning.* Available: http//.www.learningcircuits.org [February 6, 2004].

Fox, S. (2001). *Wired seniors: A fervent few, inspired by family ties.* Pew Internet and American Life Project. Washington, DC: Pew Foundation.

Fox, S., and Rainie, L. (2000). *The online health care revolution: How the Web helps Americans take better care of themselves.* Pew Internet and American Life Project. Washington, DC: Pew Foundation.

Fox, S., and Rainie, L. (2002). *Vital decisions: How Internet users decide what information to trust when they or their loved ones are sick.* Pew Internet and American Life Project. Washington, DC: Pew Foundation.

Gist, M., Rosen, B., and Schwoerer, C. (1988). The influence of training method and trainee age on the acquisition of computer skills. *Personnel Psychology, 41*(2), 255-265.

Hershey, D.A., Walsh, D.A., Read, S J., and Chulef, A.S. (1990). The effects of expertise on financial problem solving: Evidence for goal directed problem solving scripts. *Organizational Behavior and Human Decision Processes, 46*, 77-101.

Howard, J.H., and Howard, D.V. (1997). Learning and memory. In A.D. Fisk and W.A. Rogers (Eds.), *Handbook of human factors and the older adult* (pp. 2-26). San Diego: Academic Press.

Kausler, D. (1991). *Experimental psychology, cognition, and human aging* (2nd ed.). New York: Springer-Verlag.

Laberge, J., and Scialfa, C. (n.d.). *Predictors of Web navigation performance in a lifespan sample of adults.* Unpublished document.

Labouvie-Vief, G., and Hakim-Larson, J. (1989). Developmental shifts in adult thought. In S. Hunter and M. Sundel (Eds.), *Midlife myths: Issues, findings, and practice implications.* (Vol. 7, pp. 69-96). Thousand Oaks, CA: Sage.

Leventhal, E.A., Leventhal, H., Schaefer, P., and Easterling, D. (1993). Conservation of energy, uncertainty reduction, and swift utilization of medical care among the elderly. *Journal of Gerontology, 48*(2), 78-86.

Leventhal, H., and Cameron, L. (1987). Behavioral theories and the problem of compliance. *Patient Education and Counseling, 10*, 117-138.

McDowd, J.M., and Shaw, R.J. (2000). Attention and aging: A functional perspective. In F.I.M. Craik and T. Salthouse (Eds.), *The handbook of aging and cognition* (2nd ed.). Mahwah, NJ: Lawrence Erlbaum.

Mead, S.E., Spaulding, V.A., Sit, R.A., Meyer, B., and Walker, N. (1997). Effects of age and training on World Wide Web navigation strategies. *Proceedings of the Human Factors and Ergonomics Society 41st Annual Meeting* (pp. 152-156).

Meyer, B.J.F., Russo, C., and Talbot, A. (1995). Discourse comprehension and problem solving: Decisions about the treatment of breast cancer by women across the life-span. *Psychology and Aging, 10*, 84-103.

Morrell, R.W., Park, D.C., Mayhorn, C.B., and Echt, K.V. (1995). Older adults and electronic communciation networks: Learning to use ELDERCOMM. Paper presented at the 103 Annual Convention of the American Psychological Association. New York: American Psychological Association.

Reese, H.W., and Rodeheaver, D. (1985). Problem solving and complex decision making. In J. E. Birren, and K.W. Schaie (Eds.), *Handbook of the psychology of aging* (2nd ed.). New York: Van Nostrand Reinhold.

Reitman, W.R. (1964). Heuristic decision procedures, open constraints and the structure of ill-defined problems. In M.W. Shelly and G.L. Bryan (Eds.), *Human judgments and optimality.* New York: Wiley.

Rogers, W.A. (2000). Attention and aging. In D. Park and N. Schwarz (Eds.), *Cognitive aging: A primer.* Philadelphia, PA: Psychology Press.

Rogers, W.A., Cabrera, E.F., Walker, N., Gilbert, D.K., and Fisk, A.D. (1996). A survey of automatic teller machine usage across the adult life span. *Human Factors, 38*(1), 156-166.

Salthouse, T.A. (1991). *Theoretical perspectives on cognitive aging.* Mahwah, NJ: Lawrence Erlbaum.

Schaie, K.W. (2004). Cognitive aging. In National Research Council, *Technology for adaptive aging* (pp. 43-63). Steering Committee for the Workshop on Technology for Adaptive Aging. R.W. Pew and S.B. Van Hemel (Eds.). Board on Behavioral, Cognitive, and Sensory Sciences. Division of Behavioral and Social Sciences and Education. Washington, DC: The National Academies Press.

Sinnot, J.D. (1989). A model for solution of ill-structured problems: Implications for everyday and abstract problem solving. In J.D. Sinnot (Ed.), *Everyday problem solving: Theory and applications* (pp. 72-99). New York: Praeger.

Smith, A.D. (1996). Memory. In J.E. Birren and K.W. Shaie (Eds.), *Handbook of the psychology of aging* (4th ed.). San Diego, CA: Academic Press.

Staudinger, U.M., Smith, J., and Baltes, P.B. (1992). Wisdom-related knowledge in a late review task: Age differences and the role of professional specialization. *Psychology and Aging, 2,* 271-281.

Tang, B.A. (2000). E-learning 1.0: 10 tips to optimize your e-learning. *Learning Circuits: American Society for Training and Development Online Magazine. All about E-Learning.* Available: http://www.learningcircuits.org [February 6, 2004].

U.S. Department of Commerce. (2002). *A nation online: How Americans are expanding their use of the Internet.* Washington, DC: U.S. Government Printing Office.

Willis, S.L. (1996). Everyday problem solving. In J.E. Birren and K.W. Schaie (Eds.), *Handbook of the psychology of aging* (4th ed., pp. 287-307). San Diego, CA: Academic Press.

Willis, S.L., and Schaie, K.W. (1993). Everyday cognition: Taxonomic and methodological considerations. In J.M. Puckett and H.W. Reese (Eds.), *Lifespan developmental psychology: Mechanisms of everyday cognition* (pp. 33-53). Mahwah, NJ: Lawrence Erlbaum.

Zandri, E., and Charness, N. (1989). Training older and younger adults to use software. *Educational Gerontology, 15*(6), 615-631.

9

The Impact of Technology on Living Environments for Older Adults

Ann Horgas and *Gregory Abowd*

The purpose of this chapter is to discuss how technology can have a positive impact on the living environments and routine life activities of older adults. A living environment is a generic term that is used to indicate place of residence. Technology is broadly defined as the application of scientific knowledge resulting in artifacts that support the practical aims of human life. Routine life activities are a collection of activities of daily living that are needed for an individual to maintain functioning and quality of life.

In this chapter we discuss the most common types of housing available for older adults, focusing specifically on independent living, assisted living, and nursing homes. We provide definitions for each of these different living environments and discuss factors that influence housing options. In addition, we consider the technological advancements that have been made in each of these living environments and emphasize those that might be developed in the future. Finally, we discuss specific mediating and moderating factors, such as cohort effects and accessibility, that might influence the interaction of technology and living environments.

TYPES OF LIVING ENVIRONMENTS

Living environment is a generic term that is used to indicate place of residence. A word that is more commonly used to indicate residence is the word "home." At the most fundamental level, housing provides for basic human needs, as in food, clothing, and shelter. Across the life span, however, living environment, or home, takes on great personal meaning. This meaning may reflect the attainment, or lack thereof, of any of a number of different dimensions, including status and achievement (e.g., home ownership), responsibility (e.g., maintaining a family home), security (e.g., safety), and autonomy and privacy (e.g., personal choice and freedom). These different aspects of housing may take on different salience throughout an individual's life span. At the end of life, independence, autonomy, and safety are especially relevant. Older adults strive to maintain their independence and autonomy in a safe living environment. In addition to personal meaning, living environments have societal and political relevance as well. These include issues of affordability, adequacy, accessibility, and appropriateness of housing (Maddox, 2001). Thus, living environments are a critical issue for older adults, and for our society, as America ages.

There are three main types of living environments for aging adults that we discuss: independent living (e.g., private housing), assisted living, and nursing homes. According to the census of 2000, approximately 95 percent of adults aged 65 and older reside in private households (Cohen and Miller, 2000). These data also point out that the number of elders who maintain a private household declines across age groups. In addition, the proportion of elders who live alone increases across successive age groups and varies markedly by sex (see Figure 9-1). Among those aged 85+, the

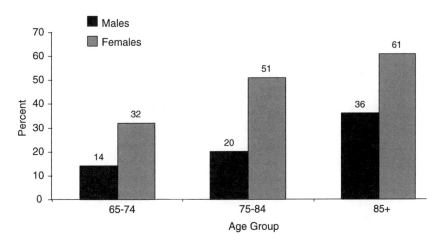

FIGURE 9-1 Percent of older adults living alone in the United States, by age group.
SOURCE: Kinsella and Velkoff (2001, p. 66).

majority of women live alone according to recent census data (Kinsella and Velkoff, 2001). Given the preference of older adults to "age in place," private homes will remain an important housing option in the future, particularly for the young-old, and will be important targets for increased technology to help elders remain there.

The second type of living environment for older adults is assisted living housing (ALH). ALH is a relatively new type of residential option that was developed in the 1990s. It is characterized as a housing-and-services setting where older adults with disabilities can live in private, disability-adapted houses and apartments and receive services tailored to their needs (Kane, Ouslander, and Abrass, 1999). ALH is actually a broad term that encompasses a variety of licensed care facilities, such as residential care facilities, personal care homes, adult foster homes, or small group homes. For the purposes of this chapter, we use the general term "assisted living" to mean a group residence, not licensed as a nursing home, that provides or arranges for personal care and routine nursing care for people with disabilities (Kane and Wilson, 1993). These facilities take many forms but most commonly consist of self-contained, private-occupancy apartments in a range of sizes, styles, and amenities. ALH typically provides access to services such as medical and nursing care, monitoring of residents (including monitoring of medications, medical conditions, falls, and so forth), meal services, and housekeeping. ALH also provides residents with a range of structured activities (such as exercise or reading groups), transportation (to stores and healthcare providers), and social activities (e.g., holiday parties, informal contact with neighbors and friends).

ALH housing is premised on the widely held personal and societal preference of older adults with functional disabilities to live independently for as long as possible in communities designed to provide the security of having reliable services available for use as needed (Maddox, 2001). ALH has emerged as a very attractive housing option for many older adults. The consumer demand for housing that is private, provides needed services, is "noninstitutional," and provides residents with choice and control has been very high. Private-sector developers have been responsive to consumer demand, and the number of assisted living facilities in the United States has grown dramatically. By 1998, there were at least 28,000 ALH facilities in the United States (Mollica, 1998). It has been estimated that as many as 1.5 million older adults currently reside in ALH (U.S. General Accounting Office, 1999), and this trend is expected to continue.

Prior to the development of ALH, nursing homes were the only option for older adults who needed healthcare services that could not be provided at home. In contrast to assisted living facilities, nursing homes are a more medical environment, characterized by minimal personal autonomy and maximal dependence on formal caregivers. Uniformed nursing assistants provide 80-90 percent of all direct care in this setting. Nursing homes were considered to be a longterm care facility; that is, older adults who were too physically frail, too cognitively impaired, or too socially isolated to remain at home moved into a nursing home, and most lived there until death. Admission to a nursing home was often feared and avoided for many reasons, including the connotation of these facilities as "the last stop" before death, the poor quality of care provided in them (Institute of Medicine, 1986), and the lack of autonomy and privacy.

Currently, there are approximately 17,000 nursing homes in the United States providing care for over 1.6 million elders (U.S. General Accounting Office, 1999). As shown in Figure 9-2, whether one is a resident of in a nursing home is highly age related. According to the 1999 National Nursing Home Survey, approximately 12 percent of older nursing home residents in the United States are in the 65-74 age range, whereas 47 percent are in the 85 and older age group (U.S. General Accounting Office, 1999). These age differences are particularly pronounced for women.

Since the 1980s, there have been dramatic changes in nursing homes. The Institute of Medicine report in 1986 drew attention to poor quality and prompted nursing home reform. This resulted in a number of changes to improve the quality of care for residents, including mandatory assessment of residents' status, care planning, and documentation, as well as mandatory training for nursing assistants. In addition, the regulatory and

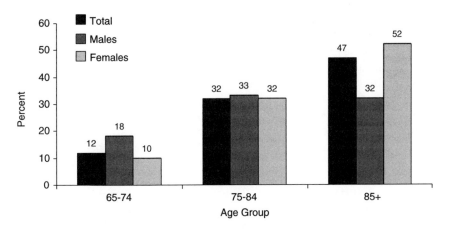

FIGURE 9-2 Age and sex distribution of nursing home residents in the United States.
SOURCE: U.S. General Accounting Office (1999, Table 13).

reimbursement climate has changed and, for the first time in decades, the rates of nursing home occupancy have begun to decrease slightly (Kane et al., 1999). This trend probably reflects an increased availability of alternative care settings, including home-based care and ALH. The nature of nursing home care has changed dramatically over the past decade or so; nursing homes have shifted to providing subacute care (e.g., care after discharge from hospital stay and care for more medically complex patients) and/or care for the most frail, most cognitively impaired elders who can no longer be cared for at home or in less-restrictive environments.

Independent living, ALH, and nursing homes are often viewed on a continuum. The most healthy, most independent elders live at home; the most frail, most dependent elders live in nursing homes. Indeed, over the past decade or so, continuing care retirement communities have been developed to capitalize on this continuum of care model. These retirement communities typically have independent living apartments or houses, assisted living facilities, and a nursing home on the same grounds. Residents can move between levels of care as their health and functioning demand. For example, they can move into a nursing home room while recovering from a fracture or acute medical event and then move back into their own home when ready; they may be guaranteed care from the time they enter the community until death. Typically, residents of continuing care retirement communities are financially advantaged (a large financial buy-in is often required) and healthy at the time of entry (medical screening prior to admission is required, and persons with some medical conditions such as stroke or cancer are often ineligible). These retirement communities are often located near, and in some cases affiliated with, major universities, thus attracting well-educated alumni as residents. Thus, they represent a highly selected living environment. Still, the continuum of care model is one that is attractive to many older adults, their families, and service providers. Recently, there has been a dramatic upswing in the development of communities that cater to elders and that provide access to a variety of services and levels of care. Many of these are rental communities that are more accessible to people of diverse financial means. These retirement communities recognize the fact that the housing demands of older adults vary over time and that aging individuals require options that enable them to move between living environments as needed.

What determines where older adults live? Most people prefer to "age in place." That is, they prefer to continue living in their private home, with their personal possessions, and their familiar community and surroundings. For many people, this is not only a preference, but also a reality. Others choose to relocate as they age. They may do this proactively, either to minimize the work and responsibility of home ownership, to pursue retirement leisure activities, or to be closer to relatives and friends. Some elders may "downsize" or move into a retirement community in anticipation of age-related declines. For the vast majority, however, the move from a private dwelling into an alternative living environment is the consequence of some event, such as a serious fall, illness, death of spouse, or gradually declining health or cognition that necessitates increased healthcare and services. Thus, they move to a living environment that provides them with services because they need to.

FUNCTIONAL STATUS AND INDEPENDENCE

Functional status is one very important determinant of a living environment. Functional status is an index of individuals' ability to perform self-care tasks in two general domains: activities of daily living (ADLs) and instrumental activities of daily living (IADLs). ADLs are basic self-care tasks such as bathing, dressing, toileting, transferring, continence, and feeding (Katz, Ford, Moskowitz, Jackson, and Jaffe, 1963). IADLs are tasks that require higher levels of functioning, such as food preparation, shopping, doing laundry, light housekeeping, using the telephone, managing medications, managing money, and using transportation (Lawton and Brody, 1969). In general, performance of IADLs is necessary for maintenance of one's household, and thus necessary for independent living in the community. Disability in IADL tasks (higher-level tasks) often precedes disability in basic tasks (ADLs). Recently, two additional types of activities of ADLs have been added to the literature. Advanced ADLs (Wolinsky and Johnson, 1991) refer to activities that require higher levels of cognitive capacity, such as telephone use, managing finances, and managing medications. Another term, enhanced activities of daily living (EADLs), denotes the behaviors of active elders who are able to adapt to new environments and exhibit the willingness to accept new challenges (Rogers, Meyer, Walker, and Fisk, 1998). EADLs include social communication, continuing education, community volunteering, and part-time work.

There are multiple assessment tools that are used to measure these important concepts of functional status and independence. Regardless of the measure used, there is a steep increase with age in the proportion of persons who report ADLs, IADLs, and EADLs limitations. In the United States as of 1996, 44 percent of community-dwelling women and 42 percent of men age 75 years and older reported difficulty or inability to perform at least one daily activity (Kramarow, Lentzner, Rooks, Weeks, and Saydah, 1999). Among community-dwelling elders age 85 and older, approximately 55 percent of women and 42 percent of men report ADLs disability. Functional disability results from both physical and cognitive conditions. Osteoarthritis, fractures, stroke, and osteoporosis are some of the specific medical conditions that limit physical functioning. Cognitive losses associated with dementia (e.g., Alzheimer's disease, multi-infarct dementia, and others) also limit functional ability. Cognitive and physical limitations often occur together in advanced age; thus elders are at increased risk for functional impairments as they age.

Functional disability is a key determinant of moving into an assisted living facility or nursing home. It has been reported that the average older adult living in an assisted living facility requires assistance in three IADLs and that about 50 percent of these residents have some level of cognitive impairment (Mollica, 1998). In contrast, nursing home residents have an average of 4.7 ADL limitations, and between 75 and 86 percent have cognitive impairment (Cohen and Miller, 2000). Thus, ALH residents have functional disabilities, largely in the IADL domain, that require supportive services whereas nursing home residents are substantially more impaired and more dependent in both IADL and basic ADL functioning.

In addition to functional status, there are other factors that influence transitions from independent living to assisted living to nursing home. These include acute illness (such as stroke), progression of chronic diseases (both cognitive and physical), and lack of social support. Indeed, it has been stated that the difference between needing and not needing nursing home care depends on the availability of social support (Kane et al., 1999). It is has been estimated that for every person over age 65 in a nursing home, there are approximately 1-3 people equally disabled living in the community (Kane et al., 1999). The people in the community, however, typically have more resources, support services, and family caregivers available to assist them. In addition, these elders may have more access to, and ability to use, the various technological means that are available to help them maintain their functioning.

Other factors that often determine placement in ALH or nursing homes are conditions that are particularly difficult to manage at home, like incontinence and behavior problems associated with cognitive and mental disorders (e.g., wandering, disruptive, or aggressive behaviors). Thus, there are a number of factors that determine the living environments of older adults. Functional status, however, plays a key role in triggering a transition from more independent housing to that offering supportive services or total care. When independently living elders can no longer manage ADLs, and lack family or resources to assist them, they require an alternative home environment that will enable them to maintain the highest level of functioning possible. Increasingly, this alternative living environment is an assisted living facility. Technology may play an important role in enabling older adults to live in a less-restrictive environment for as long as possible and may delay transitions into assisted living or nursing home facilities.

The topic of housing and living environments for older adults has been of some interest to gerontologists over the past several decades. In 1973, Lawton and Nahemow introduced the term "person-environment fit" as an important factor in determining the well-being and functioning of older adults. Person-environment fit refers to the match between individuals' personal needs and capabilities and the available resources and demands of the living environment. Later, Parmelee and Lawton (1990) emphasized the importance of balancing individuals' needs for autonomy and security in housing options for elders. Kane and Kane (2001) stressed the need for an integrated approach to meeting the needs of older adults; that is, a merging of the therapeutic (e.g., medical) and social service (e.g., rehabilitative and compensatory) models of care. Thus, technology is likely to play different roles in different living environments.

TECHNOLOGICAL DEVELOPMENTS RELATED TO LIVING ENVIRONMENTS

In this section we review a variety of technologies that have been developed to support the independence and security of an aging population in a variety of living environments. We first provide a categorization of the technologies based on the needs served. The categories of technology we consider are

• assistive devices that compensate for motor, sensory, or cognitive difficulties;

• monitor and response systems, both for emergency response to crisis situations and for early warning for less critical and emerging problems; and

• social communication aids.

Assistive Devices

As is well known, aging results in changes to many human capabilities (Mynatt and Rogers, 2002). Age-related changes in motor movement include slowing, inability to make continuous motions, and lack of or variable coordination (Vercruyssen, 1997; Ketcham and Stelmach, this volume). Sensory difficulties are also common, and much is known about changes in vision and audition (Schneider and Pichora-Fuller, 2000; Schaie, this volume). For many years, devices that replace or compensate for deficiencies in motor and sensory capabilities have been readily available, and many of these are suitable for both the young and the old.

Difficulties in gross motor movement are mitigated by devices that either perform the motor function, such as powered wheelchairs and stair climbers, or provide assistance, such as well-placed grab bars in bathrooms or power-assisted chairs that facilitate sitting and rising. Hearing aids and low-light visual cues (e.g., magnifiers, large-print materials) are available to assist those declining senses. These physical deficiencies make it hard to operate many of the small appliances and controls that are commonplace in homes today. Consider, for example, setting a digital clock for daylight saving time or programming speed dial buttons on the phone. Researchers at places like the University of Florida's Rehabilitation Engineering Research Center on Technology for Successful Aging (http://www.rerc.ufl.edu/) evaluate the effectiveness of a variety of designs for adaptive household appliances and controls. At the Georgia Institute of Technology, computer vision researchers have prototyped the Gesture Pendant as a wearable device to control a variety of home appliances through simple hand gestures (Starner, Auxier, Ashbrook, and Gandy, 2000).

Perhaps more interestingly from the perspective of this chapter, the field of cognitive aging has matured and we better understand how changes in cognitive function occur as part of the natural process of aging (Craik and Salthouse, 2000; Schaie, this volume). Declines are apparent in attributes such as the capacity of working memory, on-line reasoning, and the ability to attend to more than one source of information. Other abilities remain largely intact, such as recall of rehearsed material, vocabulary and reading, and ability to focus on a single source of information.

Technological support for cognitive aging, often referred to as *cognitive orthotics*, is a very promising direction for research, evidenced by a recent survey on assistive technology for cognition by LoPresti, Mihailidis, and Kirsch (in press). The applications of cognitive orthotics range from simple reminder systems to more-elaborate interactive robotic assistants.

LoPresti et al. provide a useful categorization of cognitive orthotics along two separate dimensions. The technological interventions are first distinguished by whether they support executive function or information processing. Executive functions include planning, task sequencing and prioritization, self-monitoring, problem solving and self-initiation, and adaptability. These executive skills are related to memory, attention, and orientation. Information processing concerns the ability of the brain to properly process and integrate sensory information, with deficiencies leading to problems in the processing of visual-spatial, auditory, sensory-motor, and language information, as well as difficulties in understanding social cues. For the purposes of this chapter, technological support for executive functions is emphasized. The second dimension for technological aids concerns whether they attempt to strengthen a person's intrinsic abilities or seek to provide extrinsic support. Intrinsic aids are often classified as rehabilitation technologies, whereas extrinsic aids are considered as compensation technologies. Our bias here is on the extrinsic, or compensation technologies, because we are trying to address issues of support for aging of otherwise healthy individuals.

This whole area of cognitive orthotics is of growing interest. For example, the reader is referred to the results of a 2002 workshop on cognitive aids from within the computer science community (see http://www. cs.washington.edu/homes/kautz/ubicog/). Also, Jorge, Heller, and Guedj (2001) report on a recent workshop relating ubiquitous computing and universal access in providing for older adults. An appendix to this chapter lists the URLs for Web sites of a number of research centers that are active in technology for application to living environments. Table 9-1 provides an overview of cognitive orthotics research, some of which we further highlight in this section. The table briefly characterizes the purpose for each technology and distinguishes between mature commercial products, emerging technologies that could soon be available commercially, and more far-reaching research visions.

Some cognitive orthotics research focuses on support for extreme cognitive dysfunction, such as Alzheimer's disease or severe dementia. For example, within the Gloucester Smart House consortium (http://www. bath.ac.uk/bime/projects/smart/), devices such as a locator for lost possessions are designed to be usable by people with dementia and their caretakers in order to prolong independent living. Mihailidis, Fernie, and Cleghorn (2000) conducted a pilot study and observed that a person with severe dementia would complete an ADL in response to a computerized device that used a recorded voice for cueing. The computerized device monitored and prompted a subject through hand washing. In response to problems discovered with their first prototype, Mihailidis, Fernie, and Barbenel (2001) used artificial intelligence to develop a new cognitive orthotic for people with moderate to severe dementia. The COACH (cognitive orthosis for assisting activities in the home) was a prototype of an adaptable device to help people with dementia complete hand washing with less dependence on a caregiver.

There is also research that aims to design systems for people in the less-severe stages of memory impairment. Many people have difficulty locating important objects around the home, so commercial versions of the Gloucester Smart House object location system are available at high-end consumer outlets like the Sharper Image. These solutions work for a small number of specialized objects, like keys. One of the research efforts at the University of Rochester's Center for Future Health (http://www. futurehealth.rochester.edu) involves computer vision researchers trying

TABLE 9-1 Categorization of Cognitive Orthotics

Technology	Impairment Addressed	Maturity
IQ Voice Organizer, from Voice Powered Technology, Inc., Burlington. N.J.	Prospective memory aid that plays back recorded messages at specified times	Commercial product
NeverMiss DigiPad, from ICP Inc., Montreal, Quebec, Canada	Prospective memory to record and play back messages without time trigger	Commercial product
CellMinder, from Institute for Cognitive Prosthetics, Bala Cynwyd, Pa.	Prospective memory aid that links personal computer calendar tasks with cell phone to send reminders	Commercial product
ISAAC, from Cogent Systems, Inc., Orlando, FLa.	Prospective memory aid consisting of a handheld unit customized with services to assist the cognitively disabled with routine tasks	Commercial product
Planning and Executive Assistant and Trainer (PEAT), from Attention Control Systems, Mountain View, Calif.	Prospective memory aid consisting of handheld reminding device with intelligent support for revising schedules	Commercial product
Easy Alarms, from Nisus Software, Inc., Solana Beach, Calif.	Prospective memory aid that provides calendar assistance with daily prompts	Commercial product
Essential Steps, from MASTERY Rehabilitation Systems, Inc. Bala Cynwyd, Pa.	Prospective memory aid with software to provide graphical and audio cues to support task completion	Commercial product
COGORTH (Levine and Kirsch, 1985)	Prospective memory aid with specialized programming language to specify multistep tasks with prompting	Emerging

System	Description	Status
ProsthesisWare (Chute and Bliss, 1994)	Prospective memory aid with object-oriented programming support for customized ADL definition to monitor and cue individual	Emerging
VIC 2.0 Recipe assistant (Steele et al., 1989)	Prospective memory to assist subject with severe aphasia to follow a simple recipe	Research
Friedman (1993)	Prospective memory aid using location-aware wearable computer to provide faded prompting for scheduled tasks.	Research
COACH (Mihailidis et al., 2000)	ADLs support for detecting hand washing, also providing prospective task support	Research
Cook's Collage (Mynatt and Rogers, 2002)	Retrospective memory aid using visual cues to provide support for resumption from interruption in cooking tasks	Research
MemoClip (Beigl, 2000)	Prospective memory aid as a wearable appliance that provides location-based reminders	Research
Memory Glasses (DeVaul et al., 2000)	Short-term retrospective memory and navigation aid based on wearable sensors	Research
Three-tiered Control Architecture (Bonasso, 1996)	Prospective memory for general ADLs using environmental and biosensors	Research
AutoMinder (Pollack et al., 2003)	General ADLs support consisting of intelligent reasoning system underlying robotic assistant	Research

to develop more flexible object tracking systems to assist with the location of a wider variety of lost objects within the home. The Nursebot Project at Carnegie Mellon University, University of Pittsburgh, and University of Michigan (http://www-2.cs.cmu.edu/~nursebot/) has been investigating ways that a robotic assistant, Pearl, can assist in eldercare (Montemerlo, Pineau, Roy, Thrun, and Verma, 2002). One of the cognitive aids being developed uses a system called Autominder, developed by Pollack and colleagues at Michigan, to remind an older person about his or her ADLs (Pollack, Brown, Colbry, McCarthy, Orosz, Peintner, Ramakrishnan, and Tsamardinos, 2003). Several commercial products provide support for prospective memory aids (see Table 9-1). Within the Aware Home Research Initiative at the Georgia Institute of Technology (http://www.awarehome.gatech.edu), researchers are focusing on short-term retrospective memory. Mynatt and Rogers (2002) proposed initial designs for a visual collage to assist one to resume routine cooking tasks after an interruption. This simulated memory aid records and displays salient near-term actions from a recipe so that, upon resumption from an interruption, the cook can determine things such as how many cups of flour have already been added to the mixing bowl.

As Table 9-1 shows, many cognitive orthotics are designed to support prospective memory, that is, remembering tasks that need to be performed and carrying out these tasks at the appropriate time (Ellis, 1996). This research has progressed from using very basic and inexpensive timing technologies (e.g., calendars, timers, and watches) to much more sophisticated and forward-thinking applications of artificial intelligence. One of the most important examples of prospective memory tasks is medication compliance. Medication compliance devices range from plastic boxes divided into sections labeled by time and day to electronic systems that provide auditory cues (Fernie and Fernie, 1996). For an individual living alone, remembering to take medication at the right time and in the right order can make the difference between remaining independent or not.

Monitor and Response Systems

We have all seen the classic "I've fallen and I can't get up!" commercials. This caricature is sometimes humorous, but it is representative of an important class of technology that provides monitoring of health and well-being status, communication to interested parties, and in some cases provides automated responses to perform some corrective action. These monitor and response systems can operate in the short term to sense a crisis situation, such as a fall, and provide a way to make a call for help. Medical alert systems like those from the American Senior Safety Agency (http://seniorsafety.com/), American Medical Alarms, Inc. (http://www.americanmedicalalarms.com/), and LifeFone (http://www.lifefone. com/) all allow a greater degree of freedom for an older person, and peace of mind for adult children, by allowing independence while providing a safety net in case of medical crisis. Some devices might automatically detect a crisis (such as a fall). Others depend on activation by the individual (or someone nearby) to initiate a call for help.

Monitoring systems can be classified along a number of dimensions:

• What information is being recorded or transmitted? It could be medical information (e.g., heart rate, respiration, blood pressure, medication compliance, incontinence), movement data (e.g., restlessness in bed, gait patterns), or simply awareness information (e.g., a video transmission to a relative).

• Over what period of time are data analyzed? The capture of information can be for instantaneous purposes only (e.g., a "GrannyCam" usually transmits images over the Internet to be viewed in real time only) or over a period of time for trend analysis, as you would expect for vital signs in a telemedicine application or in medication monitoring for compliance in a home or assisted living environment.

• How is information reported to relevant individuals? Medical alert systems provide a phone call to a response agency. Telemedicine applications report over a secure channel to an electronic patient record that can be consulted by trusted medical professionals or even by the individual being monitored. Cameras are used to provide easy monitoring for family (usually over the Internet, serving an important social communication function discussed below) or remote caregivers (at a nursing station, for example).

• What is the role of the older person in using the technology? Does the monitoring require any instrumentation or active cooperation on the part of the individual being monitored? For example, do they have to wear an infrared badge for a positioning system, or is it passive, with the environment instrumented to measure a naturally occurring phenomenon using devices such as a motion detector or face recognition system?

There are many examples of these monitoring systems for an aging population. Some address the safety and security of individuals who may wander. Devices can either prevent undesired wandering (e.g., automatically closing doors or gates to a house or community grounds to protect Alzheimer's patients) or remind others to take corrective action (e.g., at nighttime when someone inappropriately leaves the bed). A system like the Vigil Integrated Care Management System™ (http://www.vigil-inc.com/), which can detect cases of incontinence via special moisture sensors on bed sheets, allows staff to schedule preemptive nighttime wakings to prevent accidents in the future. Simple load sensors in the beds of residents at Elite Care's Oatfield Estates Cluster in Milwaukie, Oregon (http://www.elite-care.com), feed a visualization to allow caretakers to detect periods of restlessness in the night. Some of the more advanced research in this area is trying to use passive means to perform early detection of chronic, but treatable, conditions. For example, researchers at the University of Rochester's Center for Future Health (http://www.futurehealth.rochester.edu/) are using computer vision techniques to determine asymmetries in gait patterns during visits to the doctor. These data can provide early warnings of the possible onset of a wide range of common neurological and musculoskeletal disorders such as stroke, Parkinson's disease, and arthritis. Similarly, the same vision technology that underlies the Gesture Pendant (Starner et al., 2000) can detect asymmetric tremors indicative of Parkinson's disease and can be used to track the effectiveness of medication regimes to control the disease. Although monitoring technology is not used in these cases to treat the condition of an individual, early detection can increase the effectiveness of medical intervention and counseling for the afflicted.

Cognitive orthotics discussed above rely on context-sensitive reminders, and these often require a way to monitor a person's environment and activities (LoPresti et al., in press). Some research is focused on monitoring ADL tasks in the home using a variety of sensing technologies. Sensors and switches attached to various objects, or optical and audio sensors embedded in the environment, are used to detect which task a person is performing. Trials with several subjects indicate that this method of tracking a person's actions is a good way to monitor the state of a person's health and independence (Bai, Zhang, Cui, and Zhang, 2000; Nambu, Nakajima, Kawarada, and Tamura, 2000; Ogawa, Ochiai, Shoji, Nishihara, and Togawa, 2000). Friedman (1993) developed a wearable microcomputer with a location-sensing system and additional sensors to determine task-related information. Using these inputs, together with the user's schedule, the computer provided voice prompts as needed and only as needed to help the user maintain his or her schedule. Continued evidence of difficulty adhering to the schedule would cause the computer to automatically call for human assistance (Friedman, 1993). By providing prompts only as needed, the system could "fade" (gradually reduce) cues and therefore decrease the user's dependence on them. Because the system does not rely solely on a timed schedule to determine the user's possible activities, it could allow more user independence.

Social Communication Aids

Much of what has been presented so far is in the form of technological interventions to alleviate a physiological or cognitive problem that results from aging. The social aspects of aging, however, are also an important part of the equation in determining the health, safety, functioning, and autonomy of older adults. Peace of mind is an important element for the individual and a distributed family (Mynatt and Rogers, 2002). It has been stated that "geographic distance between extended family members exacerbates the problem by denying the casual daily contact that naturally occurs when families are co-located" (Mynatt, Rowan, Craighill, and Jacobs, 2001, p. 333).

Technology can connect individuals with information. Over the past decade, the burgeoning Internet has introduced a wealth of health information to many who would otherwise not have access to it. More relevant to this chapter, technology can connect individuals with other individuals or groups. Synchronous forms of communication, such as the popular instant messaging, or less popular videophones or even "smart intercoms," whole-house communication systems that leverage knowledge of where individuals are located (Nagel, Kidd, O'Connell, Dey, and Abowd, 2001), present compelling visions of seamless communication aids. Asynchronous forms of communication, such as electronic mail, newsgroups, and on-line forums (e.g., see SeniorNet at http://www.seniornet.org/php/) are all examples of communication technologies that have hit the mainstream. When elders see clear benefits of communication technologies, acceptance is likely (Melenhorst, Rogers, and Caylor, 2001), and there is evidence that they are willing and capable of learning new skills, as reported in a National Science Foundation study of SeniorNet (see http://www.seniornet.org).

One particularly novel asynchronous communication aid has been suggested by Mynatt and colleagues (Mynatt et al., 2001). A digital family portrait is an electronic equivalent of the picture of a loved one that is often found in our homes. However, the digital family portrait is also used to portray a qualitative and dynamic account of the well-being of the subject by means of icons embedded in the frame of the picture. Monitoring systems in the home of the subject are used to provide summaries of daily life. The digital family portrait shows a history of one month's activity, providing an aesthetically acceptable communication aid aimed directly at supporting awareness for a distant adult child. This use of technology will try to approximate the subtle peace of mind that comes from physical proximity.

Relating Technology Aids to Living Environments

We have presented several categories of technological aids to provide assistance to an aging population. These technologies take on different roles depending on the living environment (e.g., independent living, assisted living, or nursing home).

In the home, the goal is to maintain independent functioning, security, autonomy, and safety. Examples are safety and security devices that actively prevent day or nighttime wandering into dangerous places or outside the home for individuals who live alone or alerts of wandering for a partner or caregiver living with that individual. Communication technologies that promote social interaction are very important, providing both synchronous and asynchronous means of connecting with distant relatives and friends. Motor, sensory, and cognitive assistive devices will also be important to compensate for any age-related difficulties.

In assisted living facilities, monitoring for falls, wandering, and general safety and security continue to be important, despite the availability of nearby caregiving staff. In this context, monitoring devices can assist caregivers to provide prompt and effective care. Monitoring of medication management and medical conditions takes on greater emphasis in this setting because the older adults who live there are likely to have more health problems and to be more frail. In a nursing home setting, in which the supervision and assistance is more critical, medication and general medical monitoring are also important to help caregiving staff provide prompt and efficient care and to maximize frail elders' remaining skills, functioning, and quality of life. The need for social communication is important across all living environments, although the type, availability, and ability to use various technologies may vary across settings.

TECHNOLOGY ASSISTANCE IN OTHER ENVIRONMENTS

In this chapter the focus has been almost exclusively on living environments. We recognize, however, that not all time is spent at home. Elders go out to eat, shop, be with friends, go to church, and visit medical facilities and doctors' offices, and this desire does not suddenly disappear just because we get older. How can technology address the needs of an aging population when they are not in their own living environment? Chapter 10 in this volume addresses issues of transportation, both private and public. In public spaces, generic assistive devices, such as handicap-enabled bathroom stalls, work much like they do in a living environment and facilitate functioning in these alternative environments.

Monitoring applications and individually targeted services, however, are more difficult. In public spaces, such as hotels, shopping malls, and parks, it is more difficult to build systems based on knowledge of the individual. Many of the sensing technologies used in living environments today, such as the Vigil Dementia System (see http://www.vigil-inc.com/pdf/Room%20 Layout.pdf for a schematic), rely on knowledge of who the normal resident is. If a motion detector over the bathroom door is tripped in the middle of the night, it can be assumed that it is the lone occupant of the apartment who has entered the bathroom. This same technique will not work in a public restroom. Monitoring and perception of activity in public spaces present a greater challenge, particularly for passive forms of monitoring, in which the individual is wearing no special instrumentation (e.g., computer vision). Tagging techniques, such as radio-frequency identification used on freeways and in airports and hotels to identify frequent customers, are much more effective, although their acceptability for general-purpose tracking remains dubious.

SUMMARY AND CONCLUSIONS

Over the next few decades, the aging population will face numerous changes and challenges. Many of these will involve changes in health and functioning and will impact where older adults live. The vast majority of elderly Americans live at home, often with the assistance of family, friends, and professional home-care services to assist them as their functional abilities decline. Over the past decade, assisted living facilities have been developed and have proven to provide a desirable living environment for those who require some assistance in functional ADLs and more monitoring and security. Nursing homes remain an option for those individuals who require more-intensive assistance, especially with basic ADLs, due to cognitive or health declines. As elders age and face functional declines, they may choose, or be forced, to relocate. Thus, elders may select living environments that optimize their health, safety, and functioning.

Technology may serve as a compensatory mechanism to assist the aging population, especially in the cognitive and security domains, and also as a mechanism that optimizes their daily life (Baltes and Baltes, 1990). Technology assistance in this chapter has been categorized as (a) assistive devices that compensate for motor, sensory, or cognitive difficulties; (b) monitor and response systems, both for emergency response to crisis situations as well as for early warning of less-critical and emerging problems; and (c) social communication aids. There is substantial research being conducted in each of these domains, but we emphasize the particular importance of cognitive orthotics to support the specific needs of cognitive aging.

In addition, current evidence suggests that aging adults are receptive to technology and find it usable. In the coming decades, as the baby boomer generation ages, we can expect to see an even greater demand for technology. Cohort effects refer to differences between groups depending on when they were born. For example, the baby boomers represent a distinct cohort of individuals born between 1946 and 1964. Much has been written about this cohort, and it has been noted that compared with today's seniors, the boomer vanguard is better educated and more technologically adept. Thus, this cohort of people, as they age, may increasingly look to technology to help them maintain their health and independence and to optimize their living environments.

Some question the openness of older individuals to technological interventions. As Mynatt and Rogers (2002, p. 27) indicate, older adults "are willing to use new technologies, contrary to some stereotyped views." Older adults are more accepting if they are provided with adequate training (Rogers, Fisk, Mead, Walker, and Cabrera, 1996) and if the benefits of the technology are clear to them (Melenhorst et al., 2001). A recent study by Mann, Marchant, Tomita, Fraas, and Stanton (2002) suggests strong consumer acceptance for home health monitoring among frail elders.

A recent report from Forrester Research explains why healthcare can and should become more home centric (Barrett, 2002). The big technological enabler is residential broadband, which will reach 37 percent of U.S. households by 2004. The other technology of importance is wireless home networks. These will become increasingly important as computers become a fixture of more and more households. This trend may increase further as the baby boomer cohort ages and retires. Baby boomers are less trusting of medical authority and may look for alternatives to traditional long-term care solutions as they age. These reasons all point to a future in which the vast majority of assistance and healthcare for elders is provided in the home environment. Thus, technological improvements in the home will be increasingly important in the provision of home care. Questions remain as to the affordability of these technological advances, and thus the accessibility of these options for individuals of lower financial means.

Despite these issues, technology—both current and future—is a common feature of many living environments today and is likely to be increasingly important over the next few decades. Technology can facilitate the safety and security of older adults and can compensate for age and disease-related declines in health and functioning. Using technology, older adults may be able to delay or avoid moving from their home to alternative living environments and may maximize their ability to live independently. Specifically, technology applied across living environments can provide cognitive assistance, monitoring, and social communication, thus optimizing "home" for many older adults as they age.

REFERENCES

Bai, J., Zhang, Y., Cui, Z., and Zhang, J. (2000). Home telemonitoring framework based on integrated functional modules. Paper presented at the World Congress on Medical Physics and Biomedical Engineering. Chicago, IL.

Baltes, P., and Baltes, M. (1990). Psychological perspectives on successful aging: The model of selective optimization with compensation. In P. Baltes and M. Baltes (Eds.), *Successful aging: Perspectives from the social sciences* (pp. 1-34). Cambridge, England: Cambridge University Press.

Barrett, M.J. (2002). *Healthcare unbound*. A briefing from the Forrester Research, Inc. Cambridge, MA., March 7-8 in New Orleans.

Beigl, M. (2000). Memoclip: A location-based remembrance appliance. *Personal Technologies, 4*(4), 230-234.

Chute, D.L., and Bliss, M.E. (1994). ProthesisWare. *Experimental Aging Research, 20,* 229-238.

Cohen, M.A., and Miller, J. (2000). *The use of nursing home and assisted living facilities among privately insured and non-privately insured disabled elders*. Washington, DC: U. S. Government Printing Office.

Craik, F.I.M., and Salthouse, T.A. (2000). *The handbook of cognitive aging* (2nd ed.). Mahwah, NJ: Lawrence Erlbaum.

DeVaul, R., Schwartz, S., and Pentland, A. (2000). *The memory glasses project*. Available: http://www.media.mit.edu/wearables/mithril/memory-glasses.html [April 2003].

Ellis, J. (1996). Prospective memory or the realization of delayed intentions: A conceptual framework for research. In M. Brandimonte, G.O. Einstein, and M.A. McDaniel (Eds.), *Prospective memory: Theory and applications* (pp. 1-22). Mahwah, NJ: Lawrence Erlbaum.

Fernie, G., and Fernie, B. (1996). The potential role of technology to provide help at home for persons with Alzheimer's disease. Paper presented at the 18th Annual Conference of the Alzheimer's Society of Canada, Ottawa, ON.

Friedman, M. (1993). A wearable computer that gives context-sensitive verbal guidance to people with memory or attention impairments. In *Proceedings of the Rehabilitation Society of North America (RESNA)* (pp. 199-201). Arlington, VA: RESNA.

Institute of Medicine. (1986). *Improving the quality of care in nursing homes*. Washington, DC: National Academy Press.

Jorge, J., Heller, R., and Guedj, R. (2001). *2001 EC/NSF Workshop on Universal Accessibility of Ubiquitous Computing: Providing for the Elderly*. Setubal, Portugal: ACM Press.

Kane, R.L., and Kane, R.A. (2001). Emerging issues in chronic care. In R.H. Binstock, and L.K. George (Eds), *Handbook of aging and the social sciences* (5th ed., pp. 406-425). New York: Academic Press.

Kane, R., and Wilson, K.B. (1993). *Assisted living in the United States: A new paradigm for residential care for frail older persons*. Washington, DC: American Association of Retired Persons.

Kane, R.L., Ouslander, J.G., and Abrass, I.B. (1999). *Essentials of clinical geriatrics* (4th ed.). New York: McGraw-Hill.

Katz, S., Ford, A., Moskowitz, R., Jackson, B.A., and Jaffe, M.W. (1963). The index of ADL: A standardized measure of biological and psychosocial function. *Journal of the American Medical Association, 185,* 914-919.

Ketcham, C.J., and Stelmach, G.E. (2004). Movement control in the older adult. In National Research Council, *Technology for adaptive aging* (pp. 64-92). Steering Committee for the Workshop on Technology for Adaptive Aging. R.W. Pew and S.B. Van Hemel (Eds.). Board on Behavioral, Cognitive, and Sensory Sciences. Division of Behavioral and Social Sciences and Education. Washington, DC: The National Academies Press

Kinsella, K., and Velkoff, V.A. (2001). *U.S. Census Bureau, An aging world*. (P95/01-1.) Washington, DC: U.S. Government Printing Office.

Kramarow, E., Lentzner, H., Rooks, R., Weeks, J., and Saydah, S. (1999). *Health and aging chartbook: Health, United States, 1999*. Hyattsville, MD: National Center for Health Statistics.

Lawton, M.P., and Brody, E.M. (1969). Assessment of older people: Self-monitoring and instrumental activities of daily living. *Gerontologist, 9*, 179-186.

Levine, S.P., and Kirsch, N.L. (1985). COGORTH: A programming language for customized cognitive orthoses. In *Proceedings of the Rehabilitation Engineering Society of North America (RESNA)* (pp. 359-360). Arlington, VA: RESNA.

LoPresti, E.F., Mihailidis, A., and Kirsch, N. (in press). Technology for cognitive rehabilitation and compensation: State of the art. *Neuropsychological Rehabilitation*.

Maddox, G.L. (2001). Housing and living environments: A transactional perspective. In R.H. Binstock and L.K. George (Eds.), *Handbook of aging and the social sciences* (5th ed., pp. 426-423). New York: Academic Press.

Mann, W.C., Marchant, T., Tomita, M., Fraas, L., and Stanton, K. (2002). Elder acceptance of home monitoring devices. *Journal of Long Term Home Health Care, 3*(2), 91-98.

Melenhorst, A.S., Rogers, W.A., and Caylor, E.C. (2001). The use of communication technologies by older adults: Exploring the benefits from the user's perspective. In *Proceedings of the Human Factors and Ergonomics Society 46th Annual Meeting*. Santa Monica, CA: Human Factors and Ergonomics Society.

Mihailidis, A., Fernie, G., and Barbenel, J.C. (2001). The use of artificial intelligence in the design of an intelligent cognitive orthotic for people with dementia. *Assistive Technology, 13*, 23-39.

Mihailidis, A., Fernie, G.R., and Cleghorn, W.L. (2000). The development of a computerized cueing device to help people with dementia to be more independent. *Technology and Disability, 13*(1), 23-40.

Mollica, R. (1998). *State assisted living policy, 1998*. Portland, ME: National Academy for State Health Policy.

Montemerlo, M., Pineau, J., Roy, N., Thrun, S., and Verma, V. (2002). Experiences with a Mobile Robotic Guide for the Elderly. In *Proceedings of the AAAI National Conference on Artificial Intelligence 2002*. Menlo Park, CA: AAIA.

Mynatt, E.D., and Rogers, W.A. (2002). Developing technology to support functional independence of older adults. *Ageing International, 27*(1), 24-41.

Mynatt, E.D., Rowan, J., Craighill, S., and Jacobs, A. (2001). Digital family protraits: Providing peace of mind for extended family members. In *Proceedings of the 2001 ACM Conference on Human Factors in Computing Systems (CHI 2001)*. Seattle, WA: ACM Press.

Nagel, K., Kidd, C., O'Connell, T., Dey, A., and Abowd, G.D. (2001). The family intercom: Developing a context-aware audio communication system. In *Proceedings of Ubicomp 2001*. Atlanta, GA: Ubicomp.

Nambu, M., Nakajima, K., Kawarada, A., and Tamura, T. (2000). *A system to monitor elderly people remotely, using the power line network*. Paper presented at the World Congress on Medical Physics and Biomedical Engineering, Chicago, IL.

Ogawa, M., Ochiai, S., Shoji, K., Nishihara, M., and Togawa, T. (2000). *An attempt of monitoring daily activities at home*. Paper presented at the World Congress on Medical Physics and Biomedical Engineering, Chicago, IL.

Parmelee, P.A., and Lawton, M.P. (1990). The design of special environments for the aged. In J.E. Birren and K.W. Schaie (Eds.), *Handbook of the psychology of aging* (3rd ed., pp. 464-488). San Diego, CA: Academic Press.

Pollack, M.E., Brown, L., Colbry, D., McCarthy, C., Orosz, C., Peintner, B., Ramakrishnan, S., and Tsamardinos, I. (2003). Autominder: An intelligent cognitive orthotic system for people with memory impairment. *Robotics and Autonomous Systems, 44*(3-4), 273-282.

Rogers, W.A., Meyer, B., Walker, N., and Fisk, A.D. (1998). Functional limitations to daily living tasks in the aged: A focus group analysis. *Human Factors, 40*(1), 111-125.

Rogers, W.A., Fisk, A.D., Mead, S.E., Walker, N., and Cabrera, E.F. (1996). Training older adults to use automatic teller machines. *Human Factors, 38*(3), 425-33.

Schaie, K.W. (2004). Cognitive aging. In National Research Council, *Technology for adaptive aging* (pp. 43-63). Steering Committee for the Workshop on Technology for Adaptive Aging. R.W. Pew and S.B. Van Hemel (Eds.). Board on Behavioral, Cognitive, and Sensory Sciences. Division of Behavioral and Social Sciences and Education. Washington, DC: The National Academies Press.

Schneider, B.A., and Pichora-Fuller, M.K. (2000). Implications of perceptual deterioration for cognitive aging research. In F.I.M. Craik and T.A. Salthouse (Eds.), *The handbook of aging and cognition* (2nd ed., pp. 155-219). Mahwah, NJ: Lawrence Erlbaum.

Starner, T., Auxier, J., Ashbrook, D., and Gandy, M. (2000). The gesture pendant: A self-illuminating, wearable, infrared computer vision system for home automation control and medical monitoring. *Proceedings of IEEE International Symposium on Wearable Computing (ISWC 2000)* (pp. 87-94). Atlanta, GA: IEEE.

Steele, R.D., Weinrich, M., and Carlson, G.S. (1989). Recipe preparation by a severely impaired aphasic using the VIC 2.0 interface. In *Proceedings of the Rehabilitation Engineering Society of North America (RESNA)* (pp. 218-219). Arlington, VA: RESNA.

U.S. General Accounting Office. (1999). *Assisted living: Quality of care and consumer protection issues.* Washington, DC: U.S. General Accounting Office.

Vercruyssen, M. (1997). Movement control and speed of behavior. In A.D. Fisk and W.A. Rogers (Eds.), *Handbook of human factors and the older adult* (pp. 55-86). San Diego, CA: Academic Press.

Wolinsky, F., and Johnson, R. (1991). The use of health services by older adults. *Journal of Gerontology: Social Sciences, 46*, S345-357.

APPENDIX:
Research Centers Active in Technology for
Living Environments

Nursebot: Robotic assistants for the elderly from Carnegie Mellon University, University of Michigan. Pittsburgh, and University of Michigan (http://www-2.cs.cmu.edu/~nursebot/).

Aware Home Research Initiative at Georgia Institute of Technology (http://www.awarehome.gatech.edu).

Center for Future Health at the University of Rochester (http://www.futurehealth.rochester.edu).

Changing Places/House_n: The MIT Home of the Future Consortium (http://architecture.mit.edu/house_n/web/).

Rehabilitation Engineering Research Center on Technology for Successful Aging at the University of Florida (http://www.rerc.ufl.edu/).

Assisted Interactive Dwelling (AID) House in Edinburgh, Scotland (http://www.dinf.ne.jp/doc/english/Us_Eu/conf/tide98/77/bonner_steve.html).

Gloucester Smart Home for People with Dementia (http://www.bath.ac.uk/bime/projects/smart/).

Extending Quality of Life for Older People (EQUAL) initiative in the United Kingdom (http://www.equal.ac.uk).

Helen Hamlyn Research Centre, Royal College of Art in London, England (http://www.hhrc.rca.ac.uk/).

Research Group for Inclusive Environments, University of Reading, England (http://www.rdg.ac.uk/AcaDepts/kc/nhe/).

Institute of Human Ageing, Department of Primary Care, University of Liverpool (http://www.liv.ac.uk/HumanAgeing/).

Age Concern Institute of Gerontology, King's College London, England (http://www.kcl.ac.uk/kis/schools/life_sciences/health/gerontology/top.html).

Honeywell Independent LifeStyle Assistant™ (http://www.htc.honeywell.com/projects/ilsa/). For a list of related projects and products, see http://www.htc.honeywell.com/projects/ilsa/content/weblinks_researcherTechnology.html.

Assisted Cognition project at the University of Washington (http://www.cs.washington.edu/assistcog/).

10

Personal Vehicle Transportation

Joachim Meyer

The face of aging is rapidly changing. Although older age in the past was mainly considered as a transient period in which abilities and activities decline, today more and more older people hope to spend their later years filled with activity and meaningful and enjoyable involvement. A crucial precondition for well-being in older age is independence. A condition for this, in turn, is the ability to move easily from place to place, i.e., the ready availability of means of transportation. Older people in urban settings may have access to various forms of public transportation. Some of these are particularly adapted to the needs of older travelers (e.g., "kneeling" buses that facilitate entrance and exit, paratransportation services that pick up people at their homes). Many mass-transit systems in metropolitan areas are also designed to accommodate older passengers. These forms of transportation have obvious societal and environmental value, and their use should be encouraged. However, transportation for the majority of older adults in the United States, and increasingly in other parts of the world, means using a privately owned and driven car (Coughlin, 2001a). The issue of well-adjusted aging is therefore closely related to the ability to continue to drive for as long as possible and to maintain the independence provided by a car. However, an older person's driving at an advanced age may cause concern if the person has some limitations that affect driving safety.

Numerous questions need to be answered regarding older drivers' continuing to drive. Government and regulatory agencies, car manufacturers, healthcare providers, families, and society at large must address these questions. The answers to these questions and the solutions provided by the different agencies should be based on sound scientific research rather than on guesswork and unfounded beliefs. Some of the relevant data are already available from the large body of research on aging and driving, but many questions remain open. These issues should be at the focus of the research agenda for the coming years.

In this chapter I address a number of relevant issues. I begin by discussing the transportation needs and driving patterns of older drivers. I review some of the reasons why older drivers might differ from other driver populations and focus on vision as one of the fields in which there is compelling evidence for age related decline in abilities that can affect driving. I then discuss whether older drivers constitute a safety risk (and for whom) and under which conditions they do so. I then review some of the changes that older drivers make to cope with the potential safety problems. I then discuss technologies and new in-vehicle devices and their potential to help older drivers, as well as some of the possible problems that may be associated with these technologies. I end the chapter with a brief discussion of some of the necessary research directions on older drivers in view of the new technologies that are available.

CONTINUED DRIVING AT AN ADVANCED AGE

The wish to be able to drive for as long as possible is understandable, given the fact that especially in rural and suburban communities there is often no alternative form of transportation other than a car. A person must use a car to go shopping, to access medical services, to attend social functions, and to visit friends and family (Rosenbloom, 1993). The loss of a driver's license thus implies losses in many aspects of life, including personal freedom, independence, and the possibility of making useful contributions to society (Waller, 1991; Coughlin, 2001b). For the importance of mobility for the well-being of older people, see also Carp (1988).

Indeed, an increasing number of people continue to drive up to an advanced age, leading to a steady growth in the number of "older old" drivers, those aged 75+ or 80+ according to different definitions (Barr, 1991). Kosnick et al. (1988) report that people 65 years and older use the automobile for 80 percent of their errands and trips. Similarly, Jette and Branch (1992) found that older drivers continue to drive for as long as possible and they resist any change in the preferred mode of travel, although they may lower the frequency of travels. Chipman, Payne, and McDonough (1998) report that 37.5 percent of a sample of Ontario, Canada, drivers aged 80 and over reported that they still drove. Relatively healthy older people were especially likely to drive. Although most of the drivers and the nondrivers suffered from two and more chronic diseases and more than 84 percent of both groups suffered from at least one chronic disease, the drivers had fewer chronic diseases than the nondrivers.

Given the importance of driving, driving cessation can have strong adverse effects on a person. For example, Marottoli et al. (1997) showed an increase in depressive symptoms among older adults who stopped driving. The continuing ability to drive seems to be a precondition for some older people's well-being. However, this is not a general need. Chipman et al. (1998) found in their study of 80+ years old drivers in Canada that driving cessation did not lead to a significant decrease in contacts with relatives and friends. Thus, driving, at least for this group, was not necessary for maintaining social relations.

WHAT MAKES OLDER DRIVERS DIFFERENT?

Discussing the issue of older drivers assumes that this group differs in some way from other groups of drivers. Obviously, one variable on which older drivers differ from other drivers is their age. However, it is not at all clear at what age a person becomes an "older driver." Visual capabilities begin to decline in the 20th year, whereas other skills and abilities remain often practically unimpaired up to an advanced age. There is no general age criterion to define older drivers, and different studies have adopted different definitions.

In spite of the lack of a universal criterion for defining older drivers, a fairly large number of studies show systematic differences between drivers as a function of age. The cause for these differences is not always clear. Below I discuss four possible reasons for differences between age groups.

Cohort Effects

Drivers from different age groups belong to different generations. These generations grew up in different cultural, social, and technological environments. Consequently the differences between members of the age groups may be due to these generational effects, which caused them to be exposed to different environments during critical phases of their development. One cohort effect that affects driving is the progressive motorization of Europe and the United States. Whereas most 20-year-old people today have access to cars, the same was not true 60 years ago. Women in particular had less driving experience. These differences can still affect older women's current driving behavior. If this is the case, then differences between today's older men and women in the frequency of trips and the use of cars will disappear in the future when the baby boom generation approaches retirement. Also, overall car use and trip frequency of older drivers will increase for the older drivers of the future. This will lead to an even greater increase in the presence of older drivers on the road, beyond the increase due to changes in demographics.

Changing Lifestyles

The aging process is not only a physiological process in which biological systems undergo changes, but it is also a social process in which a person changes involvement in activities and obligations. One major change that affects the driving habits of many older drivers is the fact that older people cease to commute regularly after they retire from work. This relieves them of the need to drive daily without considering the traffic and weather conditions. After retirement, these drivers are likely to limit their driving in adverse conditions, and after some time they may feel less confident driving at all in these conditions. Thus the exit from the work force (or other changes in lifestyle) may be a cause for changes in driving patterns. Here, too, future older drivers will differ from today's older drivers because of the expected continuing involvement of older people in the work force beyond the current retirement age.

Disease and Medication

The aging process is related to an increase in the frequency of chronic and acute diseases that have adverse effects on a person's functioning in general and driving in particular. The most extreme cases are degenerative diseases, such as Alzheimer's disease, that limit a person's ability to function to an extent that eventually requires constant supervision and care. More frequent are other diseases with less severe impacts. It is not quite clear how chronic disease affects driving ability. For example, Gresset and Meyer (1994) found in a study on Canadian drivers that only arrhythmia (from among a number of medical problems) was associated with a significant increase in the risk of being involved in a crash. In addition to the possible adverse effects of the diseases themselves, there are also possible adverse effects of medication that is taken to control chronic or acute health problems. Some types of medication may impair driving ability to an extent that makes continued driving unsafe.

Age-Related Changes

The fourth possible cause for differences between age groups is changes that are due to the physiological aging process itself. With increasing age certain basic functions change, and in most cases these changes are in the direction of lessened abilities. An extensive review of age-related sensory, cognitive, and motor changes is presented in Chapters 2 and 3 of this report (Schaie, and Ketcham and Stelmach, this volume). I concentrate in the following sections on those changes most likely (or actually demonstrated) to affect driving. With respect to driving, Planek (1972), in one of the earliest larger reviews of the literature on older drivers, identified three interconnected areas of deficiencies: (1) sensory reception, (2) neural processing and transmission, and (3) motor response. Later studies put greater emphasis on cognitive aspects of driving that are related to decision making (Hakamies-Blomqvist, 1996). Llaneras, Swezey, Brock, and Rogers (1993) and Shaheen and Niemeier (2001) summarize some of the age related sensory and cognitive changes that affect driving.

SOME AGE-RELATED CHANGES THAT AFFECT DRIVING

Vision

One domain in which there is compelling evidence for age-related changes is vision. This sensory ability is particularly important, because driving is a continuous control task that is largely guided by visual information. Malfetti and Winter (1986) suggest that 85-95 percent of the sensory cues in the driving task are visual. It is therefore reasonable to assume that changes in visual performance are likely to affect driving.

The decrease in visual abilities begins after the age of 20 and continues throughout a person's life. Shinar and Schieber (1991) reach a number of general conclusions regarding the effect of normal aging on visual perception. First, apparently all visual functions deteriorate with age. Second, the amount, rate, and onset of deterioration vary widely between individuals and functions. Third, whereas static acuity begins to deteriorate in the 60s, other visual abilities deteriorate earlier. Fourth, performance differences between individuals increase with age. Table 10-1 presents a list of some of the major visual abilities that are relevant for driving. It also lists changes that occur with age in each of these abilities and the impact that these changes are likely to have on driving.

The importance of vision for driving and the relative ease of administering vision tests led to the almost universal screening of drivers according to their visual ability. Tests of visual acuity are standard in the licensing procedure of most countries, and many countries require periodic retesting of acuity after a certain age. However, a closer inspection of the aging-related changes in visual performance shows that the changes in static acuity (which is measured in most vision evaluations) are by no means the only changes that occur. Also, it appears that static acuity may not be the visual ability that is most relevant for safe driving. Groeger

TABLE 10-1 Age-Related Changes in Visual Abilities

Ability	Major Changes	Some Implications for Driving	Selected References
Visual acuity: Ability to resolve small details when viewed from a distance	Decline of visual acuity (myopia, near sightedness); can be partly corrected with lenses	Need for corrective lenses while driving	Anderson and Palmore (1974), Kline et al. (1992), Kosnick et al. (1988), Reuben et al. (1988)
Dynamic visual acuity: Ability to correctly observe the direction and speed of a moving object	Decline in dynamic visual acuity	Difficulty in determining rate of approach and time to collision of moving objects	Sekuler et al. (1982), Wist et al. (2000)
Focusing on near objects: Ability to resolve small details in a near object (farsightedness or presbyopia when related to age)	Difficulty in focusing on near objects due to the loss of elasticity in the lens of the eye; can be corrected with reading glasses or bifocal lenses	Need for-bifocal lenses or reading glasses to see in-vehicle displays or to locate smaller controls	Bruckner (1967), Kline et al. (1992)
Contrast sensitivity: Ability to detect changes in the lightness of a surface	Decline in contrast sensitivity	Difficulty in detecting objects or changes in the road that appear as changes in shading	Fozard (1990), Owsley et al. (1983)
Night vision: Ability to see in poor lighting conditions	Cataracts and senile miosis limit the amount of light that reaches the receptors	Difficulty in seeing objects in dim lighting (at night, in tunnels, or garages)	Charness and Bosman (1992), Kline et al. (1992)
Disability glare resistance: Poor vision in glare conditions	Less luminance is required to produce disability glare	Difficulty in night driving and in changing levels of illumination	Olson (1988), Olson and Sivak (1984), Sanders et al. (1990)

Recovery from glare: Time required to regain night vision after exposure to bright light	Increased susceptibility to glare and slower recovery from glare	Difficulty in night driving and driving in changing levels of illumination	Charness and Bosman (1992), Pulling et al. (1980), Sloane et al. (1988), Wolf (1960)
Peripheral vision: Angular width of field of view in which motion information is perceived	Decrease in size of horizontal peripheral visual field	Late detection of events that develop in the periphery, such as approaching cars	Burg (1968), Retchin et al. (1988)
Useful field of view: Width of visual field over which information can be acquired in a quick glance	Decline in spatial and peripheral vision	Difficulty in detecting events that develop at the sides of the visual field (merging cars, etc.)	Haegerstrom-Portnoy et al. (1999), Sekuler et al. (2000)
Color vision: Differential perception of light with different wavelengths	Loss of sensitivity to shorter wavelengths resulting in reduced ability to discriminate blues, greens and violets	Responses to color-coded displays may be affected	Botwinick (1984)
Visual scan: Speed and efficiency of movement of fixations in the visual field	Slowing of visual scan	Difficulty taking in complex traffic situations	Maltz and Shinar (1999)

(1999) points out that, in spite of the long history of research on vision and driving, very little is known about the role of different visual parameters in driving.

This fact that it is not at all clear what visual abilities are actually crucial for safe driving points to one of the major issues that require research and clarification in the future. Driving ability is likely to depend on factors that are difficult to measure. Also, drivers can be highly adaptive and can compensate for deficiencies in certain areas by changing their behavior (use different driving techniques, change the conditions in which they drive, use technology to help them deal with some of the problems, etc.). It will therefore be difficult to come up with a valid, objective test that can predict who can and who cannot continue to drive safely. Clearly, simply measuring visual acuity is not enough.

The age-related changes in vision presented in Table 10-1 are by no means isolated phenomena. Rather, many of these changes are connected and may affect driving performance in similar conditions. One condition in which many of the changes will lower the older driver's ability to obtain the necessary visual information for driving is at dusk and dawn and in darkness. Here a decrease in contrast sensitivity, general diminished night vision, and prolonged recovery from glare make driving more difficult and stressful. Older adults' vision in low illumination is impaired, relative to younger adults, even if they are in good eye health (Owsley and Sloane, 1987; Sloane, Owlsey, and Alvarez, 1988). The decrease in contrast sensitivity in older adults can be attributed to age-related reduction in pupil size and the loss of lens transparency (Owsley, Sekuler, and Siemsen, 1983; Sloane et al., 1988). The effects of aging and decreased retinal illumination (for example, because of tinted glass) are not additive. It seems that aging enhances the effects of limited illumination. Levels of transmittance of tinted glass that have no effect on younger drivers can impair vision for older drivers (LaMotte, Ridder, Yeung, and DeLanel, 2000). Thus when any manipulation or condition can lower the retinal illumination, special attention should be given to the evaluation of its effect on older drivers.

Changes in vision are obviously not the only age-related changes. In addition to the aging-related changes in visual abilities, a number of other major changes in sensory, motor, and cognitive functions are likely to occur with age. I briefly review the other major changes and point out their potential relevance for driving.

Hearing

Hearing acuity decreases progressively, beginning as early as age 40 (e.g., Stelmachowicz, Beauchaine, Kalberer, and Jesteadt, 1989). The main changes are in the higher frequency range. The causes for these changes can be structural changes with aging, the cumulative effects of noise exposure, the result of traumatic events or disease, or side effects of certain types of medication. The hearing loss itself does not necessarily have direct implications on driving performance. However, it needs to be considered when auditory stimuli are intended to guide the driver or to provide warning information. The design of these auditory displays may have to take the changing hearing abilities of older drivers into account.

Attention

The effects of aging on attention are complex. There exists a distinction between different attention skills. One is focused attention, which is the ability to concentrate resources on a single task or information source without being distracted by other sources of information or cognitive processes. A second skill is divided attention—the ability to divide attention between a number of concurrent tasks and the monitoring of different concurrent stimuli. A third skill is attention control, which is a person's ability to switch the allocation of attentional resources from one task to another. There is evidence that older adults have greater difficulties dividing attention effectively compared with middle-aged and younger adults (Brouwer, Waterink, van Wolfelaar, and Rothengatter, 1991). The problem is particularly pronounced when two tasks require the same output modality (e.g., motor responses) and is reduced when the tasks employ different modalities (Brouwer, Ickenroth, Ponds, and van Wolfelaar, 1990). In a study on selective attention, Mihal and Barrett (1976; see also Barrett, Mihal, Panek, Stern, and Alexander, 1977) found a correlation between selective attention and accident rates for drivers 45-64 years old, and they found no such correlation for drivers 25-43 years old.

Memory

The existence of aging-related changes in memory is well established (e.g., Jacoby and Hay, 1998). Problems with short-term memory may cause difficulties in retaining information over short periods of time (e.g., instructions on route choice). Problems with long-term memory may be in the encoding of information (people may find it difficult to learn new names, routes, or information). Other problems with long-term memory may be in the retrieval of information, where information that was encoded in the past (which is evident by the fact that at some time in the past a person remembered this information) is now temporarily unavailable. Although these problems can occur at any age, they become increasingly common when a person ages. The memory difficulties may affect the use of new in-vehicle technologies, for example, by making it more difficult to remember procedures for using the system or by interfering with the recall of names and codes that are used in speech-activated systems.

Another domain where aging-related changes may impact performance is skill acquisition (Craik and Jacoby, 1996). Generally skill acquisition becomes slower with age, and a person will find it difficult to alter familiar ways of performing certain tasks. On the other hand, the procedural memory for familiar tasks and skills may remain intact up to a very advanced age. Thus a person can perform complex sets of actions, such as playing a musical instrument or driving a car. However, they may find it difficult to acquire some new skills that require changes in well-established routines.

Information Processing

The major change in information processing is a general slowing in processing speed. This causes a lengthening of response times and slower actions and, in particular, slower responses to unexpected events (e.g., Falduto and Baron, 1986). One study that dealt with simple and choice response times as a function of age showed that simple response times were relatively little affected by age, whereas choice response times were much more severely affected (Fozard, Vercruyssen, Reynolds, Hancock, and Quilter, 1994). With respect to driving, it appears that there are only small differences in response times to hazards on the road as a function of age. It seems that older drivers are able to brake rapidly when they encounter a problematic situation as long as they expect it (Korteling, 1990; Lerner, 1993; Olson and Sivak, 1986).

Decision Making

Some age-related differences in decision making have been identified (see Schaie, this volume), but decision processes that are relevant for driving seem to be relatively little affected by age. For instance, a study by Dror, Katona, and Mungur (1998) showed no effect of age on the speed of risk-taking decisions. However, one difference that seems to exist is that with increasing age people become more safety conscious (Boyle, Dienstfrey, and Sothorn, 1998). This may be due to the fact that the consequences of adverse events, such as traffic accidents or falls, are likely to be more severe for older people than for younger ones.

Actions and Motor Behavior

In addition to the cognitive changes that occur with age, there are also motor changes. Together with the cognitive slowing of responses, there often occurs a motor slowing of responses, which causes an older person to perform a movement more slowly than a younger person. Under certain conditions this may delay responses to safety hazards.

Muscular strength decreases approximately 12-15 percent between the ages of 30 and 70 (Blocker, 1992). Overall there is clear evidence for a loss of strength with age, especially after the age of 65. This loss of strength is more pronounced in women than in men (Bassey and Harries, 1993). There is also a loss in the speed of muscle contractions and coordination with age (Blocker, 1992). Thus an older driver is likely to have less strength than a younger person and may consequently have more need of power steering or power brakes.

A third characteristic related to aging is lowered flexibility. Approximately half of the population over age 75 experiences some degree of arthritis (Adams and Collins, 1987). This makes vehicle ingress and egress more difficult. It also limits a person's ability to turn the head and trunk, causing difficulty looking toward the sides and rear of the car. In particular the flexibility of the neck diminishes with age, leading older drivers to have less flexion and extension and rotation capability in the neck compared to younger people (Kuhlman, 1993). This lowered motility of the neck and head is a likely cause for accidents in which an older driver either collides with an object that is behind the car when backing up or fails, when changing lanes, to see a vehicle that comes up from behind in a parallel lane.

ARE OLDER DRIVERS A PROBLEM AND, IF SO, WHAT IS THE PROBLEM?

The age-related changes listed above seem to indicate that older drivers are likely to constitute a traffic safety problem. However, contrary to common beliefs, it is not at all clear whether older drivers are indeed a safety risk. There are some undisputable facts. For one, the fatality rate of older drivers is high compared with other age groups. It is close to the rate of 16-24-year-old drivers. Thus older drivers are at a greater risk of dying in an accident than most younger drivers.

There are two possible causes for the increased fatality rate. First, older drivers may be more likely to die in accidents because of their frailty and fragility. Impact forces that are negligible for a younger person can lead to severe and even fatal injuries for an older person (e.g., Evans, 2000). Therefore the increased fatality rate is not an indication that older drivers constitute a safety risk unless we consider their exposure to risks to themselves as a problem.

The second possible reason for the increased fatality rate of older drivers is that they are more likely to have an accident than younger drivers. There is some evidence that there is an increase in accident involvement for older drivers, but the strength of this evidence is not clear. It is also unclear at what age this increase occurs. Different studies point to different ages. For example, in a Florida accident database Abdel-Aty, Chen, and Schott (1998) found that drivers over age 64 (as well as drivers under 25) were more likely to be involved in crashes. In contrast, Kweon and Kockelman (2003) analyzed crash involvement and severity for different age groups, controlling for vehicle type, accident type, and driver exposure. They found that overall crash involvement was lower for 60+ year old drivers or equal to that for middle-aged drivers. Male older drivers had 4.74 crashes per million miles, whereas male middle-aged drivers had 6 crashes per million miles. For female drivers the corresponding numbers of crashes were 5.52 for the older drivers and 5.59 for middle-aged drivers. These numbers were much lower than the crash rates for drivers up to the age of 20, which were 21.79 for males and 20.24 for females.

Li, Braver, and Chen (2003) attempted to determine the relative importance of older drivers' fragility and their increased crash involvement for the increase in the fatality rates for older drivers. Their analysis showed an increase in the rate of deaths for 1,000 drivers involved in crashes, beginning with age 60. The increase continued with advanced age, and at age 80 or older the chances of dying when involved in a crash were 4.3 times higher for males and 5.2 times higher for females than the chances for 30-59-year-old drivers. Crash involvement (as indicated by the number of crashes per vehicle miles traveled) also increased with age. However, this increase began later and was smaller. The accident involvement for the 70-74-year-old group of drivers was still very close to the accident involvement rates for middle aged drivers. In the 75-79-year-old drivers the accident rate was 1.7 times the rate for middle aged drivers. A noticeable increase is evident for the 80+ year-old drivers. They had 3 times (for males) or 2.6 times (for females) the crash involvement of middle aged drivers. These rates were still smaller than the rates for 16-19-year-old drivers, who had accident rates that were 4 times the rates for middle aged drivers.

Older drivers have an increased chance of being involved in certain types of accidents. They are overrepresented in collisions in intersections where they are usually hit when entering the intersection without giving the right of way (Hakamies-Blomqvist, 1993). A disproportionately large number of accidents occur when driving across traffic (as in left turns in countries where people drive on the right side of the road). Evans (1991) mentions that older drivers are also particularly likely to be involved in accidents during backing and parking maneuvers, which are probably caused by older drivers' limited flexibility and ability to turn and their limited peripheral fields of view. When involved in an accident, older drivers are more likely to be considered the party at fault and legally responsible (Cooper, 1990; Hakamies-Blomqvist, 1994).

One reason why it is so difficult to answer the question whether older drivers constitute a safety risk is the great variety of ways in which one can compare the data for different age groups. Each comparison has certain advantages and disadvantages (see Hakamies-Blomqvist, 1998, for an in-depth discussion of the issue). Computing crash rates by adjusting to the number of licensed drivers (as was, for example, done by Evans, 2000) will lead to an underestimation of crash rates for older drivers because a fairly large number of older drivers maintain a driver's license but have in fact stopped driving. Other ways to compare data have different problems. For example, computations of the number of crashes per 1 million miles driven for different age groups (as well as other measures of crash involvement) have to be based on the number of crashes in some database. A crash is more likely to be reported if it leads to severe injury or a fatality. Given that older drivers are more vulnerable, crashes in which they are involved should have a greater chance to be reported in an accident database. Consequently the crash rate for older drivers will seem to be high.

The issue is further complicated by the fact that the older driver population is highly diverse. Even if the crash rate for older drivers is indeed higher than for younger drivers, it is not clear what drivers cause this increase. With age, a growing percentage of people suffer from severe debilitating diseases, the most frequent being Alzheimer's disease (Evans, 1990). It has been shown that Alzheimer's disease leads to an increase in accident risks (e.g., Drachman and Swearer, 1993; Dubinsky, Williamson, Gray, and Glatt, 1993; Hunt, Morris, Edwards, and Wilson, 1993). Part of the increase in accident rates for older drivers could be due to greatly increased accident risk for a fairly small group of older drivers who suffer from dementia or severe sensory problems (of which they may not be aware). Unimpaired older drivers may not constitute a risk.

DRIVING CHARACTERISTICS OF OLDER DRIVERS

Older drivers are obviously aware of the fact that they are aging and that some of their sensory, cognitive, and motor abilities change. They tend to respond to these changes by driving differently from when they were younger. They mainly tend to limit their driving to conditions with which they feel comfortable. The selective limitation of driving in adverse conditions is essentially a process of self-regulation. This adaptive response is highly appropriate (Eberhard, 1996). As early as 1968, a study showed that older drivers are less likely as a group to drive at night or in heavy traffic (Planek, Condon, and Fowler, 1968). More recently Ball and colleagues (1998) studied a sample of drivers in seven age categories from 55 up (mean age 70) and three categories of accident involvement (none, 1-3, and 4 and more). More than 80 percent of the sample reported often or always avoiding driving at night, about 70 percent avoided driving during rush hour, and almost 70 percent avoided driving on high-speed interstates. About 30 percent avoided driving in high-traffic roads. About 20 percent reported avoiding driving alone and turning left across traffic. Less than 20 percent often or always avoided driving in rain. Older drivers who were more visually or cognitively impaired reported more avoidance and fewer driving days. There were small correlations between crash involvement in the past 5 years and avoidance of driving during rain, driving in rush hour, and left turns.

Another adaptive response that is evident in various studies is that older drivers tend to drive more slowly than younger drivers (Boyle et al., 1998; Hakamies-Blomqvist, 1994; Planek, 1981). This is true even when they are involved in an accident (Hakamies-Blomqvist, 1993). Thus it is reasonable to conclude that the driving style of older drivers differs to some extent from that of younger drivers (Cooper, 1990; Rothe, 1990).

Older drivers are aware that they drive differently, and they tend to consider themselves as a group to be cautious, courteous, and safe drivers compared with younger drivers (Nelson, Evelyn, and Taylor, 1993). The impression that older drivers tend to be more cautious is supported by research. Shinar, Schechtman, and Compton (2001) analyzed self-reports of driving behavior in the U.S. driving population. They showed that women report observing speed limits more than men and that older drivers (over age 50) report observing speed limits more (48 percent) than 26-50-year-old drivers (42 percent) or drivers under the age of 26 (34 percent). Older male drivers reported more use of seat belts all the time than younger drivers (79, 66, and 54 percent for the three groups, respectively). There was no such effect for female drivers, among whom 78 percent overall reported using the seat belt all the time. The increased use of seat belts by older drivers supports the notion that caution increases with age and is not a cohort effect. Most older drivers began driving when seat belt use was rare, and they adopted it relatively late in life. Younger drivers, in contrast, were generally exposed to the message to "buckle up" from the time they began to drive.

The self-regulation of older drivers affects their accident patterns. They were found to be comparatively less involved in accidents at night, during bad weather, or in bad road surface conditions than younger drivers, and they were less likely to be in a hurry, to be intoxicated, or to be distracted by nondriving activities (Hakamies-Blomqvist, 1994).

The self-regulation that older drivers apply to their own driving is probably the main reason for the relatively small increase in crash risk with age in spite of the numerous age-related changes that should have an adverse effect on traffic safety. Older drivers actively lower their exposure to problematic situations and are thereby able to maintain crash risks that are comparable to those of younger drivers.

Keskinen, Ota, and Katila (1998) and Hakamies-Blomqvist (1996) consider the possibility that many accidents involving older drivers are in fact due to their defensive and slower driving, combined with faster driving by younger drivers. These young drivers may actually cause the accidents, although the older driver is often considered at fault in the accident report. One study assessed the behavior of young (<30), middle aged (30-60), and older (over 60) drivers while turning at intersections (Keskinen et al., 1998). It showed that older drivers took longer to make a turn across traffic (which were in this case right turns, as the study was conducted in Japan). This left less time for the oncoming vehicles compared with cases in which a younger driver drove the turning vehicle.

Driver self-regulation seems to be an effective way to alleviate some of the problems that arise with age. However, it is by no means perfect. For example, in studies on visual field deficiencies one study found that 56.7 percent of the participants who had abnormal visual fields were unaware of the problem (Johnson and Keltner, 1983). In another study 48 percent of the participants for whom a test showed visual field loss had not been aware of the problem before the test (Bengtsson and Krakau, 1979). Apparently some drivers are unaware of their limitations and may fail to take the proper precautions. This problem is particularly severe for older drivers with dementing diseases, such as Alzheimer's disease. Their limited capability for judgment makes it impossible for them to adjust their driving to their impairments.

NEW TECHNOLOGIES AND THE OLDER DRIVER

Until quite recently, innovations in cars were mainly related to the physical aspects of vehicle design, propulsion, and control. Over the past few years, new technologies have been introduced into the car that affect driving and the driver's actions in the car. The new devices with which drivers directly interact can broadly be divided into three categories:

• **Vehicle control devices** are immediately tied into the perceptual-motor cycle of vehicle control. One group of devices enhances the sensory capabilities of the driver, for example, by providing visual information that may otherwise be less available. Examples are night vision systems, as are currently available in various high-end cars, and rear-view or blind-spot cameras that display views of the surroundings of the car on dedicated monitors. In the future there may also be enhanced-vision systems that superimpose images or icons on a visual scene so that, for example, a car with which there could be a possible conflict receives some visual salient marking that makes it easier to detect and to follow. Other devices that provide critical information are various forms of alerts and warnings, such as collision warning systems. Some devices that are already installed in cars or are developed take an active part in the control of the vehicle. Examples are adaptive cruise control systems that adjust vehicle acceleration and deceleration to the distance from other vehicles to maintain a constant headway.

• **Driving assistance devices** provide the driver with information that is relevant for driving but does not immediately affect vehicle control. The information can be useful for the driver, but it is usually not safety critical. Examples of such devices are traffic information systems and navigation systems.

• **Driver infotainment and comfort devices** provide entertainment for the driver and other occupants of the car, allow communication, or support driver comfort. These devices are unrelated to the driving task itself. They do, however, engage some of the driver's attentional capacity and can thereby indirectly affect driving. Examples of these systems are car entertainment systems, cellular phones, e-mail, web access, and climate control in the vehicle.

These three categories of devices are not necessarily installed as separate pieces of equipment. Instead, the general trend in the industry in recent years is to integrate a number of different devices in one entity, for example, using a single display and control unit for communication, entertainment, and navigation systems.

Some of the new technologies that are introduced into the car can have particular value for older drivers, considering that they can alleviate some of the effects of age-related changes. This can facilitate driving, allowing older people to drive in conditions in which they may otherwise have refrained from driving. These devices can also make driving safer for an older person by improving the protection in case of an accident and lowering the risk for accidents (Coughlin and Tallon, 1999).

Other systems (such as entertainment and communication systems) are not intended to help with driving. These systems often have no special value for older drivers. However, these devices are also installed in the older driver's car and need to be designed in view of the characteristics of older users if they are to be of any use for them.

Design of Technology for Older Drivers

The introduction of new technologies for older drivers should be based on the notion of "user-centered design" (e.g., Owens, Helmers, and Sivak, 1993). It requires the entire design process to be driven by the attempt to address the needs of the user and to adapt the product to the user characteristics. Usability considerations are of major importance for consumer acceptance and satisfaction with almost all consumer products. However, in the context of in-vehicle technologies they are particularly important because of the inherent safety issues related to these devices (Flyte, 1995). Below I provide a brief overview of some of the major design issues relevant for older drivers. Of course, the design for an older user will often improve a device for all users, regardless of age.

Physical Design

The physical changes that occur with aging should be considered when designing a car that can accommodate older drivers and passengers. At one level, the increased fragility of older drivers and passengers requires the design of safety systems that are adjusted to their specific needs. Seat belts, precrash seat belt tightening and seat adjustment, and airbags should adapt automatically to the weight and height of the person occupying a seat. Such measures can potentially lower the severity of injuries for older drivers.

In normal use of the car, steps should be taken to facilitate ingress and egress. Turning seats and large doors can help with this. Considering the increasing number of older adults in the population who not only drive but also often ride as passengers in cars, such design changes are likely to have definite appeal to a large section of the population.

It is also possible to use technological solutions to help cope with age-related physical difficulties. One problem that many older drivers experience is limited ability to rotate the neck and upper body, making it difficult to look to the side and back when backing up. A rear-view system that displays a wide-angle view of the area behind the car can help an older driver back up safely. Another system that is already installed in many larger vehicles is a backup warning system that alerts drivers when they approach an object while backing up.

Visual Design

The visual design of the vehicle interior and of in-vehicle devices should take into consideration the changes in vision that occur with age. As mentioned above, lowered acuity and contrast sensitivity are common among older drivers. The contrast between display elements and the background should therefore be maximal. Displays should use digital or analog indicators that are at a brightness level that differs as much as possible from the background. It is also beneficial to provide adequate lighting of the information and to avoid reflectance. The introduction of digital displays into the car makes it possible to adjust the display properties to the needs of the individual driver. The same "real estate" in the driver's field of view can be used to present more detailed information for a younger driver and less information (in larger displays) with greater contrast for an older driver.

Older drivers also benefit from relatively low-tech improvements in the car that can help alleviate some aging-related changes. For example, providing better lighting can reduce some of the problems with night vision. This can be done by improving headlights, which should be designed to illuminate longer stretches of road while lowering the likelihood of glare (Shinar and Schieber, 1991). In addition, a simple headlight washing device that helps to remove dirt from the lights and restore their full lighting potential will have particularly great benefits for older drivers (Mortimer and Fell, 1989). Using more-sophisticated technologies, older drivers can benefit from the augmented vision in darkness that is provided by night vision systems, such as GM's infrared system. Such systems can help older drivers extend their driving beyond daylight and maintain mobility in limited visual conditions. However, these systems can also cause new problems, in particular for older drivers. For one, the position of the displayed image may require the driver to accommodate to a closer distance, a process that becomes slower and more difficult with age. Also, the position of the image in the visual field differs from the position at which the image would usually be in the driver's field of view. This requires the driver to adopt new ways of visual scanning. This may be confusing, particularly for older drivers.

Auditory Design

Auditory displays are an alternative to visual information displays. However, hearing difficulties are fairly common among older adults, and they need to be considered when auditory displays are designed. Care should be taken not to create an overload in the auditory modality. This modality is relatively little used today in driving, but may become easily overloaded if a variety of devices, such as warning systems, cell phones, entertainment systems, traffic information systems, and navigation systems, provide the driver with various kinds of stimulation.

The properties of the auditory display should be adapted to the hearing abilities of the older driver. This is not a simple adjustment, because the loudness and frequency range of the displayed information should ideally be tuned to the existing acoustic situation in the car. When it is quiet, the windows are closed, and there is no source of auditory stimulation in the car, the displays can be less loud. Stimuli that are too loud will be perceived as annoying. Also, sudden loud stimuli could cause a startle response that may be dangerous. However, in conditions of strong auditory stimulation, such as when the driver listens to music or drives with open windows, the displays should be louder and adjust the information accordingly. The sound systems that present information from navigation, communication, or information devices should be individually tuned to the properties of a specific older driver's hearing. It may also be possible to improve the acoustic environment for hearing these messages, for example, by lowering the volume of all other auditory stimuli (e.g., the entertainment system) when a message is given.

Visual and auditory designs obviously need to go hand in hand. A recent study on the response to visual, auditory, and combined in-vehicle information systems by older (65-73-year-old) and younger (18-25-year-old) drivers showed that older drivers benefit from the use of multimodal displays that employ both visual and auditory modalities (Liu, 2000).

Cognitive Design

In addition to the more obvious sensory and motor aspects of aging that need to be considered when designing for older drivers, there are also cognitive aspects that must be addressed. The increasing availability of in-vehicle devices that provide the driver with various types of information can impose severe demands on the driver's attentional capabilities. The design of systems for older drivers needs to take into consideration the issue of information overload and allow the older driver to limit his or her information input as desired.

One important aspect of the cognitive design of new in-vehicle technologies for older drivers is mode awareness and situation awareness with respect to automated components (Sarter and Woods, 1995). For example, an adaptive cruise control system that adjusts the vehicle speed to the speed of another car in the same lane is actually a form of automation. It automates the driver's acceleration and deceleration required to maintain a constant distance from the car ahead. To use this system safely the driver needs to be aware of the mode in which the system is at each moment in time. For example, the system can be turned on or off and, if on, it can be engaged or not engaged. Older drivers may have more problems maintaining appropriate mode awareness and may therefore find automated systems less reliable, more confusing, and less useful. As a result, such systems, even if they could be particularly useful for an older driver, can go unused.

Design of the Driving Environment

In addition to design changes in the vehicle that can make driving easier and safer for older drivers, there are also various changes in the driving environment that can be made and that can be very beneficial for older drivers. The Federal Highway Administration has recently published a report pointing to ways in which roadways, intersections, signs, and markings can be designed to help older drivers (Staplin, Lococo, Byington, and Harkey, 2001). Older drivers are particularly likely to benefit from improved lighting, especially at intersections. Signs and pavement markings should be large and clearly visible. Longer merge and exit lanes will make it easier to cope with fast-flowing traffic. Adjusting roadways to the needs of older drivers will obviously also benefit other drivers, especially in difficult driving conditions such as heavy rain and fog.

What Technologies Are Good for Older Drivers?

The brief discussion of design issues and technologies for older drivers should make it clear that the introduction of a new device into the car is not always easy and will not necessarily constitute an improvement. Some of the new technologies that are introduced into the car require the driver to change behavior patterns that have served the older driver for decades. This change may be difficult, and the need to adopt new behaviors may rob older drivers of one of their main advantages—the extensive driving experience they have acquired over the years.

The notion that a device makes sense on the drawing board does not ensure that it will have the desired effect once it is introduced into the car. A number of reasons make it difficult to predict the effects of introducing a new system.

Users Do Not Necessarily Accept Innovation

It is by no means assured that a technologically sound device that provides definite benefits for the user will eventually be adopted. The most effective protective system against injury in a crash is a properly fastened seat belt (e.g., Rivara, Koepsell, Grossman, and Mock, 2000). In spite of the fact that this was widely known, it took decades for seat belts to become accepted by the majority of drivers, and this only after major efforts on the part of government agencies involved with traffic safety.

Good Intentions, Bad Outcomes

It is also often difficult to predict how a device will affect driving, especially because the effects of new technologies can change greatly over time. Expectations based on preliminary testing during the development phase may be unjustified. For example, the antilock braking system promised to have major safety benefits, but the actual benefits turned out to be very small. In fact, the system had an initial negative effect on safety, and some time had to pass before the accident rate returned to its level before the system was introduced (Farmer, 2001).

There are at least four reasons why a system that should improve safety can yield smaller than expected benefits and may at times even lead to negative effects. First, users may not use the device correctly and therefore may fail to obtain the safety benefits (e.g., drivers with an antilock braking system may cease to apply force to the brakes when the system is active and the brake pedal vibrates).

Second, the introduction of a device can create a feeling of safety that can induce a person to take a greater risk than he or she would without the device. This notion is expressed in models, such as Wilde's (1988) risk homeostasis theory, according to which people maintain a fairly constant level of risk and expose themselves to greater danger when they are protected by some safety device.

Third, a device that should benefit older drivers may not have the desired effect because it does not fit the specific driving characteristics of older drivers. For example, because older drivers may be less likely to detect possible hazards (because of diminished vision, distraction, etc.), they should particularly benefit from warning systems that provide an alert for possible problems. Indeed, older drivers respond to in-vehicle warnings in the same way as younger drivers (Cottè, Meyer, and Coughlin, 2001). However, warning systems tend to have false alarms, and the proportion of false alarms out of all alarms increases as the driver becomes more cautious (Meyer and Bitan, 2002). To demonstrate this point, consider two drivers who drive with the same collision warning system. The system has a certain detection rate when a collision is genuinely imminent and a detection rate when a collision is unlikely, the so-called false alarm rate. One driver takes great risks and therefore has many near collisions. This driver will encounter frequent warnings, and most will be justified. This driver is likely to view the warning system as useful. The second driver is very cautious, and collisions can almost never occur. This driver will encounter fewer warnings, and most warnings will be false alarms. Consequently this driver will believe that the warning system has only limited value. Considering that older drivers tend to drive more cautiously than younger drivers, they are likely to experience an unacceptably high false alarm rate in warning systems, causing the system to appear annoying and leading to its eventual rejection.

Fourth, the user may develop new behavioral patterns following the introduction of the new technology. A backup collision warning system can serve as an example. Backup collisions are particularly likely when a person has difficulties turning the head, which is rather common for older drivers. The installation of such a system should help drivers avoid many of these collisions and should make driving safer. However, the system can also change the way a person drives. In extreme cases the user may come to back up without even bothering to look back, waiting for the warning system to cue them when to stop. This turns the warning system from being a safety device into a device for primary vehicle control. As long as the warning serves only as a safety device, a malfunction in the warning usually has no severe consequences. When the warning serves as the information source for vehicle control, its reliability becomes crucial and any malfunction can lead to an accident.

The complex interplay of factors that determine the outcome of the introduction of a new device makes it necessary to develop new models and methodologies to predict the user's reactions to a new technological system. It cannot be simply assumed that a certain system analysis that applies for the current use patterns of a device will also apply when the device is altered. The benefits that are to be expected from a new technology have to be considered very carefully. New technologies need to be evaluated over time, in conditions that are as close as possible to the actual use conditions, and with people who represent the future user population.

The evaluation of devices also must take into account that the device will not be used in isolation. Rather, combinations of devices will be installed in the car and can at times be used together. For example, the driver may use a cellular phone to contact a person whom he or she intends to meet and at the same time look at the navigational system to receive directions on how to get to the meeting. The joint use of devices may create interactions that affect the utility and safety of using each of the separate devices.

The prediction of the effects of new technologies is further complicated because more than the driver's response to a system needs to be considered when evaluating the likelihood of its successful introduction. Legal and political issues are also crucial. For example, no system is perfect, and even with a very good system some collisions may occur. Some of them will likely be blamed on the system, and the manufacturer may be held liable. In view of this possibility, the manufacturer may take various steps to lower the chances of litigation, but these steps may also limit the usefulness of the system. Thus, the introduction of these systems requires a careful analysis of all aspects of the use of such a system, an analysis that requires the development of adequate predictive tools.

CONCLUSIONS

The question of how to provide older drivers with the opportunity to drive for as long as possible, while minimizing the risks due to incapacitated and unsafe drivers, is a crucial topic that will require even more attention in the future. There are numerous topics that need to be addressed to adjust for the aging driving population. For one, it is still largely unknown what causes the differences between older and younger drivers. We need to obtain a clearer picture of age-related driving characteristics. In particular it may be important to see how these characteristics change over cohorts and which of these characteristics will persist in the future. Also, the diversity of older drivers needs to be better understood, and more information must be collected on driving with different levels of impairment.

At a second level we need to determine how we can change driving so that older drivers will find it easier to fit into the driving population. Some of the necessary means may involve training older drivers to become aware of age related changes and to cope effectively with safety issues. We may also want to consider changes in the driving environment. Some of these changes can be related to changes in the road infrastructure that will make it friendlier for older drivers. For example, older drivers tend to have difficulties making left turns across traffic. Left-turn traffic lights or the use of traffic circles can solve this problem. Also, at some places older drivers may have trouble merging with traffic because other drivers drive at excessive speeds. The use of traffic control devices to lower the speed of oncoming vehicles can help to cope with this problem.

In the design of in-vehicle technologies, we are facing many unknowns regarding the effects of these technologies on drivers in various situations. The design of the device, the allocation of functions to it, and the design of the interface all require a thorough understanding of the interaction between users and technologies. This goes clearly beyond current knowledge in this field. The empirical basis for our research needs to be expanded by collecting both field and laboratory data. In addition, researchers need to develop appropriate design methodologies that take into account the unique characteristics of the driving situations and the needs and properties of the driver. This will be particularly important for older drivers, who may have less ability to adapt to a nonoptimal design of the system. Finally, models of the use of the automation and devices are needed for predicting how users will respond to a certain system design. Such models will allow us to move from the unsystematic engineering of human-vehicle systems that is practiced today to a more systematic and model-driven technique that approaches the methods used in other fields of engineering.

The introduction of the new technologies into cars for older drivers also makes it necessary for car manufacturers to reconsider their roles. More attention will have to be paid to the familiarization of the new driver with the technologies in the car. The best ways to do this are still fairly unclear. Because the use of many new in-vehicle devices is not entirely intuitive, companies will need to invest resources in the training of users in order to teach them how to maximize the utility of the system and how to deal with adverse situations. This need for training is particularly important for safety-critical systems, which are usually used only rarely and in conditions in which a very rapid and almost automatic response is required. Training will be particularly important when the system requires the relearning of some well-established skills. This is likely to be a greater problem for older drivers who, on the one hand, have much experience with older systems, and who are, on the other hand, usually somewhat slower in the learning of new skills.

Possibly car sales will have to include the use of simulator or test track driving to teach the driver how to respond to different events with the complex technologies. In addition, older drivers in particular will need to have the technologies customized to their particular needs. Drivers themselves can do this, but, in all likelihood, optimal customization should be based on the objective evaluation of the individual driver's needs by a specialist. This will require the development and validation of techniques to determine the optimal configuration for a driver. Also, specialists for customizing cars to the needs of individual customers may have to be trained. It is unlikely that current sales personnel can be expected to do this job appropriately, unless they receive the tools and knowledge for this additional service.

Thus the introduction of new in-vehicle technologies for older drivers requires us to expand the boundaries of our knowledge and our understanding in a wide variety of fields. It is likely that the insights gained here will be important in various domains, beyond the design of vehicles. Thus, this may be an opportunity to develop some of the major technologies for the twenty-first century, while helping an increasing number of people maintain independence, involvement, and quality of life.

REFERENCES

Abdel-Aty, M.A., Chen, C.L., and Schott, J.R. (1998). An assessment of the effect of driver age on traffic accident involvement using log-linear models. *Accident Analysis and Prevention, 30,* 851-861.

Adams, P.F., and Collins, G. (1987). Measures of health among older persons living in the community. In R.J. Havlik, B.M. Liu, and M.G. Kovar (Eds.), *Health statistics on older persons, United States, 1986. Vital and Health Statistics* (DHHS Publication No. 87-1409). Washington, DC: U.S. Government Printing Office.

Anderson, D., and Palmore, E. (1974). Longitudinal evaluation of ocular function. In E. Palmore (Ed.), *Normal aging: II. Reports from the Duke longitudinal studies, 1970-1973* (pp. 166-230). London: Butterworth.

Ball, K., Owsley, C., Stalvey, B., Roenker, D.L., Sloane, M.E., and Graves, M. (1998). Driving avoidance and functional impairment in older drivers. *Accident Analysis and Prevention, 30,* 313-322.

Barr, R.A. (1991). Recent changes in driving among older adults. *Human Factors, 33,* 597-600.

Barrett, G.V., Mihal, W.L., Panek, P.E., Stern, H.L., and Alexander, R.A. (1977). Information processing skills predictive of accident involvement for younger and older commerical drivers. *Industrial Gerontology, 4,* 173-182.

Bassey, E.J., and Harries, U.J. (1993). Normal values for handgrip strength in 920 men and women aged over 65 years, and longitudinal changes over 4 years in 620 survivors. *Clinical Science, 84,* 331-337.

Bengtsson, B., and Krakau, C.E.T. (1979). Automatic perimetry in a population survey. *Acta Ophthalmologica, 57,* 929-937.

Blocker, W. (1992). Maintaining functional independence by mobilizing the aged. *Geriatrics, 47*(1), 42-56.

Botwinick, J. (1984). *Aging and behavior: A comprehensive integration of research findings.* New York: Springer-Verlag.

Boyle, J., Dienstfrey, S., and Sothorn, A. (1998). *National survey of speeding and other unsafe driving actions.* (Report No. NHTSA DOT HS 808 749). Washington, DC: U.S. Department of Transportation.

Brouwer, W., Ickenroth, J.G., Ponds, R.W.H.M., and van Wolfelaar, P.C. (1990). Divided attention in old age. In P. Drenth, J. Sergeant, and R. Takens (Eds.), *European perspectives in psychology* (Vol. 2, pp. 335-348). Indianapolis, IN: John Wiley and Sons.

Brouwer, W., Waterink, W., van Wolfelaar, P., and Rothengatter, T. (1991). Divided attention in experienced young and older drivers: Lane tracking and visual analysis in a dynamic driving simulator. *Human Factors, 33,* 573-582.

Bruckner, R. (1967). Longitudinal research on the eye. *Gerontologia Clinica, 9,* 87-95.

Burg, A. (1968). Lateral vision field as related to age and sex. *Journal of Applied Psychology, 52,* 10-15.

Carp, F.M. (1988). Significance of mobility for well-being of the elderly. In *Transportation in an aging society: Improving mobility of older persons.* (Special Report 218). Washington, DC: Transportation Research Board.

Charness, N., and Bosman, E. (1992). Human factors and age. In F.I.M. Craik and T.A. Salthouse (Eds), *Handbook of aging and cognition* (pp. 495-552). Mahwah, NJ: Lawrence Erlbaum.

Chipman, M.L., Payne, J., and McDonough, P. (1998). To drive or not to drive: The influences of social factors on the decision of elderly drivers. *Accident Analysis and Prevention, 30,* 299-304.

Cooper, P.J. (1990). Elderly drivers' view of self and driving in relation to the evidence of accident data. *Journal of Safety Research, 21,* 103-113.

Cottè, N., Meyer, J., and Coughlin, J.F. (2001). Older and younger drivers' response to collision warning systems. In *Proceedings of the Human Factors and Ergonomics Society 45th Annual Meeting*. Santa Monica, CA: Human Factors and Ergonomics Society.

Coughlin, J.F. (2001a). Beyond health and retirement: Placing transportation on the aging policy agenda. *Public Policy and Aging, 11*(4), 1-23.

Coughlin, J.F. (2001b). *Transportation and older persons: Needs, preferences and activities*. Washington, DC: AARP Public Policy Institute.

Coughlin, J.F., and Tallon, A. (1999). Older drivers and ITS: Technology, markets and public policy. *ITS Quarterly, 7*, 123-134.

Craik, F.I.M., and Jacoby, L.L. (1996). Aging and memory: Implications for skilled performance. In W.A. Rogers, A.D. Fisk, and N. Walker (Eds.), *Aging and skilled performance: Advances in theory and applications* (pp. 113-137). Mahwah, NJ: Lawrence Erlbaum.

Drachman, D.A., and Swearer, J.M. (1993). Driving and Alzheimer's disease: The risk of crashes. *Neurology, 43*, 2448-2456.

Dror, I.E., Katona, M., and Mungur, K. (1998). Age differences in decision making: To take a risk or not. *Gerontology, 44*, 66-71.

Dubinsky, R.M., Williamson, A., Gray, C.S., and Glatt, S.L. (1993). Driving in Alzheimer's disease. *Journal of the American Geriatric Society, 40*, 1112-1116.

Eberhard, J. (1996). Safe mobility for senior citizens. *IATSS Research, 20*, 29-37.

Evans, D.A. (1990). Estimated prevalence of Alzheimer's disease in the United States. *Milbank Quarterly, 68*(2), 267-289.

Evans, L. (1991). *Traffic safety and the driver*. New York: Van Nostrand Reinhold.

Evans, L. (2000). Risks older drivers face themselves and threats they pose to other road users. *International Journal of Epidemiology, 29*, 315-322.

Falduto, L.L., and Baron, A. (1986). Age-related effects of practice and task complexity on card sorting. *Journal of Gerontology, 41*, 659-661.

Farmer, C.M. (2001). New evidence concerning fatal crashes of passenger vehicles before and after adding antilock braking systems. *Accident Analysis and Prevention, 33*, 361-369.

Flyte, M. (1995). The safe design of in-vehicle information and support systems: The human factors issues. *International Journal of Vehicle Design, 16*, 158-169.

Fozard, J. (1990). Vision and hearing in aging. In J.E. Birren and K.W. Schaie (Eds.), *Handbook of the psychology of aging* (3rd ed., pp. 150-170). San Diego, CA: Academic Press.

Fozard, J.L., Vercruyssen, M., Reynolds, S.L., Hancock, P.A., and Quilter, R.E. (1994). Age differences and changes in reaction time: The Baltimore Longitudinal Study of Aging. *Journal of Gerontology, 49*(4), P179-189.

Gresset, J., and Meyer, F. (1994). Risk of automobile accidents among elderly drivers with impairments or chronic disease. *Canadian Journal of Public Health, 85*(282-285).

Groeger, J.A. (1999). Expectancy and control: Perceptual and cognitive aspects of the driving task. In P.A. Hancock (Ed.), *Human performance and ergonomics* (pp. 243-264). San Diego, CA: Academic Press.

Haegerstrom-Portnoy, G., Scheck, M.E., and Brabyn, J.A. (1999). Seeing into old age: Vision function beyond acuity. *Optometry and Vision Science, 76*, 141-158.

Hakamies-Blomqvist, L. (1993). Fatal accidents of older drivers. *Accident Analysis and Prevention, 25*, 19-27.

Hakamies-Blomqvist, L. (1994). Compensation in older drivers as reflected in their fatal accidents. *Accident Analysis and Prevention, 26*, 107-112.

Hakamies-Blomqvist, L. (1996). Research on older drivers: A review. *Journal of the International Association of Traffic and Safety Sciences, 20*, 91-101.

Hakamies-Blomqvist, L. (1998). Older drivers' accident risk: Conceptual and methodological issues. *Accident Analysis and Prevention, 30*, 293-304.

Hunt, L., Morris, J.C., Edwards, D., and Wilson, B.S. (1993). Driving performance in persons with mild senile dementia of the Alzheimer type. *Journal of the American Geriatric, 41,* 747-753.

Jacoby, L.L., and Hay, J.F. (1998). Age-related deficits in memory: Theory and application. In M.A. Conway, S.E. Gathercole, and C. Cornoldi (Eds.), *Theories of memory* (Vol. 2 pp. 111-134). East Sussex, England: Psychology Press.

Jette, A.M., and Branch, L.G. (1992). A ten-year follow-up of driving patterns among the community-dwelling elderly. *Human Factors, 34,* 25-31.

Johnson, C.A., and Keltner, J.L. (1983). Incidence of visual field loss in 20,000 eyes and its relationship to driving performance. *Archives of Ophthalmology, 101,* 371-375.

Keskinen, E., Ota, H., and Katila, E. (1998). Older drivers fail in intersections: Speed discrepancies between older and younger male drivers. *Accident Analysis and Prevention, 30,* 323-330.

Ketcham, C.J., and Stelmach, G.E. (2004). Movement control in the older adult. In National Research Council, *Technology for adaptive aging* (pp. 64-92). Steering Committee for the Workshop on Technology for Adaptive Aging. R.W. Pew and S.B. Van Hemel (Eds.). Board on Behavioral, Cognitive, and Sensory Sciences. Division of Behavioral and Social Sciences and Education. Washington, DC: The National Academies Press.

Kline, D.W., Kline, T.J.B., Fozard, J.L., Kosnick, W., Schieber, F., and Sekuler, R. (1992). Vision, aging, and driving: The problems of older drivers. *Journal of Gerontology: Psychological Sciences, 47,* 27-34.

Korteling, J.E. (1990). Perception-response speed and driving capabilities of brain-damaged and older drivers. *Human Factors, 32,* 95-108.

Kosnick, W., Winslow, L., Kline, D., Rasinski, K., and Sekuler, R. (1988). Vision changes in daily life throughout adulthood. *Journal of Gerontology, 43,* 63-70.

Kuhlman, K.A. (1993). Cervical range of motion in the elderly. *Archives of Physical Medicine and Rehabilitation, 74,* 1071-1079.

Kweon, Y.J., and Kockelman, K.M. (2003). Overall injury risk to different drivers: Combining exposure, frequency and severity models. *Accident Anaylsis and Prevention, 35,* 441-450.

LaMotte, J., Ridder, W., Yeung, K., and DeLanel, P. (2000). Effect of aftermarket automobile window tinting films on driver vision. *Human Factors, 42,* 327-336.

Lerner, N.D. (1993). Brake reaction times of older and younger drivers. In *Proceedings of the Human Factors Society 37th Annual Meeting* (pp. 206-210). Santa Monica, CA: Human Factors Society.

Li, G., Braver, E.R., and Chen, L.H. (2003). Fragility versus exessive crash involvement as determinants of high death rates per vehicle-mile of travel among older drivers. *Accident Analysis and Prevention, 35,* 227-235.

Liu, Y. C. (2000). Effect of advanced traveler information system displays on younger and older drivers' performance. *Displays, 21,* 161-168.

Llaneras, R.E., Swezey, R.W., Brock, J.F., and Rogers, W.C. (1993). Human abilities and age-related changes in driving performance. *Journal of the Washington Academy of Sciences, 83,* 32-78.

Malfetti, J.L., and Winter, D. (1986). *Drivers 55 plus: Test your own performance.* Washington, DC: AAA Foundation for Traffic Safety.

Maltz, M., and Shinar, D. (1999). Eye movements of older and younger drivers. *Human Factors, 41,* 15-25.

Marottoli, R.A., Mendes de Leon, C.F., Glass, T.A., Williams, C.S., Cooney, L.M.Jr., Berkman, L.F., and Tinetti, M.E. (1997). Driving cessation and increased depressive symptoms: Prospective evidence from the New Haven EPESE (Established Populations for Epidemiological Studies of the Elderly). *Journal of the American Geriatric Society, 45,* 202-206.

Meyer, J., and Bitan, Y. (2002). Why better operators receive worse warnings. *Human Factors, 44,* 343-354.

Mihal, W.L., and Barrett, G.V. (1976). Individual differences in perceptual information processing and their relation to automobile accident involvement. *Journal of Applied Psychology, 61,* 229-233.

Mortimer, R.G., and Fell, J.C. (1989). Older drivers: Their night fatal crash involvement and risk. *Accident Analysis and Prevention, 21,* 273-282.

Nelson, T.M., Evelyn, B., and Taylor, R. (1993). Experimental intercomparisons of younger and older drivers' perceptions. *International Journal of Aging and Human Development, 36,* 239-253.

Olson, P. (1988). Problems of nighttime visibility and glare for older drivers. In *Society of Automotive Engineers, Effects of Aging on Driver Performance* (SP-762, pp. 53-60). Warrendale, PA: Society of Automotive Engineers.

Olson, P.L., and Sivak, M. (1984). Glare from automobile rear-vision mirrors. *Human Factors, 26,* 269-282.

Olson, P.L., and Sivak, M. (1986). Perception-response time to unexpected roadway hazards. *Human Factors, 28,* 91-96.

Owens, A., Helmers, G., and Sivak, M. (1993). Intelligent vehicle highway systems: A call for user-centered design. *Ergonomics, 36,* 363-369.

Owsley, C., Sekuler, R., and Siemsen, D. (1983). Contrast sensitivity throughout adulthood. *Vision Research, 23,* 689-699.

Owsley, C., and Sloane, M.E. (1987). Contrast sensitivity, acuity, and the perception of "real world" targets. *British Journal of Ophthalmology, 71,* 791-796.

Planek, T.W. (1972). The aging driver in today's traffic: A critical review. In T. W. Planek, W. A. Mann, and E. L. Wiener (Eds.), *Aging and highway safety: The elderly in a mobile society* (pp. 1-38). Chapel Hill, NC: North Carolina Symposium on Highway Safety.

Planek, T.W. (1981). The effects of aging on driver abilities, accident experience, and licensing. In H.C. Foot, A.J. Chapman, and F.M. Wade (Eds.), *Road safety: Research and practice* (pp. 171-179). New York: Praeger.

Planek, T.W., Condon, M.E., and Fowler, R.C. (1968). *An investigation of the problems and opinions of aged drivers.* Chicago: National Safety Council.

Pulling, N.H., Wolf, S.P., Sturgis, D.R., Vaillancourt, D.R., and Dolliver, J.J. (1980). Headlight glare resistance and driver age. *Human Factors, 22,* 103-112.

Retchin, S.M., Cox, J., Fox, M., and Irvin, L. (1988). Performance-based measurements among elderly drivers and non-drivers. *Journal of the American Geriatric Society , 36,* 813-819.

Reuben, D.B., Stillman, R.A., and Traines, M. (1988). The aging driver. *Journal of the American Geriatric Society, 36,* 1135-1142.

Rivara, F.P., Koepsell, T.D., Grossman, D.C., and Mock, C. (2000). Effectiveness of automatic shoulder belt systems in motor vehicle crashes. *Journal of the American Medical Association, 283,* 2826-2827.

Rosenbloom, S. (1993). Transportation needs of the elderly population. *Clinical Geriatric Medicine, 9,* 297-310.

Rothe, J.P. (1990). *The safety of elderly drivers.* London: Transaction.

Sanders, M., Shaw, B., Nicholson, B., and Merritt, J. (1990). *Evaluation of glare from center-high-mounted stop lights.* Washington, DC: National Highway Traffic Safety Administration.

Sarter, N.B., and Woods, D.D. (1995). How in the world did we ever get into that mode? Mode error and awareness in supervisory control. *Human Factors, 37*(1), 5-19.

Schaie, K.W. (2004). Cognitive aging. In National Research Council, *Technology for adaptive aging* (pp. 43-63). Steering Committee for the Workshop on Technology for Adaptive Aging. R.W. Pew and S.B. Van Hemel (Eds.). Board on Behavioral, Cognitive, and Sensory Sciences. Division of Behavioral and Social Sciences and Education. Washington, DC: The National Academies Press.

Sekuler, R., Kline, D., and Dismukes, K. (1982). Aging and visual function of military pilots: A review. *Aviation, Space and Environmental Medicine, 53*(8), 747-758.

Sekuler, A.B., Bennett, P.J., and Mamelak, M. (2000). Effects of aging on the useful field of view. *Experimental Aging Research, 26,* 103-120.

Shaheen, S.A., and Niemeier, D.A. (2001). Integrating vehicle design and human factors: Minimizing elderly driving constraints. *Transportation Research Part C, 9,* 155-174.

Shinar, D., and Schieber, F. (1991). Visual requirements for safety and mobility of older drivers. *Human Factors, 33,* 507-519.

Shinar, D., Schechtman, E., and Compton, R. (2001). Self-reports of safe driving behaviors in relation to sex, age, education and income in the U.S. adult driving population. *Accident Analysis and Prevention, 33,* 111-116.

Sloane, M.E., Owsley, C., and Alvarez, S.L. (1988). Aging, senile miosis and spatial contrast sensitivity at low luminance. *Vision Research, 28,* 1235-1246.

Staplin, L., Lococo, K., Byington, S., and Harkey, D. (2001). *Guidelines and recommendations to accommodate older drivers and pedestrians* (Report No. FHWA-RD-01-051). Washington, DC: Federal Highway Administration.

Stelmachowicz, P.G., Beauchaine, K.A., Kalberer, A., and Jesteadt, J. (1989). Normative thresholds in the 8- to 20-kHz range as a function of age. *Journal of the Acoustical Society of America, 86,* 1384-1391.

Waller, P.F. (1991). The older driver. *Human Factors, 33,* 499-505.

Wilde, G.J.S. (1988). Risk homeostasis theory and traffic accidents: Propositions, deductions and discussion of recent commentaries. *Ergonomics, 31,* 441-468.

Wist, E.R., Schrauf, M., and Ehrenstein, W.H. (2000). Dynamic vision based on motion-contrast: Changes with age in adults. *Experimental Brain Research, 134,* 295-300.

Wolf, E.W. (1960). Glare and age. *Archives of Ophthalmology, 64,* 502-514.

Appendix A
Workshop Materials

WORKSHOP ON TECHNOLOGY FOR ADAPTIVE AGING
JANUARY 23-24, 2003
PROGRAM AND SCHEDULE

National Academy of Sciences Lecture Room
2101 Constitution Avenue, NW
Washington, DC 20418
Sponsored by:

The National Institute on Aging—Behavioral and Social Research Program

The National Research Council, with sponsorship from the National Institute on Aging, will hold a workshop on **Technology for Adaptive Aging** at the National Academy of Sciences building in Washington, DC, on January 23 and 24, 2003. The workshop will address some of the ways in which technology can be developed and applied to improve the lives of an aging population. Nationally recognized experts will discuss potential applications of technology to the domains of Living Environments, Health, Communication, Education and Learning, Transportation, and Employment. Special emphasis will be given to the challenges of translating laboratory successes into useful, marketable products and services. Speakers will highlight technologies that are promising candidates for SBIR and other support of translational research and development.

DAY 1—THURSDAY, JANUARY 23, 2003

	Topic	Paper authors
9:00	**Welcome and Introduction to Program**	**Richard Suzman**, NIA Behavioral and Social Research, Sponsor
		Richard Pew, BBN Technologies, Steering Committee Chair
9:20	**Overview of Changes with Aging**	**K. Warner Schaie**, Pennsylvania State University **George Stelmach**, Arizona State University

10:20 *Discussion* (**Arthur Kramer**,* University of Illinois, discussant)

10:50 *Break*

11:00	**Methodological and Measurement Considerations in RGD of Technology for Adaptive Aging**	**Leah Light**, Pitzer College **Christopher Hertzog**, Georgia Institute of Technology

12:00 *Discussion* (**Melissa Hardy**,* Florida State University, discussant)

12:30 *Lunch Break*

1:30	**Living Environments**	**Ann Horgas**, University of Florida
		Gregory Abowd, Georgia Institute of Technology

2:30 *Discussion* (**Martha Pollack**,* University of Michigan, discussant)

3:00 *Break*

3:10	**Health**	**Jackie Dunbar-Jacob** and **Judith Matthews**, University of Pittsburgh **Eric Dishman**, Intel Corporation

4:10 *Discussion* (**Richard Schulz**,* University of Pittsburgh, and **Jonathan Skinner**, Dartmouth College, discussants)

---

*Member of Steering Committee

DAY 2 — FRIDAY, JANUARY 24, 2003

Topic	Paper authors

9:00 **Employment**   **Phyllis Moen**, Cornell University

Sara Czaja, University of Miami

10:00 *Discussion* (**Scott Bass**,* University of Maryland, Baltimore County, and **Joseph Quinn**, Boston College, discussants)

10:45 *Break*

11:00 **Communications**   **Susan Kemper**, University of Kansas

Jose Lacal, Motorola, Inc.

12:00 *Discussion* (**Wendy Rogers**,* Georgia Institute of Technology, discussant)

12:30 *Lunch Break*

1:30 **Transportation**   **Patricia Waller**, University of North Carolina

Brian Repa, General Motors Corporation

2:30 *Discussion* (**Joseph Coughlin**,* Massachusetts Institute of Technology, discussant)

3:00 *Break*

3:10 **Education, Learning**   **Sherry Willis**, Pennsylvania State University

James Sullivan and **Gerhard Fischer**, University of Colorado

4:10 *Discussion* (**Charles Scialfa**,* University of Calgary, discussant)

4:40 **Summary, Closing Remarks**   (**Thomas Sheridan**,* Massachusetts Institute of Technology)

---

*Member of Steering Committee

WORKSHOP ON TECHNOLOGY FOR ADAPTIVE AGING
JANUARY 23-24, 2003
LIST OF ATTENDEES

NAME	TITLE	ORGANIZATION

Steering Committee and Staff

Richard W. Pew, Chair	Principal Scientist	BBN Technologies
Scott A. Bass	Dean and Vice Provost	Univ. of Maryland, Baltimore County
Joseph Coughlin	Director	MIT
Melissa Hardy	Director and Professor	Florida State University
Arthur Kramer	Professor	University of Illinois
Wendy Rogers	Professor	Georgia Institute of Technology
Richard Schulz	Director	University of Pittsburgh
Charles Scialfa	Professor	University of Calgary
Thomas Sheridan	Professor	MIT
Susan Van Hemel	Study Director	National Research Council

Workshop Speakers and Authors Attending

Sara J. Czaja	Professor	University of Miami
Eric Dishman	Manager	INTEL
Jacqueline Dunbar-Jacob	Professor	University of Pittsburgh
Christopher Hertzog	Professor	Georgia Institute of Technology
Ann Horgas	Associate Professor	University of Florida
Susan Kemper	Professor	University of Kansas
Jose Lacal	Senior Management	Motorola
Leah Light	Professor	Pitzer College
Judith Matthews	Assistant Professor	University of Pittsburgh
Phyllis Moen	Professor	Cornell University

Joseph F. Quinn	Professor and Dean	Boston College
Brian Repa	Princ. Research Engineer	General Motors Inc.
K. Warner Schaie	Director	Pennsylvania State University
Jonathan S. Skinner	Professor	Dartmouth College
George Stelmach	Professor and Director	Arizona State University
James Sullivan	Senior Research Scientist	University of Colorado
Sherry Willis	Professor	Pennsylvania State University

Authors not Attending

| Gregory Abowd | Associate Professor | Georgia Institute of Technology |
| Gerhard Fischer | Professor, Director | University of Colorado |

Guests*

Mira Ahn		Virginia Tech
Nancy Aldrich	Editor	Aging Research & Training News
Mark Baard		Wired News
Ann Benbow	Director	SPRY Foundation
Sandy Berman	Consumer Safety Officer	FDA
Russell Bodoff	VP Technology & Business Dev.	American Association of Homes & Services for the Aging
Lona Choi	Project Manager	SPRY Foundation

---

*NOTE: Guest titles and affiliations are given as found on workshop registration forms or on sign-in sheet at the workshop.

Rita K. Chow	Director	National Interfaith Coalition on Aging, National Council on Aging
Margaret Chu	USEPA	ORD
Arthur Ciarkowski	Associate Director, DCD	CDRH/FDA
Kenneth Cook		
Jennifer Cornman	Senior Research Scientist	Madlyn and Leonard Abramson Center for Jewish Life
Shelia Cotten		University of Maryland Baltimore County
Stephanie Dailey	Education Research Specialist	National Institute on Aging
Skip DeRosier	Rehabilitation Technologist	Abramson Center for Jewish Life
Deborah DiGilio	Aging Issues Officer	American Psychological Association
Gerald M. Eggert	Executive Director	Monroe County Long Term Care Program, Inc
David Gamse	Executive Director	Jewish Council for the Aging
Daryle Gardner-Bonneau	Principal	Bonneau and Associates
Sarah Geitz	Sr. Human Factors Engineer	Micro Analysis and Design
Michael E. Gluck	Research Associate Professor	Georgetown University
Darlene Howard	Professor	Georgetown University
James Howard		
Robert Jaeger	Interagency and International Affairs	National Institute for Disability and Rehabilitation Research

Michael-David Kerns	Health Scientist Administrator	National Institute on Aging
Jim Kling		Web MD
Laura Kolb		EPA
Kara Latorella	Human Factors Engineer	NASA Langley
Lila Laux		Micro Analysis and Design
Alex Libin	Research Associate	Research Institute on Aging
Lena Libin	Director	Research Institute on Complex Interactive Systems
Rose Li	Senior Management	Analytical Sciences, Inc.
Diane F. Mahoney	Director and Senior Research Scientist	Hebrew Rehabilitation Center for Aged
Giorgio Mattiello		Embassy of Italy
Joan McIntrie	Writer	Washington Post
Susan Meadows	Senior Advisor	FDA
Jeannine Mjoseth	Public Affairs Specialist	NIA/NIH
Russell Morgan	President	SPRY Foundation
Gregg O'Neill	Director	National Academy on an Aging Society
David Padgham		National Academy of Sciences
Sital Patel		CBS MarketWatch
David Pick	Professor	Purdue University Calumet
Irae Raskin		
George Rebok	Associate Research Professor	Johns Hopkins University

Jane Saczynski		Johns Hopkins University
John Schumacher	Assistant Professor	Univ. of Maryland, Baltimore County
John Senders	Professor Emeritus	University of Toronto
Arthur Sherwood	Science and Technology Advisor	National Institute on Disability and Rehabilitation
Laura Shrestha		NIA/NIH
Sidney Stahl	Chief, Behavioral Medicine	NIA/NIH
Jeannette Steeves	Doctoral Candidate	Virginia Tech
Richard Suzman	Associate Director	National Institute on Aging/NIH
Yvette Tenney		BBN Technologies
Pamela Tsang	Associate Professor	Wright State University
Nancy Valley	Disability Access Coordinator	Motorola
Kathleen Wiseman	Board Member	JCA
Steven Zaleznick		

Appendix B
Biographical Sketches

BIOGRAPHICAL SKETCHES OF
STEERING COMMITTEE MEMBERS

Richard W. Pew (*Chair*) holds a bachelors degree in electrical engineering from Cornell University (1956), a master of arts degree in psychology from Harvard University (1960), and a Ph.D. in psychology with a specialization in engineering psychology from the University of Michigan (1963). He has been at BBN Technologies since 1974 where he is a Principal Scientist. From 1976 to 1997 he was also Manager of the Cognitive Sciences and Systems Department. He is currently working part time for BBN. He has 35 years of experience in human factors, human performance and experimental psychology as they relate to systems design and development. Throughout his career he has been involved in the development and utilization of human performance models and in the conduct of experimental and field studies of human performance in applied settings. Before joining BBN, he spent 11 years on the faculty of the psychology department at Michigan where he was involved in human performance teaching, research and consulting. The University has recently created a collegiate chair in his name. He was the first chair of the National Research Council Committee on Human Factors, and has been president of the Human Factors Society and president of Division 21 of the American Psychological Association, the division concerned with engineering psychology. He has also been chair of the Biosciences Panel of the U.S. Air Force Scientific Advisory Board and was recently chair of the Soldier Systems Panel of the U.S. Army Research Laboratory Technical

Advisory Board. In 1999 he was awarded the Arnold M. Small Distinguished Service Award of the Human Factors and Ergonomics Society for career-long contributions to the field and to the society. Dr. Pew has more than 70 publications as book chapters, articles, and technical reports.

Scott Bass is dean of the Graduate School and vice provost for research and planning at the University of Maryland, Baltimore County (UMBC), where he holds academic appointments of distinguished professor of sociology and public policy. His responsibilities involve the development and expansion of research and graduate education at this selective, midsized, public research university. Dr. Bass was formerly a professor at the University of Massachusetts, Boston, as well as director of the University's Gerontology Institute. He was founding director of the Ph.D. program in gerontology—the second such Ph.D. program in the United States. Most recently, Dr. Bass helped to establish a new Ph.D. program in gerontology at UMBC in cooperation with faculty at the University of Maryland, Baltimore. A Gerontological Society of America Fellow, he was a visiting associate at the Lincoln Gerontology Centre, La Trobe University, Australia, in 1989, a distinguished visiting professor at Yokohama City University, Japan, in 1994, and was awarded a Fulbright Research Scholarship to study in Japan in 1994. Dr. Bass' recent written work has focused on the social and economic roles of older people. He is the editor of *Older and Active* (1995) and coeditor of *Challenges of the Third Age: Meaning and Purpose in Later Life* (2002), *Public Policy and the Old Age Revolution in Japan* (1996), and three additional books. He is also founding coeditor of the *Journal of Aging & Social Policy* and has published approximately 50 book chapters and articles and over 30 monographs or research reports regarding aging policy. Dr. Bass received a combined doctorate in psychology and education in 1976 from the University of Michigan, from which he also earned an M.A. in clinical psychology and a B.A. in psychology.

Joseph F. Coughlin, Ph.D., is founding director of the Massachusetts Institute of Technology (MIT) AgeLab—a partnership among MIT, industry, and the aging community to engineer innovative approaches and technologies to improve the quality of life of older adults and those who care for them. AgeLab conducts multidisciplinary research addressing the problems and opportunities of global aging, including housing, transportation, health, communications, leisure and the workplace. AgeLab's industry sponsors are from around the world and include information technology and telecommunications firms, pharmaceutical companies, consumer products manufacturers, financial services, and the automotive industry. Dr. Coughlin's own research seeks to develop new business models that respond to the demands of today's and tomorrow's older adults by seamlessly integrating technology and consumer services. He is recognized around the world as a leader in the field of aging and technology. Dr. Coughlin has published in a variety of aging, business, and policy research journals. He recently completed a book on the transportation needs of an aging society along with Roger W. Cobb, Brown University, forthcoming from Johns Hopkins University Press. Dr. Coughlin is currently writing a second book that envisions how business and society will leverage the convergence of technology and graying demographics to reshape how all of us will live, work, and play tomorrow. He frequently speaks to a wide range of audiences including those in the healthcare, automotive, insurance, travel, and computer industries, lecturing on the business and public policy implications of aging, changing lifestyles, and technology in Europe, Japan, and North America. Dr. Coughlin has served as a keynote speaker at national and international events including the annual meetings of the American Geriatrics Society, AARP Board of Directors, COMDEX, and the White House Conference on Technology and Aging. His research has been featured in *Business Week,* the *Wall Street Journal, New York Times, Le Monde,* and ABC News, CBS Evening News, NBC Nightly News, and CNN World. Dr. Coughlin consults regularly and has assisted numerous organizations including AT&T, IBM, the American Business Collaborative for Quality Dependent Care, Johnson & Johnson, and the White House Office of Science and Technology Policy. Dr. Coughlin was recently named to lead the 35-nation Organization for Economic Cooperation and Development's study on new transportation technologies and services for older people. Prior to joining MIT, Dr. Coughlin was with EG&G (now PerkinElmer) for 12 years. He teaches strategic management and public policy within the MIT School of Engineering's Engineering Systems Division. He has a B.A. from the State University of New York in international politics, an A.M. in public policy from Brown University, and a Ph.D. in public policy from Boston University.

Melissa A. Hardy is director of the Gerontology Center and professor of human development/family studies and sociology at the Pennsylvania State University and the former director of the Pepper Institute on Aging and Public Policy at Florida State University (1995-2003). She was recently elected chair of the Behavioral and Social Sciences Section of the Gerontological Society of America for 2005. Professor Hardy received a Ph.D. in sociology, with a minor in economics, from Indiana University in 1980. She has been a member of the Council of the American Sociological Association's Section on Aging, a member of the Section on Human Development and Aging for the National Institutes of Health, executive director of Florida's Panel for End-of-Life Care, one of the U.S. representatives to the International Comparative Research Group addressing public and private policies that affect older workers, and a consultant to the

Commission on Long-Term Care in Florida. She has served on the editorial boards of the *American Sociological Review*, the *Journal of Gerontology, Research on Aging*, and *Social Forces*. In addition to her administrative duties, Professor Hardy maintains an active research agenda, specializing in studies of social stratification, income inequality, labor-force behavior, health, and public policy. Her projects have been supported by funding from agencies such as the National Institute on Aging and the Andrus Foundation.

Arthur Kramer received a Ph.D. in 1984 in cognitive and experimental psychology at the University of Illinois. Since then he has spent a good deal of time working on a variety of research topics in cognitive psychology, cognitive neuroscience and human factors at the University of Illinois and elsewhere. He currently holds appointments in the Department of Psychology, the University Neuroscience program, the Institute of Aviation, and the Beckman Institute, where he has served as the cochair for the Human-Computer Interaction main research theme since 1998. Dr. Kramer served as an associate editor of *Perception and Psychophysics* from 1993 to 1999 and is currently a member of seven editorial boards. His research is currently funded by the National Institute on Aging, the Institute for the Study of Aging, the National Science Foundation, the U.S. Army Research Laboratory, the Federal Aviation Administration, and General Motors. His research on aging is concerned with both (a) explicating the changes in a variety of cognitive processes that occur during the course of normal aging and (b) designing interventions to slow the detrimental cognitive effects experienced during the process of aging. For example, Dr. Kramer and his research group have been investigating changes in the processes that support executive control (and more specifically multitask performance and task switching) that occur during aging. To that end they have found age-related deficiencies in the ability to suppress previously relevant but currently irrelevant stimulus-response mappings as well as in the ability to rapidly shift priorities among concurrently performed tasks. However, they have also found that such deficiencies can be reduced, in part, by both training interventions and programs of aerobic fitness. In a recently completed series of studies, they found that not only do adaptive training strategies that emphasize cognitive flexibility reduce age-related performance differences on the trained tasks, but the performance strategies that are learned transfer to novel sets of concurrently performed tasks. Dr. Kramer and his colleagues are also interested in the relationship among aging, fitness, cognition and brain function—a relationship that they have been examining through the use of event-related functional magnetic resonance imaging (fMRI).

Martha E. Pollack is professor of electrical engineering and computer science at the University of Michigan. She was previously professor of computer science and director of the Intelligent Systems Program at the University of Pittsburgh, and before that, senior computer scientist at the AI Center, SRI International. Professor Pollack received her B.A. from Dartmouth College and her M.S.E. and Ph.D. degrees from the University of Pennsylvania. She is a recipient of the Computers and Thought Award (1991), a National Science Foundation (NSF)Young Investigator's Award (1992), and the University of Pittsburgh Chancellor's Distinguished Research Award (2000), and she was elected to be a fellow of the American Association for Artificial Intelligence in 1986. She has served on numerous editorial boards and program committees, and is currently executive editor of the *Journal of Artificial Intelligence Research*. Her research interests are in artificial intelligence: For many years, she has conducted research on plan generation, plan management, temporal reasoning, and cognitive models of rationality. More recently she has been interested in the uses of Artificial Intelligence technology to support elderly and disabled people, and in particular she has been developing assistive technology for people with memory impairment, with funding from the NSF and the Intel Corporation.

Wendy A. Rogers is a professor in the School of Psychology at Georgia Institute of Technology in the engineering and experimental psychology programs. She received her B.A. from the University of Massachusetts, Dartmouth, and her M.S. (1989) and Ph.D. (1991) degrees from Georgia Institute of Technology. Prior to returning to the Georgia Institute of Technology for her current position, she was a member of the faculty of the University of Memphis (1991-1994) and the University of Georgia (1994-1998). Her research interests include skill acquisition, human factors, training, and cognitive aging. Her research is currently funded by the National Institute on Aging (NIA) as part of two centers: the Center for Aging and Cognition: Health, Education, and Technology and the Center for Research and Education on Aging and Technology Enhancement. She also has a grant funded by NIA to study cognitive strategies and aging. Dr. Rogers has published extensively in the field of human factors and cognitive aging with over 60 journal articles and book chapters. Dr. Rogers serves on the editorial boards of *Experimental Aging Research*, *Ergonomics in Design*, and *Human Factors;* she just completed a term on the editorial board of *Psychology and Aging*. She is past president and fellow of Division 21 (Applied Experimental and Engineering Psychology) and a fellow of Division 20 (Adult Development and Aging) of the American Psychological Association. She also served a term as an at-large member of the Executive Council of the Human Factors and Ergonomics Society, and is now President-elect of the society.

Richard Schulz is currently professor of psychiatry and director of the University Center for Social and Urban Research at the University of

Pittsburgh. He has spent most of his career doing research and writing on adult development and aging. His research has focused on social-psychological aspects of aging, including the role of control as a construct for characterizing life-course development, and the impact of disabling late-life disease on patients and their families. Much of his recent research has focused on issues of health and aging and family caregiving. This body of work is reflected in more than 200 publications, which have appeared in major medical, psychology, and aging journals. He is also author of numerous books and has served as editor of the *Journal of Gerontology: Psychological Sciences*. He is the year 2000 recipient of the Kleemeier Award for research on aging given by the Gerontological Society of America, and in 2003 he received the Developmental Health Research Award from the American Psychological Association.

Charles T. (Chip) Scialfa received a Ph.D. in experimental psychology from the University of Notre Dame (1987) and subsequently spent several years as a postdoctoral fellow in both developmental methodology and visual function at Pennsylvania State University. He has been on the faculty at the University of Calgary since 1989. His research focus is on perceptual and cognitive aging. This interest includes clinical and applied aspects of spatial vision, eye movements, visual attention, skill acquisition, human factors, and driving performance.

Thomas B. Sheridan received a B.S. degree from Purdue University, an M.S. degree from the University of California at Los Angeles, a Sc.D. degree from the Massachusetts Institute of Technology (MIT), and the Doctor (honorary) from Delft University of Technology, the Netherlands. For most of his professional career he has remained at MIT, where currently he is Ford Professor of Engineering and Applied Psychology Emeritus in both the Department of Mechanical Engineering and Department of Aeronautics and Astronautics. He has also served as a visiting professor at the University of California at Berkeley, Stanford, Delft (the Netherlands), Kassel (Germany), and Ben Gurion (Israel). Currently he is senior research fellow at the Department of Transportation Volpe Center and a consultant for patient safety to Harvard's Risk Management Foundation. As director of the MIT Human-Machine Systems Laboratory his research activities have included experimentation, analysis, modeling, and design to enhance human performance and safety for air, highway and rail transportation, space and undersea robotics, nuclear power systems, medical systems, arms control, and virtual reality. He has published over 200 technical papers in these areas. He is co-author of *Man-Machine Systems* (MIT Press 1974, 1981; USSR, 1981); coeditor of *Monitoring Behavior and Supervisory Control* (Plenum, 1976); author of *Telerobotics, Automation, and Human Supervisory Control* (MIT Press, 1992); coeditor of *Perspectives on the Human Controller* (Erlbaum, 1997); and author of *Humans and Automation*

(Wiley, 2002). He is currently senior editor of the MIT Press journal *Presence: Teleoperators and Virtual Environments* and serves on several editorial boards. He chaired the National Research Council's Committee on Human Factors and has served on numerous government and industrial advisory committees. Dr. Sheridan served as president of the IEEE Systems, Man and Cybernetics Society, and editor of *IEEE Transactions on Man-Machine Systems*. He was elected to the National Academy of Engineering in 1995.

BIOGRAPHICAL SKETCHES OF WORKSHOP PARTICIPANTS

Gregory D. Abowd is an associate professor in the College of Computing and the Graphics, Visualization, and Usability (GVU) Center at the Georgia Institute of Technology. His research interests include software engineering for interactive systems, with particular focus on mobile and ubiquitous computing applications. He leads a research group in the College of Computing focused on the development of prototype future computing environments that emphasize mobile and ubiquitous computing technology for everyday uses. The general themes he investigates include automated capture environments, context-aware computing, and natural interaction. He has focused his applications research in the domains of university education (the Classroom 2000 and eClass projects), the office (CyberDesk,) and the home (the Aware Home). Dr. Abowd has affiliations with several campus research groups, including the GVU Center and the Broadband Institute. He currently serves as director for the Aware Home Research Initiative. Dr. Abowd received a B.S. in mathematics from the University of Notre Dame in 1986 and the degrees of M.Sc. (1987) and D.Phil. (1991) in computation from the University of Oxford, where he attended as a Rhodes Scholar. Before coming to the Georgia Institute of Technology in 1994, Dr. Abowd held postdoctoral positions with the Human-Computer Interaction group at the University of York in England and with the Software Engineering Institute and Computer Science Department at Carnegie Mellon University.

Sara J. Czaja has a B.S. in psychology and an M.S. and Ph.D. in industrial engineering from the State University of New York at Buffalo. She is currently a professor in the departments of Psychiatry and Behavioral Sciences and Industrial Engineering at the University of Miami and is the director of the Center on Research and Education for Aging and Technology Enhancement (CREATE) and the Research Director of the Center on Adult Development and Aging at the University of Miami School of Medicine. CREATE, funded by the National Institute on Aging, involves collaboration with the Georgia Institute of Technology and Florida State University. The focus of CREATE is on making technology more accessible, useful, and usable for older adult populations. Prior to joining the faculty at Miami in 1990, Dr. Czaja was an associate professor of industrial engineering at the State University of New York at Buffalo. Dr. Czaja has a long commitment to developing strategies to improve the quality of life of older adults. Her research interests include aging and cognition, caregiving, human-computer interaction, training, and functional assessment. She has received funding for her research from the Administration on Aging, the National Institute on Aging (NIA), the National Institute of Nursing Research, the Markel Foundation, and Pfizer Inc. She is currently the principal investigator of a project, funded by NIA, concerned with the ability of older adults to use technology for information search and retrieval. She is also the Principal Investigator of the Miami site of the Resources for Enhancing Alzheimer's Caregiver Health program, a multisite clinical trial evaluating the efficacy of a multicomponent psychosocial intervention in enhancing the quality of life and reducing burden and distress among family caregivers of Alzheimer's patients. The intervention involves the use of a computer-integrated communications system. She is also the principal investigator of a project concerned with the impact of Aricept on the functional performance of patients with Alzheimer's disease, and is leading a project concerned with evaluating the feasibility of applying engineering and operations research analytic techniques to psychosocial intervention research. Dr. Czaja has written numerous book chapters and scientific articles. She is currently coauthoring a book with other members of the CREATE team concerning the design of technology for older adult populations. She is also very active at the national level in promoting aging research. Dr. Czaja served as the cochair of the Committee on Aging and Human Factors of the National Research Council and National Science Foundation. She was the cochair of the November 2002 meeting of the International Society of Gerontechnology. She also served as the chair of the Technical Group on Aging of the Human Factors and Ergonomics Society and is the chair-elect of the Council on Technical Groups of the Human Factors and Ergonomics Society. She is a member of the external advisory board of the Center on Aging at the University of Alabama at Birmingham. In addition, she is a fellow of the American Psychological Association and the Human Factors and Ergonomics Society. She is the current chair of the Risk Prevention and Behavior Scientific Review Panel of the National Institute on Health. She is a recognized leader within the university community in aging research. In 1996 she was selected as the researcher of the year within the College of Engineering and received the provost's award for scholarly activity in 1998.

Eric Dishman, senior social scientist at Intel Corporation, was trained as a communication scholar but has been leading qualitative research studies for the past 10 years in technology companies. He received an

M.S. in speech communication from Southern Illinois University and is a Ph.D. candidate in communication at the University of Utah. His research centers on the development of ubiquitous computing technologies by studying the everyday lives of people in their natural environments. Mr. Dishman currently directs several healthcare efforts in Intel Research, including the Proactive Health research laboratory to develop aging-in-place technologies for the baby boomer cohort. He is the chair of the Intel Research Council Health Subcommittee, which funds university grants on consumer health and wellness technologies. His team's current field-work and technology prototyping efforts focus on the home activities of elder and boomer populations who are dealing with cognitive disability, physical disability, cancer, cardiovascular disease, and nutrition and fitness concerns. In partnership with the American Association of Homes and Services for the Aging (www.aahsa.org), Mr. Dishman is also the inaugural chair of the Center for Aging Services Technology (www.agingtech.org). He is a frequent speaker on the topics of aging and home health care technologies.

Jacqueline Dunbar-Jacob is currently professor of nursing, epidemiology, and occupational therapy and dean of the School of Nursing at the University of Pittsburgh. She received her B.S. in nursing from Florida State University, an M.S. in psychiatric nursing from the University of California at San Francisco, and a Ph.D. in counseling psychology at Stanford University. She is licensed as both a registered nurse and a psychologist. Dr. Dunbar-Jacob has been studying adherence to treatment in primarily chronic conditions since the mid-1970s and currently has studies in type 2 diabetes supported by the National Institute of Diabetes and Digestive and Kidney Diseases, and rheumatoid arthritis supported by the National Institute of Nursing Research. She is a co-principal investigator in the multi-university National Science Foundation-supported Nursebot project and is director of the NINR-supported Center for Research in Chronic Disorders. The majority of her studies have included older adult populations. She had a particular interest in both the behavioral and the technological strategies that may improve older adults' ability to manage and adhere to their healthcare regimen.

Christopher Hertzog received A.B., A.M., and Ph.D. degrees from the University of Southern California, with a specialization in adult development and aging. His Ph.D. dissertation, done under the supervision of K. Warner Schaie, was completed in 1979. After a 2-year postdoctoral fellowship at the University of Washington, he was an assistant professor of human development at the Pennsylvania State University from 1981 to 1985. He then moved to the Georgia Institute of Technology, where he has remained and is currently a professor of psychology. He has received several research grants from the National Institute on Aging, including a

MERIT (Method to Extend Research in Time) award for his research program on aging, metacognition, and strategy use during learning. His published research has spanned a broad range of interests, including longitudinal methods; multivariate statistics; individual differences in human cognition; effects of aging on memory, intelligence, and problem solving; metacognition; and social cognition. He is a fellow of the American Psychological Association, the American Psychological Society, and the Gerontological Society of America.

Ann Horgas is an associate professor in the College of Nursing at the University of Florida. She received a B.S. and M.S. in nursing, and a Ph.D. in human development and family studies (1992) from the Pennsylvania State University. Dr. Horgas completed her postdoctoral fellowship in the Gerontology and Geriatrics department at Free University of Berlin in Germany, where she worked on the Berlin Aging Study. Dr. Horgas has been the recipient of many awards including the Harriet H. Werley New Investigator Award from the Midwest Nursing Research Society, an Undergraduate Mentorship Recognition Award from Wayne State University, and a Junior Scholar Fellowship to attend the Sapio Summer School of Methodology and Research Strategies in Developmental Studies at the Sapio Research Institute in Sofia, Bulgaria. Most recently, she was the recipient of the Springer Award for outstanding contributions to geriatric nursing through the Gerontological Society of America. Dr. Horgas is the principal investigator or coinvestigator on a large number of research projects funded by the National Institute on Aging, National Institute of Nursing Research, and the American Nurses Foundation. Her program of research focuses on chronic pain in late life and its impact on physical health, mental health, and everyday functioning. She has done extensive research in nursing homes and assisted living facilities, focusing primarily on strategies for improving care, dealing with behavior problems, and managing pain.

Susan Kemper is the Roberts Distinguished Professor of Psychology and Gerontology at the University of Kansas. She is a participating faculty member in the Gerontology Doctoral program as well as in the Child Language Doctoral program in addition to that in cognitive psychology. In the Language Across the Lifespan Project, she addresses how aging affects the processing of spoken and written language and includes comparative studies of healthy older adults and adults with Alzheimer's disease. Her research ranges from studies of how working memory affects older adults' speech to studies of how to enhance older adults' comprehension through "elderspeak," a set of special speech modifications designed for older adults. Recently, she has established an eye tracking laboratory for age-comparative studies of reading and visual information processing. Along with other researchers, she examined early language abilities as a predictor of late-life cognitive impairment and Alzheimer's disease as part of the Nun Study. Her research has been supported by a series of grants from the National Institute on Aging. Dr. Kemper earned her doctorate at Cornell University, Ithaca, New York, in 1978 and her bachelor's degree from Macalester College, St. Paul, Minnesota, in 1974. She has received a 5-year research career development award from the National Institute of Aging and the Balfour Jeffery Research Achievement Award at the University of Kansas.

Caroline J. Ketcham received an B.A. degree from Colby College in 1996 in biology and psychology. She completed an M.S. in 1999 with her research focus on bradykinesia in Parkinson's disease patients under the direction of Professor George E. Stelmach at Arizona State University. She continued on towards her Ph.D. with Dr. Stelmach and was awarded her Ph.D. in December 2003. Her current research is some of the seminal data on the pattern of oculomotor control in the production of multijoint movements. Caroline has received such honors as an Achievement Reward for College Scientists (ARCS), Outstanding Graduate Student, Graduate College Accolades, Graduate Academic Scholar, has received numerous travel awards both internal and external to present her research. Caroline has 5 peer-reviewed publications, 5 published chapters, and has presented her research at 15 national and international conferences. Caroline, in addition to her work at ASU, spent the summer of 2000 abroad conducting research at the Imperial College School of Medicine-Charing Cross Hospital in London collaborating with neuroscientists on spatial memory in Parkinson's disease patients. Caroline has been a research assistant on, and an integral part in writing, several NIH grants awarded to Dr. Stelmach. These grants have addressed control and regulation of upper extremity movements in young, elderly and Parkinson's disease patients. Dr. Ketcham is now assistant professor in the Department of Health and Kinesiology at Texas A&M University in College Station, TX.

Jose C. Lacal is senior manager, Tele-Health Solutions with the iDEN Subscriber Group of Motorola. He has a B.A. in economics from Florida International University in Miami, Florida. Prior to joining Motorola, Mr. Lacal spent 5 years with high-tech companies in Germany, Mexico and the United States. His areas of responsibility at iDEN include the identification and definition of new strategic market opportunities, including disabilities, healthcare, and seniors. Mr. Lacal is looking for new markets where iDEN could re-combine its core competencies in order to develop new solutions for emerging markets. Mr. Lacal is personally interested in using technology to develop solutions for the disabilities, healthcare, and seniors markets, both in the United States and in Western Europe.

Leah L. Light is professor of psychology at Pitzer College in Claremont, California. She received a B.A. in psychology from Wellesley

College and a Ph.D. from Stanford University. Her research interests lie in memory and aging, with a particular focus on differentiating aspects of memory that are relatively preserved in old age from those that are more affected. Her research has been supported by grants from the National Institute on Aging, including a MERIT award, since 1981. Dr. Light is a fellow of the American Psychological Association, the American Psychological Society, and the Gerontological Society of America, and is a member of the Psychonomic Society and the Memory Disorders Research Society. She has just completed a 6-year term as editor of *Psychology and Aging* and continues to serve on the board of that journal and also on the board of the *Journal of Experimental Psychology: Learning, Memory, and Cognition.*

Judith Tabolt Matthews is an assistant professor in the Department of Health and Community Systems at the University of Pittsburgh School of Nursing. Dr. Matthews received her B.S. in nursing from the Pennsylvania State University and an M.S. in community health nursing, with an emphasis in gerontology, from Boston University. She holds both a Ph.D. in nursing and an M.P.H. in epidemiology from the University of Pittsburgh. Dr. Matthews's focus over the past 25 years has been on community health nursing practice, education, and research, with particular interest in the use of technology to support the caregiving skills and preventive health practices of family caregivers. She is also a member of the Nursebot Project, a multidisciplinary collaboration involving the University of Pittsburgh, Carnegie Mellon University, and the University of Michigan that is funded by the National Science Foundation. The project focuses on developing personal robotic assistants for older adults. Dr. Matthews coteaches a project-based, robotic applications course with faculty from the Robotics Institute at Carnegie Mellon University, bringing together students from the health sciences and students in technology to design and evaluate robotic devices that may help community-residing, frail older adults and persons with disabilities sustain their independence.

Joachim Meyer is an associate professor at the Department of Industrial Engineering and Management at Ben Gurion University in Beer Sheva, Israel, and a research scientist at the Massachusetts Institute of Technology (MIT) AgeLab, where he helped to establish the driving simulator laboratory. He holds an M.A. in psychology and a Ph.D. in industrial engineering from Ben Gurion University. Before returning to Ben Gurion University, he had an appointment at the Technion-Israel Institute of Technology. He specializes in cognitive engineering and, in particular, the modeling of decision processes in settings that involve complex systems and social interactions. His recent research deals with the potential benefits and the possible problems of using technology to support older users. He has published in scientific journals dealing with cognitive psychology, human-computer interaction, ergonomics, human factors engineering and management information systems.

Phyllis Moen holds the McKnight Presidential Chair in Sociology at the University of Minnesota. For many years prior to that, she held the Ferris Family Professorship in Life Course Studies at Cornell University, serving also as founding director of the Bronfenbrenner Life Course Center, codirector of Cornell Gerontology Research Institute, and director of the Cornell Careers Institute. Her research (published in six books as well as in leading academic journals) focuses on careers, families, gender, aging, and health over the life course. She is especially interested in work-related status transitions and trajectories as they play out in particular historical, community, corporate, and policy contexts. Dr. Moen's recent scholarship addresses the mismatch between work and retirement rules and regulations, on the one hand, and characteristics of the new work force and the new, growing retired force, on the other. The Alfred P. Sloan Foundation and the National Institute on Aging have funded the bulk of her scholarship. Dr. Moen just published *It's About Time: Couples and Careers* (Cornell University Press, 2003). Two other volumes are in the works: *The Career Mystique* (Rowman and Littlefield) and *Uncertain Futures*.

K. Warner Schaie is the Evan Pugh Professor of Human Development and Psychology at the Pennsylvania State University. He also holds an appointment as affiliate professor of psychiatry and behavioral science at the University of Washington. He received a Ph.D. in psychology from the University of Washington, an honorary Dr.Phil. from the Friedrich-Schiller-University of Jena, Germany, and an honorary Sci.D. degree from West Virginia University. He was honored with the Kleemeier Award for Distinguished Research Contributions from the Gerontological Society of America and the Distinguished Scientific Contributions Award from the American Psychological Association. He is author or editor of 36 books including the textbook *Adult Development and Aging* (with S. L. Willis) and the *Handbook of the Psychology of Aging* (with J. E. Birren), both of which are now in their 5th editions. He has directed the Seattle Longitudinal Study of cognitive aging since 1956 and is the author of more than 250 journal articles and chapters on the psychology of aging. His current research interest is the life course of adult intelligence, its antecedents and modifiability, as well as methodological issues in the developmental sciences.

George E. Stelmach's teaching and research interests are in the areas of movement control and learning, aging, human factors, and neurosciences. His current research examines human movement coordination and seeks to understand how the central nervous system controls and regulates movement in normal individuals and in those with neurological impairments. Of special interest is how motor control strategies are altered through normal aging and pathology. Dr. Stelmach began his academic career in 1967 at the University of California-Santa Barbara (UCSB) in the Department of Ergonomics. After 4 years at UCSB, he left to accept the position as professor and director of the Motor Behavior Laboratory at the University of Wisconsin, Madison, where he spent the next 19 years in various academic and administrative positions. While in Madison, he was a faculty member in the Department of Kinesiology (1986-1990) and from 1984-1990 he was also a faculty member in the Department of Rehabilitation Medicine in the Clinical Science Center. From 1991 to the present he has been a professor of kinesiology and director of the Motor Control Laboratory at Arizona State University. Dr. Stelmach's collaborative research and training programs address questions pertinent to the general area of motor neuroscience. The disciplines involved in this research and training effort are neurophysiology, biomechanics, experimental psychology, engineering, computer science, and kinesiology. During the 12 years that he has been at Arizona State University, he has built a strong research program that supports nine postdoctoral and three predoctoral trainees. Professor Stelmach's extramural grant awards currently exceed $6.5 million. In addition, Dr. Stelmach is codirector of a 5-year National Science Foundation Integrated Graduated Education Research and Training Award (2000-2004). Professor Stelmach has been externally funded through peer-reviewed grant applications in the neuroscience area throughout his 35-year career. Consistent with the interdisciplinary nature of his research, grant support has come from diverse funding agencies such as the National Institute of Neurological Diseases and Stroke, National Institute of Aging, National Institute of Mental Health, National Institute of Education, American Parkinson's Disease Association, Burroughs-Wellcome Trust, RS Flinn Foundation, and the U.S. Air Force Office of Scientific Research. During the course of his career, he has also received numerous academic awards. The following reflect some of the most prestigious: University of California President's Fellow (1970); Royalty Fund Fellow, University of Wisconsin (1977); National Academy of Science Exchange Fellow (1978); Senior Fulbright Fellow (1981); Deutscher Akademischer Austauschdienst Award (1987); Netherlands Institute of Advanced Study Fellow (1989); French National Institute of Medicine Fellow (1990); German Research Council Fellow (1992); Austrian Institute of Space Neurology Fellow, (1993-94); and Max Planck Research Fellow, Munich (1999). He also has received several Wellcome Trust Awards to allow him to conduct research at the University of London (1996), the University of Oxford (1998), and the Imperial College of Medicine (2000). Dr. Stelmach has also been elected to fellow in the American Psychological Association—Divisions of Experimental Psychology and Engineering Psychology, American Psychological Society, and American Society of

Kinesiology. He has also been honored with invitations to be a visiting scholar at some of the most renowned institutes of neurology in Europe: University of Dusseldorf, University of Tubingen, University of Innsbruck, University of London, and the Imperial College of Medicine in London.

Sherry L. Willis is a professor of human development at the Pennsylvania State University. She has a Ph.D. from the University of Texas at Austin. Dr. Willis's research, funded by the National Institute on Aging for over 25 years, focuses particularly on developing and evaluating training programs to help older adults compensate for age-related declines. She also looks at practical intelligence—how people solve everyday problems, such as understanding the instructions on prescription labels. Dr. Willis serves as consulting editor for *Gerontology Review, Cognition and Aging, Journals of Gerontology: Psychological Sciences,* and as a reviewer for several other journals. She is a coauthor, with K. Warner Schaie, of the textbook *Adult Development and Aging,* now in its 5th edition, plus she is the author or coauthor of numerous journal articles and chapters related to cognitive training in the elderly. She was president of Division 20 (1993-1994) and holds fellow status in two divisions of the American Psychological Association, as well as fellow status in the Gerontological Society of America. She was honored by the Pennsylvania State University's College of Health and Human Development in 1992 with the Pattishall Distinguished Research Award; in 1999 she was awarded the Pennsylvania State University's Faculty Scholar Medal for Outstanding Achievement, and in 2001 she was honored with the Pennsylvania State University's College of Health and Human Development Pauline Schmitt Russell Distinguished Research Career Award.